Kidney Disorders in Children and Adolescents

T0172796

Kidney Disorders in Children and Adolescents

A Global Perspective of Clinical Practice

Edited by

Ron Hogg MBChB, DCH
St Joseph's Hospital & Medical Center, Phoenix, Arizona, USA

Foreword by

Chester M Edelmann, Jr, MD

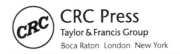

CRC Press
Taylor & Francis Group
Boca Raton London New York

CRC Press is an imprint of the
Taylor & Francis Group, an **informa** business

CRC Press
Taylor & Francis Group
6000 Broken Sound Parkway NW, Suite 300
Boca Raton, FL 33487-2742

First issued in paperback 2019

© 2006 by Taylor & Francis Group, LLC
CRC Press is an imprint of Taylor & Francis Group, an Informa business

No claim to original U.S. Government works

ISBN-13: 978-1-84184-250-9 (hbk)
ISBN-13: 978-0-367-39129-4 (pbk)

Contents

List of contributors   vii

Foreword   xi

Preface   xiii

The color plates will be found between pages xv and 1

1. Normal kidney function and development and choice of laboratory studies in children   1
   Susan Furth, Adeera Levin, George Schwartz

2. Radiographic studies in children with kidney disorders: what to do and when   15
   Michael Riccabona, Richard Fotter

3. Congenital abnormalities of the kidney and urinary tract   35
   Alan R Watson

4. Neonatal kidney problems   53
   Jean-Pierre Guignard

5. Mass screening for kidney disease in children – should it be done? If so, when?   67
   Pyung-Kil Kim, Young-Mock Lee, Kyo Sun Kim

6. Hematuria and proteinuria   75
   Juan Rodríguez-Soriano

7. The nephrotic syndrome   85
   Raymond AMG Donckerwolcke, Johan Vande Walle

8. Acute nephritis   95
   Rosanna Coppo, Allessandro Amore

9. Chronic nephritis in children – with emphasis on IgA nephropathy   103
   Norishige Yoshikawa, Koichi Nakanishi

10. Hypertension: evaluation, monitoring, and therapy   117
    Vera Hermina Koch, Ronald Portman

CONTENTS

11. Cardiovascular disease in patients with kidney disorders in childhood and adolescence   131
    Rulan Parekh, Mark Mitsnefes, Stephen Daniels

12. Urinary tract infections and vesico-ureteral reflux in children   139
    Tommy Linné

13. Nocturnal enuresis and voiding disorders   153
    Søren Rittig

14. Renal tubular disorders   165
    Israel Zelikovic

15. Acute renal failure and hemolytic uremic syndrome   181
    Rajendra Bhimma, Bernard Kaplan

16. Chronic renal failure and dialysis options   193
    Kai Rönnholm, Christer Holmberg

17. The effects of kidney disorders on the endocrine system   203
    Franz Schaefer, Otto Mehls

18. Nutritional and growth aspects of the care of children with kidney disease   215
    Constantinos J Stefanidis

19. Immunization and anti-microbial therapy for children with chronic kidney disease   225
    Ching-Yuang Lin, Yee-Hsuan Chiou

20. Social and developmental consequences of chronic kidney disease in children   235
    Ken Jureidini, Paul Henning

21. Renal transplantation in childhood   243
    Patrick Niaudet

22. Transition of children with renal diseases into adulthood   253
    J Stewart Cameron

Index   261

Contributors

Allessandro Amore
Ospedale Infantile Regina, Margherita
Piazza Polonia
Torino
Italy

Rajendra Bhimma
Department of Paediatrics & Child Health
Congella
Durban
Kwazulu/Natal
South Africa

J Stewart Cameron
Elm Bank
Melmerby
Penrith
Cumbria
UK

Yee-Hsuan Chiou
Department of Pediatrics
Kaohsiung Veterans General Hospital
Taiwan
Republic of China

Rosanna Coppo
Ospedale Infantile Regina, Margherita
Piazza Polonia
Torino
Italy

Stephen Daniels
Department of Pediatrics
Cincinnati Children's Hospital Medical Centre
Division of Cardiology
Cincinnati, OH
USA

Raymond AMG Donckerwolcke
University Hospital Maastricht
Department of Pediatrics
Maastricht
The Netherlands

Richard Fotter
Department of Radiology
Division of Pediatric Radiology
University Hospital Graz
Auenbruggerplatz
Austria

Susan Furth
Johns Hopkins University
Department of Pediatrics
Baltimore, MD
USA

Jean-Pierre Guignard
Centre Hospitalier Universitaire Vaudois (CHV)
Service de Pediatrie
Unite de Nephrologie
Centre Hospitalier Universitaire Vaudois
Lausanne
Switzerland

Paul Henning
Renal Unit
Women's and Children's Hospital
North Adelaide, SA
Australia

Christer Holmberg
Hospital for Children and Adolescents
University of Helsinki
Stenbackinkatu
Helsinki
Finland

Ken Jureidini
Renal Unit
Women's and Children's Hospital
North Adelaide, SA
Australia

Bernard Kaplan
Children's Hospital of Philadelphia
Pediatric Nephrology
Philadelphia, PA
USA

Kyo Sun Kim
Division of Nephrology, Department of Pediatrics
Konkuk University College of Medicine
Seoul
Korea

Pyung-Kil Kim
Division of Nephrology, Department of Pediatrics
Yonsei University College of Medicine
Seoul
South Korea

Vera Hermina Koch
Department of Pediatric Nephrology Unit
Instituto da Criança
Hospital das Clinicas
Universidade de São Paulo
São Paulo
Brazil

Young-Mock Lee
Division of Nephrology, Department of Pediatrics
Yonsei University College of Medicine
Seoul
South Korea

Adeera Levin
Division of Nephrology
University of British Columbia
St Pauls Hospital
Vancouver, BC
Canada

Ching-Yuang Lin
Changhua Christian Hospital
College of Health Sciences
Institute of Medical Research
Chang Jung Christian University
Taiwan
Republic of China

Tommy Linné
Astrid Lindgren Children's Hospital
Karolinska University Hospital
Solna
Stockholm
Sweden

Otto Mehls
Division of Paediatric Nephrology
University Children's Hospital
Heidelberg
Germany

Mark Mitsnefes
Cincinnati Children's Hospital
Division of Nephrology and Hypertension
Cincinnati, OH
USA

Koichi Nakanishi
Wakayma Medical University Hospital
Department of Pediatrics
Wakayama City
Wakayama
Japan

Patrick Niaudet
Hospital Necker-Enfants Malades
Service de Nephrologie Pediatrique
Paris
France

Rulan Parekh
Johns Hopkins University
North Wolfe Street
Baltimore, MD
USA

Ronald Portman
Division of Pediatric Nephrology and Hypertension
University of Texas–Houston Medical School
Houston, TX
USA

Michael Riccabona
Department of Radiology
Division of Pediatric Radiology
University Hospital Graz
Auenbrugger
Austria

Søren Rittig
Department of Paediatrics
Nephrology Section
Skejby University Hospital
Aarhus N
Denmark

Juan Rodríguez-Soriano
Basque University School of Medicine
Department of Pediatrics
Hospital de Cruces
Baracaldo
Spain

Kai Rönnholm
Hospital for Children and Adolescents
University of Helsinki
Helsinki
Finland

Franz Schaefer
Division of Paediatric Nephrology
University Children's Hospital
Heidelberg
Germany

George Schwartz
University of Rochester
Rochester, NY
USA

Constantinos J Stefanidis

"P. & A. Kyriakou" Children's Hospital

Pediatric Nephrology

Goudi

Athens

Greece

Johan Vande Walle

University Hospital Gent

Department of Pediatrics

Gent

Belgium

Alan R Watson

Department of Paediatric Nephrology

Children & Young People's Kidney Unit

Nottingham City Hospital

Nottingham

UK

Norishige Yoshikawa

Department of Pediatrics

Wakayama Medical University Hospital

Wakayama City

Wakayama

Japan

Israel Zelikovic

Rambam Medical Center

Pediatric Nephrology

Technion – Faculty of Medicine

Haifa

Israel

Foreword

Knowledge is of two kinds. We know a subject ourselves, or we know where we can find information on it.
James Boswell, *The Life of Samuel Johnson*

My excuse for agreeing to write this foreword stems from my life-long involvement in pediatric nephrology and recognition of the critical importance of reference materials for both the beginner as well as the seasoned clinician or researcher. In the face of the increasing complexity of clinical medicine, with the ever-expanding number of diagnostic procedures and therapeutic agents, *Kidney Disorders in Children and Adolescents* provides an up-to-date resource for all those caring for children with renal disease.

Renal disease and renal physiology/pathophysiology attracted my interest from the beginning of my residency experience. When I pursued further training in these areas, long before formal fellowships were established, I was appalled by the lack of textbooks. The sections on renal disease in pediatric texts were brief. Pitts' *Renal Physiology* was a gem, but obviously limited to physiology. Homer Smith published *The Kidney: Structure and Function in Health and Disease* in 1951. This was a monumental contribution, but did not deal with clinical subjects. Comprehensive texts that included renal physiology, pathophysiology, diagnosis, and treatment were nonexistent. Nephrology was a term yet to be introduced. The specialists in renal disease and renal physiology were referred to as 'the salt and water boys', reflecting a major interest in fluid and electrolyte metabolism and disturbances.

In many other ways the field was primitive. The clinical study of renal disease, in addition to family history and physical examination, involved measurement of blood chemistries and urinalysis, including calculation of the clearances of urea and creatinine. Homer Smith had demonstrated that the clearance of inulin provided an accurate measurement of GFR, of particular relevance to the study of developmental nephrology. However, this was, and has remained, a research tool. The technique of percutaneous renal biopsy was only slowly being adopted, permitting for the first time the elucidation of the major histologic abnormalities associated with various renal diseases, which radically changed the taxonomy of these disorders and, ultimately, affected the approach to therapy.

New techniques for uncovering the complexities of renal physiology were emerging, including the methods to study active and passive transport mechanisms, stop-flow techniques, single nephron micropuncture, and the use of isotopes to measure renal blood flow, glomerular filtration rate, and tubular function.

The publication of *Diseases of the Kidney* in 1963 by Maurice Strauss and Louis Welt was a signal event for us neophytes attempting to achieve competence in this rapidly expanding field. It seemed to be the stimulus for the publication of a continuing stream of texts, some providing a comprehensive coverage of all aspects of nephrology, while others focused on specialty areas such as renal pathology, acid-base disorders, tubular disorders, hypertension, nephrolithiasis, urinary tract infection, and the like. Since the major nephrology tomes dealt primarily with conditions relevant to the adult population, I was stimulated to edit the first comprehensive (two-volume) text devoted to infants and children, *Pediatric Kidney Disease*, published in 1978.

With the expanding numbers of textbooks of nephrology, the needs of the nephrologist, beginner or expert, were completely satisfied. What the generalist needed, however, were small treatises dealing with the clinical aspects of pediatric nephrology. Apart from chapters in general pediatric texts, one of the first of these, *Problèmes Actuels de Néphrologie Infantile*, was compiled in 1953 by Pierre Royer, Henri Mathieu, and Renée Habib. Unfortunately, it remained available only in French.

Renal Disease in Childhood was written by John James in 1968. In the preface, he wrote 'This book is intended to serve as a concise practical guide for pediatricians, urologists, general practitioners, and residents in training who may be called upon to care for children with renal diseases. I have therefore emphasized diagnosis and treatment rather than etiology, pathology, and pathogenesis.' This has been the unstated guide for clinically oriented texts that have followed. Royer and co-workers published an update of their original volume, now titled *Pediatric Nephrology*, written in French but translated into English in 1974. Other comprehensive texts of pediatric nephrology followed, most notably *Pediatric Nephrology*, originally edited by Mitchell Rubin and Martin Barratt, and subsequently revised several times under the direction of other editors. A complete collection of pediatric nephrology texts would now fill many shelves.

What then spurred Ron Hogg to undertake still another text of pediatric nephrology? He undoubtedly was aware of the comment made by Royer in the preface to the second edition of his book that the amount of work involved was such that he guaranteed he would never undertake such a task again!

Kidney Disorders in Children and Adolescents adds importantly to the large array of texts already available. It, like others, is a text of clinical nephrology, aimed at introducing students, residents, and fellows first approaching the complexities of pediatric nephrology and providing a comprehensible guide for practitioners in their clinical practice. As in every field of medicine, not every patient can be under the care of the specialist. Pediatricians and family physicians care for the majority of children. In most cases, the pediatric nephrologist is not needed, and the primary care physician can provide totally competent care. *Kidney Disorders in Children and Adolescents* is a much needed, up-to-date guide to clinical management, providing the essentials of diagnosis and treatment, with an indication when referral to or consultation with the pediatric nephrologist is needed. The text is user-friendly in

that there has been a deliberate effort to minimize discussion of underlying basic physiology and pathophysiology other than what is needed to understand clinical management. Although the management of all children with chronic renal failure should be in the hands of the nephrologist, such expertise is not available in every locale. Furthermore, the ideal is joint management by the primary care physician and the nephrologist. The chapters on chronic renal failure, hypertension, and transplantation will be of great help to the non-nephrologist in understanding the details of management as prescribed by the specialist.

More and more children with chronic renal disease are surviving beyond the pediatric age range, The final chapter in this volume, appropriately placed, deals with the transition of children into adulthood, a subject of vital interest and importance as our internist colleagues assume responsibility for our grown-up patients.

Finally, medical practice has become international. The International Pediatric Nephrology Association has recognized this by taking the initiative to support establishment of training programs in developing countries. As demonstrated so clearly by the International Study of Kidney Disease in Children, we must use common language, common diagnostic standards, and common management protocols, while recognizing appropriate regional differences in clinical practice. Basic textbooks of clinical nephrology are essential for this endeavor. By including experts from many countries, writing within their own area of expertise, *Kidney Disorders in Children and Adolescents* presents the authoritative voice of the international community. It will be of great value to pediatricians all over the world.

Chester M Edelmann, Jr, MD
Professor of Pediatrics
Senior Associate Dean Emeritus
Albert Einstein College of Medicine

Preface

When the prospect of editing a textbook on pediatric nephrology was first presented to me, I was initially reluctant because of the presence of many excellent texts already available. However, a series of subsequent discussions led to the conclusion that an up-to-date book, mainly oriented towards primary care physicians, pediatric residents, and other 'non-nephrologists' would be a valuable addition. The concept that the chapters would be authorized by experts from around the world was 'the clincher'. Indeed, the contributors to this book literally span the globe. Many of them have had a significant impact on the development of pediatric nephrology in the global sense.

Readers should be aware that a certain degree of duplication has been allowed, and to some extent encouraged, in the various chapters. In this way, it is anticipated that readers will be able to complete their reading of a given subject without frequently being directed to a complementary chapter for further details or explanations. It will also be apparent that we have not 'standardized' the units of measurement but chose to permit the contributors to use the units that they use in their part of the world. In contrast, a decision was made to use 'American English' throughout the book. This was not an easy decision for me to make because I spent the first 25 years of my life in England, and hence the decision was made by the publishers!

Finally, I would like to thank the contributors who have participated in the production of this book as well as the many friends and colleagues who have helped me over the years, especially those who are from distant places. The 'globalization' of pediatric nephrology has resulted from the efforts of many people, too numerous to mention. In addition, it is important to acknowledge the continued efforts of many excellent organizations to improve the kidney care that is available for children and adults around the world. In this regard, the contributions made by the International Study of Kidney Disease in Children, the International Society of Nephrology, the International Pediatric Nephrology Association and the National Kidney Foundation, via its 'Kidney Disease – Improving Global Outcomes' (KDIGO) initiative, deserve special mention. It is my hope that this textbook will add to these efforts, albeit in a small way.

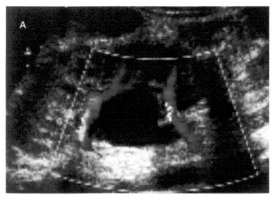

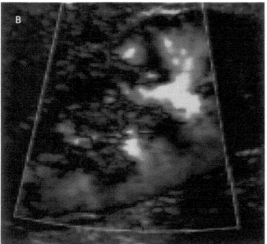

Figure 2.1. Doppler sonography in renal disease

1A) Accessory renal artery depicted by CDS in a hydronephrotic kidney with uretero-pelvic junction obstruction.
1B) Focal renal perfusional disturbance in acute pyelonephritis seen as an area of reduced color signals on amplitude coded color Doppler sonography

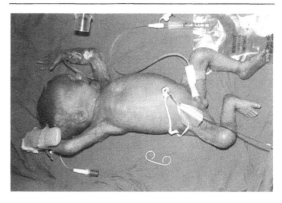

Figure 3.2 Newborn male infant with posterior urethral valves and antenatally inserted vesicoamniotic shunt which was floating free and not draining

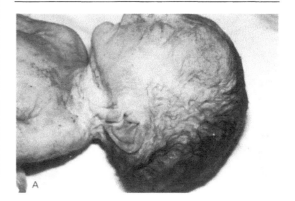

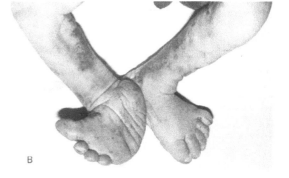

Figure 3.4 (A) Oligohydramnios sequence with low set ears, micrognathia, small chest (B) Rocker bottom feet and equinovarus deformity

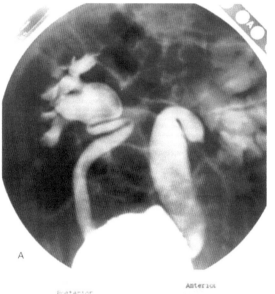

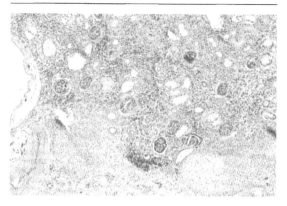

Figure 3.13 Features of renal dysplasia in kidney removed from asyptomatic infant with non-functioning kidney and gross VUR

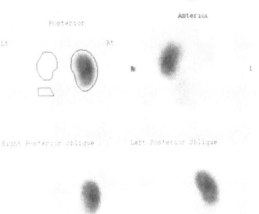

Figure 3.12 (A) Gross bilateral vesicoureteric reflux in asymptomatic newborn evaluated for antenatal hydronephrosis. (B) DMSA scan in same patient showing little function on left side

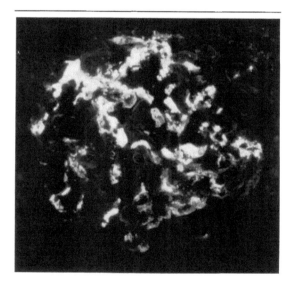

Figure 9.1 Immunofluorescence micrograph showing mesangial IgA deposits in a patients with IgA nephropathy

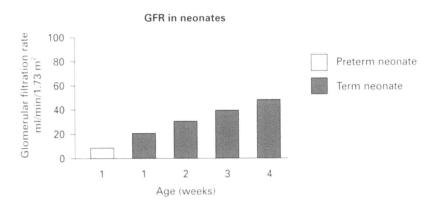

Figure 4.1 Maturation of GFR during the first month of life. The dark columns represent values found in neonates. The 100 ml/min*1.73 m² level represents normal mature levels

(adapted from ref. 1 and 2)

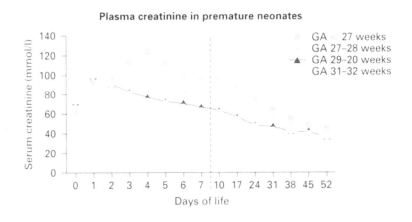

Figure 4.4 Plasma creatinine concentrations during the first 52 days of life of premature infants

(adapted from ref. 8)

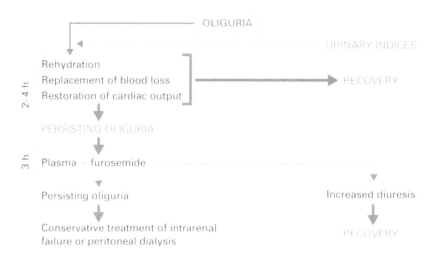

Figure 4.6 Management of acute oliguric renal failure

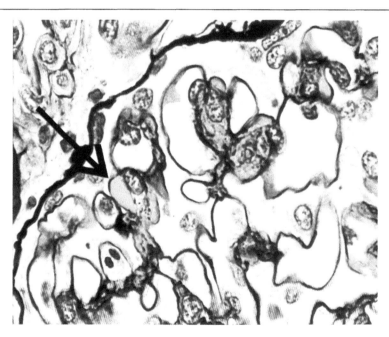

Figure 9.8 Eosinophilic nodular 'fibrinoid' mesangial deposits (arrow) (PASM)

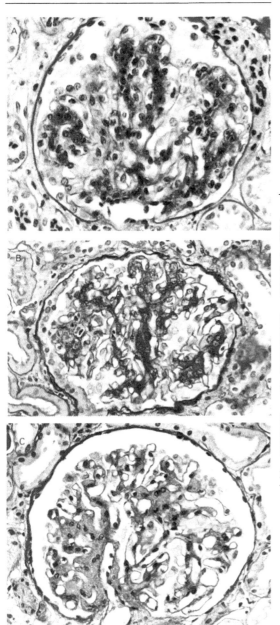

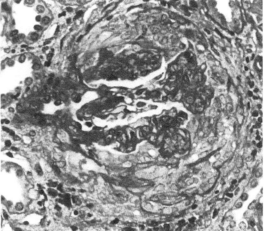

Figure 9.5 Fibrocellular crescent (PAS)

Figure 9.4 Light micrograph showing mesangial proliferation in patients with IgA nephropathy

Three types of mesangial change are identified; (A) mesangial hypercellularity is more prominent than the increase in matrix. (PAS); (B) the degrees of mesangial hypercellularity and matrix increase are similar (PAS stain), and (C) the increase in matrix is more prominent than the mesangial cellularity (PAS stain)

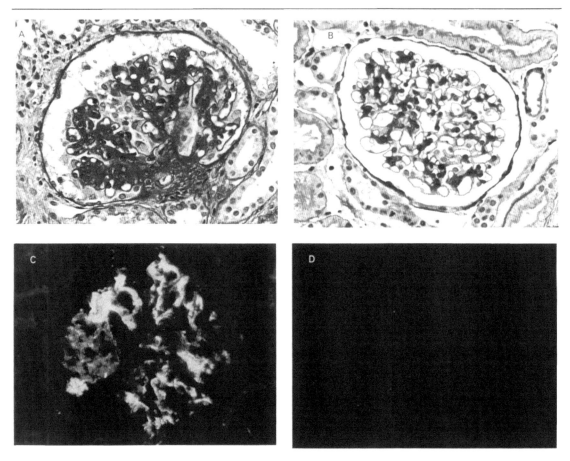

Figure 9.9 Sequential renal biopsies in a patient with IgA Nephropathy treated with combination therapy

(A) First renal biopsy from patient treated with prednisolone, azathioprine, heparin-warfarin, and dipyridamole, glomerulus showing moderate mesangial proliferation (PAS). (B) Second renal biopsy from the same patient. The extent of mesangial proliferation decreased (PAS). (C) First renal biopsy from the same patient with intense mesangial IgA deposits. (D) Second renal biopsy from the same patient showing that the mesangial IgA deposits completely disappeared.

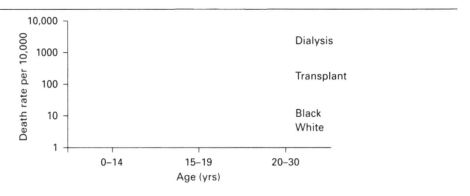

Figure 11.1. Cardiovascular mortality in pediatric ESRD patients: relationship with mode of therapy, age and race (1990–96)

Adapted from Parekh RS, Carrol C, Wolfe RA, Port FK,[8] with permission from Elsevier

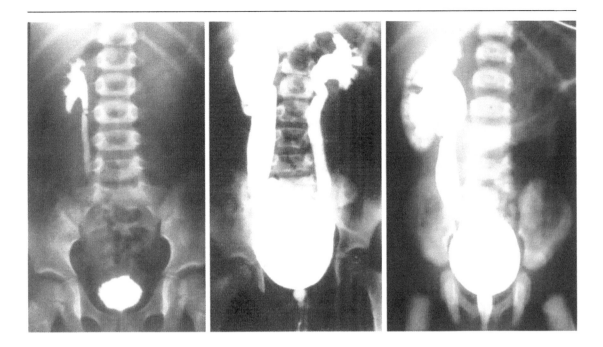

Figure 12.2 Vesico-ureteral reflux (VUR)

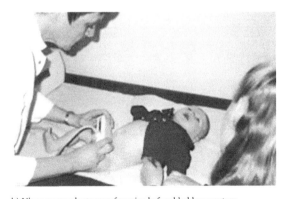

b) Ultrasonography to scan for urine before bladder puncture

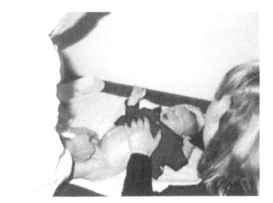

c) Suprapubic aspiration

Figure 12.3 Suprapubic aspiration

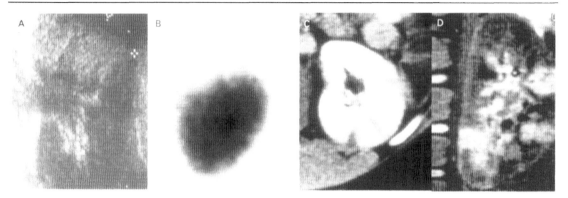

Figure 12.5 Acute pyelonephritic changes visualized by different techniques:

(A) Ultrasonography: Changed echogenicity in the upper pole, not possible to separate cortex and medulla; (B) DMSA scintigraphy: Large uptake defect in the upper pole of the kidney. (C) CT scan with contrast: Note the two areas with reduced circulation. (D) MRI: Multiple areas with changed water content = pylonephritic areas

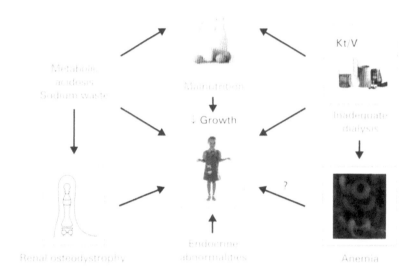

Figure 18.4 Etiology of growth failure in children with chronic renal failure

1. Normal kidney function and development and choice of laboratory studies in children

Susan Furth, Adeera Levin and George Schwartz

INTRODUCTION

"The complex function of the kidney in man and other vertebrates would suggest that this organ has an extraordinarily complex structure. On close examination, however, it is found to be made up of a very large number of structurally similar and anatomically simple functional units. Each of these units, or nephrons, consists of a glomerulus attached to an unbranched tubule, the latter being differentiated into three anatomically distinct portions. In each human kidney there are about one million nephrons, which drain by way of a series of collecting tubules into the renal pelvis and thence by the ureter into the bladder."

Homer W. Smith. *The Kidney: Structure and Function in Health and Disease.*

Oxford University Press. December 1951.

With this simple and elegant description, Homer Smith introduced one of the early definitive texts on the kidney. Since the publication of that text, dramatic advances have furthered our understanding of the morphologic and functional development of the kidney. Additionally, we have come to recognize the importance of normal kidney development and function on the health of the child and that of the future adult. In this chapter we will briefly discuss normal kidney development, and the measurement of kidney function in children outside the newborn period. The definition of kidney damage and staging of chronic kidney disease in children and adults will also be discussed. Additionally, we will present algorithms for the choice of laboratory studies for common kidney problems presenting in children. Early markers of kidney damage and/or decreased function in children should be identified and treated to protect the long-term health of the child and the adult he or she will become.

NORMAL KIDNEY DEVELOPMENT AND FUNCTION

Kidneys remove waste liquid and potentially harmful end products of metabolism from the body. Equally important is the kidney's role as a regulatory organ that selectively excretes and conserves water and other substances essential to life.[1] In humans, the development of the kidney is complex, as essentially three different kidneys form in sequence: the pronephros, mesonephros and metanephros. Development of the metanephric kidneys (the ones that persist into adult life) begins during the fifth week of gestation.[2] The primitive glomeruli appear at approximately nine weeks of gestation. Kidney organogenesis is initiated and maintained by a series of inductive interactions between different tissues derived from the intermediolateral mesoderm to form the nephrons and collecting system of the metanephric kidney.[3] Figure 1.1, adapted from a review by Gomez and Norwood,[4] shows a schematic representation of the process of nephrogenesis. Although in humans a full complement of nephrons is present at 34 weeks of gestation, glomerular and tubular functions continue to mature during the first year of life.

Recent evidence, both from epidemiologic and animal experimental studies, suggest that an unfavorable prenatal environment can affect the kidneys. In rat models, many factors, such as exposure to excess glucocorticoids, insufficient vitamin A, protein/calorie malnutrition, and alterations in the intrarenal renin angiotensinogen system, can affect fetal kidney development and ultimately produce hypertension in the adult rat.[5] Additionally, when nephron number is compromised during kidney development, maladaptive functional changes occur and can lead, eventually, to hypertension and/or

1

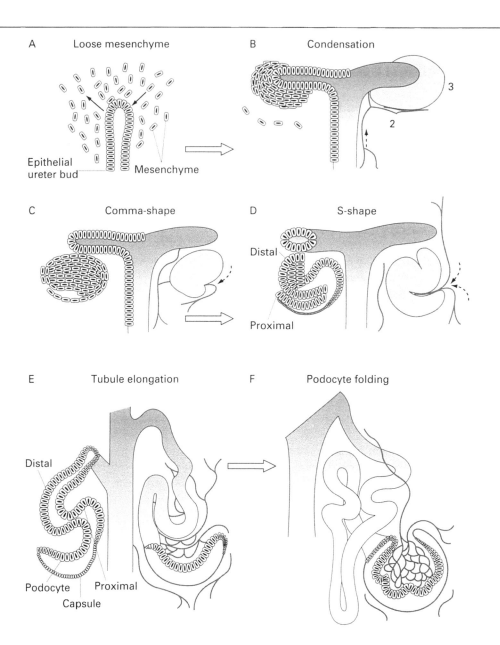

Figure 1.1 Schematic representation of nephrogenesis

A. The branching ureteric epithelium interaction with loose metanephric mesenchyma results in condensation of the mesenchyma in B. Cell lineages shown include: 1) ureteric epithelium, 2) vasculature, 3) undifferentiated mesenchyma, and 4) condensed mesenchyma differentiating into epithelia. C and D. These stages are followed by infolding of the primitive glomerular epithelium to form comma- and S-shaped bodies. E. Elongation of the proximal and distal tubular elements subsequently occurs along with further infolding of the glomerular epithelium and vascular structures to form the mature glomeruler capilliary network seen in F. The initial phases of glomerular vascularization are believed to occur during the early stages of glomerular differentiation in C and D. Figure reprinted from Gomez and Norwood, Recent advances in renal development. Current Opinion in Pediatrics 1999; 11: 135–140[4] with permission. Data from Ekblom[48]

chronic kidney disease in adulthood. Epidemiologic evidence suggests this is also true in the human kidney.[6] Substantial data indicate that maternal diet during pregnancy, as well as perinatal events, has an impact on organogenesis and may affect the function of the mature kidney. This concept, called perinatal programming, or the fetal origins of adult disease, suggests that adverse intrauterine events may determine whether an individual is prone to a variety of health problems including hypertension, cardiovascular disease, or kidney dysfunction.[5] In epidemiologic studies, the combination of small size at birth, followed by accelerated weight gain, has been shown to predict large differences in the cumulative incidence of coronary heart disease, type 2 diabetes, and hypertension in adults.[7]

GLOMERULAR FILTRATION RATE (GFR)

The most useful measure of kidney function is the glomerular filtration rate (GFR). The total kidney GFR is equal to the sum of the filtration rates in each of the functioning nephrons. GFR is measured indirectly through the concept of clearance. The clearance of a substance refers to the volume of plasma that is cleared of that substance per unit time by renal excretion. The clearance of a substance is calculated by dividing the excretion rate of a substance by its plasma concentration ($C_x = U_x V / P_x$) where U_x and P_x are urine and plasma concentrations of substance x, and V is urine flow rate. When the substance is inulin, which is freely filtered and not protein-bound, and is not reabsorbed, secreted or metabolized by the kidney, then $C_x = C_{In} = GFR$.[8] The renal clearance of inulin has become the 'gold standard' for determining GFR.[9] However, there are a number of reasons why this is seldom used – as will be discussed later.

KIDNEY FUNCTION IN THE NEWBORN, INFANT AND CHILD

The kidney of the newborn and young infant has several functional limitations, including a relatively low glomerular filtration rate (GFR). The GFR increases from 13–15 ml/min/1.73 m^2 in the prema-

ture infant, to 15 to 60 ml/min/1.73 m^2 in the full term infant, to 63–80 ml/min/1.73 m^2 at eight weeks of life. GFR, when corrected for BSA, reaches adult values between 12 and 18 months of age (Table 1.1). Although the low GFR of the newborn kidney is sufficient for growth and development under normal conditions, the newborn kidney has limited ability to adapt functionally to endogenous or exogenous stress. The newborn kidney has immature acidification capabilities, which can promote the development of metabolic acidosis when challenged by an acid load. Additionally, the decreased concentrating and diluting capacity of the newborn and infant kidney can lead to abnormal water balance. Along with the increase in GFR, tubular functions of the kidney gradually mature and reach adult levels by 1–2 years of life.[10] Premature babies waste more sodium in the urine than term infants and frequently require oral sodium supplements. The rate of decrease in fractional excretion of sodium from up to 5% immediately after birth to 1% in the more mature individual proceeds more slowly in infants of low gestational age than in term infants in whom the process is quite rapid.[11]

MEASUREMENT OF GFR

INULIN CLEARANCE (C_{In})

The classical (standard) inulin clearance to measure GFR requires an intravenous priming dose followed

Table 1.1 Normal GFR in the infant and child

Age (Gender)	Mean GFR $\pm$ SD (ml/min/1.73 m^2)
1 week (male & female)	40.6 $\pm$ 14.8
2–8 weeks (male & female)	65.8 $\pm$ 24.8
> 8 weeks (male & female)	95.7 $\pm$ 21.7
2–12 yrs (male & female)	133 $\pm$ 27.0
13–21 yrs (males)	140 $\pm$ 30.0
13–21 yrs (females)	126.0 $\pm$ 22.0

Reprinted from: Hogg et al., National Kidney Foundation's Kidney Disease Outcome Quality Initiative Clinical Practice Guidelines for Chronic Kidney Disease in Children and Adolescents, Pediatrics 2003; 111:1416–1421 with permission.[47] Data summarized from Heilbron et al[49]

by a constant infusion to establish a steady-state plasma inulin concentration.[12] After equilibration for approximately 45 min, serial urine samples are collected every 10–20 min through an indwelling bladder catheter, or by frequent urine collections (obtained every 20–30 min), as dictated by the urge of the patient to void. In this case, a high urine flow rate is maintained by providing an initial oral fluid load of 500–800 ml water per m^2 and replacing urine output with water on a ml-per-ml basis.[13] There are technical difficulties encountered in performing inulin infusions such as reaching a steady state of inulin distribution, and measuring inulin concentrations in plasma; these problems have practically rendered the standard inulin clearance obsolete in children. In cases where an accurate measure of GFR is needed, other external markers to measure kidney function have been introduced. These include exogenous radioactive tracers, such as iothalamate, ^{125}I-iothalamate, ^{51}Cr-EDTA, and ^{99m}Tc-DTPA. These substances, however, yield clearance values exceeding those derived from standard inulin clearances due to renal tubular secretion.[14,15] Moreover, the use of radioactive tracers raises ethical concerns in children. A number of other problems related to urine collection must be recognized in children with potential kidney disease when using inulin or other exogenous tracers to measure GFR. The first problem is that children may not be toilet trained and are therefore unable to provide accurate collections of timed urine unless an indwelling catheter is used. Second, urologic problems are common causes of chronic kidney disease in infants and young children,[16] and many such children will have significant vesico-ureteral reflux (VUR), neurogenic bladders, and bladder dyssynergias. Collecting timed urines in these patients is problematic and fraught with error.

Recently, a potential alternative to inulin clearance has been introduced which avoids both the use of radioactivity and the problems related to timed urination and continuous infusion of the marker. Iohexol, a non-ionic, low osmolar, X-ray contrast medium (Omnipaque) that is safe and non-toxic, and used for angiographic and urographic procedures, is eliminated from plasma exclusively by glomerular filtration.[17] Iohexol is excreted completely unmetabolized in the urine with 100% recovery within 24 hours after injection.[18] Most studies indicate close agreement between GFR (measured by inulin clearance) and clearance of iohexol.[14,18–21] Although studies utilizing these exogenous tracers to measure GFR are rarely performed in clinical practice, they are important for research purposes, when precise measures of GFR are necessary.

CREATININE CLEARANCE (C_{Cr})

Because of the difficulties with administering and measuring inulin and other exogenous markers, standard endogenous creatinine clearances are more often used to estimate GFR. However, creatinine is secreted by the kidney tubules, as well as being filtered, so the C_{Cr} exceeds C_{In}, particularly at low levels of GFR.[12] The administration of cimetidine results in a decrease in creatinine secretion by the tubules, which leads to a reduction in C_{Cr}.[22] A protocol for cimetidine treatment has been developed for children, which results in a C_{Cr} that more accurately reflects the true GFR.[23] While the cimetidine protocol is a convenient and inexpensive procedure for estimating GFR, there are still likely to be inaccuracies in timed urine collections in children, especially those with severe VUR, neurogenic bladders, and bladder dyssynergias, as outlined above.

LIMITATIONS OF SERUM CREATININE TO ESTIMATE GFR

In the clinical setting, the serum creatinine is frequently used as a marker of kidney function. However, it is problematic for the clinician to use serum creatinine alone to estimate GFR in children and adolescents. Serum creatinine concentrations are affected by dietary intake of meat, exercise, pyrexia, and a variety of substances. In the steady state, creatinine production is equal to its excretion, but creatinine production is not constant during growth, more than doubling from term infancy to adolescence.[24,25] The consequence of the increasing creatinine production is a steady increase in plasma creatinine as a function of age, along with a further increase with the increment in muscle mass in adolescent males.[26] Thus, the practitioner cannot use plasma creatinine to estimate the GFR without a table of age- and sex-specific normal values.

In adults, as well as children, the use of serum creatinine is widely acknowledged as an inaccurate measure. It is well known that over 50% of functioning nephron mass must be lost prior to a perceivable change in serum creatinine, and that the absolute levels need to be interpreted within the context of muscle mass and gender. As early as 1976, this caveat has been acknowledged and attempts at developing estimating equations for GFR or creatinine clearance have been published.[27,28]

GFR ESTIMATION IN CHILDREN AND ADOLESCENTS

Because of the limitations of serum creatinine to estimate GFR in children, Schwartz et al[28,29] developed a formula to estimate GFR from the plasma creatinine and body length, using an empirically derived constant, k, i.e.

$$\text{GFR} = \frac{kL}{Scr} \text{ where k = constant, L = length (or height) in cm,}$$

and Scr = serum creatinine in mg/dl.

The use of urine collections has not been shown to increase the accuracy of this estimate of GFR based on the serum creatinine. The value of k is 0.45 for term infants during the first year of life,[24] 0.55 for children and adolescent girls,[28] and 0.7 in adolescent boys.[29] This formula generally provides a good estimate of GFR (r ~ 0.9) when compared with creatinine and inulin clearance data.[23,28] At high values of GFR the variation between inulin clearance and GFR estimated by the Schwartz formula is about 20–30%, but it is much smaller at lower levels of GFR.[23,28]

GFR ESTIMATION IN ADULTS

In individuals aged 19 years and above, GFR should be estimated from serum creatinine by using equations that take into account the patient's age, gender, race, and body size. Two such equations are shown below:

a)   Cockcroft-Gault equation.[27]

$$C_{Cr} \text{ (ml/min)} = \frac{(140 - Age) \times Weight}{72 \times S_{Cr}} \times (0.85 \text{ if female})$$

b)   Abbreviated Modification of Diet in Renal Disease (MDRD) Study equation.[30]

$$GFR \text{ (ml/min/1.73m}^2\text{)} = 186 \times (S_{Cr})^{-1.154} \times (Age)^{-0.203}$$
$$\times (0.742 \text{ if female}) \times (1.210 \text{ if African American})$$

where C_{Cr} = creatinine clearance; S_{Cr} = serum creatinine in mg/dL; age in years; weight in kg.

Studies reviewed in the National Kidney Foundation's Chronic Kidney Disease Outcomes Quality Initiative (NKF K/DOQI) guidelines indicate that the MDRD Study equation is more accurate and precise than the Cockcroft-Gault equation for individuals with GFR less than approximately 90 ml/min/1.73 m². In addition, the MDRD Study equation has the advantages of having been derived based on GFR measured using an accepted method (urinary clearance of ^{125}I-iothalamate), a large development database (n > 1000) with a variety of kidney diseases, a large validation database (n > 500) separate from the development database, not requiring measurement of height or weight, and having been validated in kidney transplant recipients and African Americans with nephrosclerosis. The K/DOQI guidelines review other limitations to estimating GFR from serum creatinine based equations and identify clinical conditions wherein one may need to measure GFR using clearance methods. Important clinical examples where the equations may misrepresent the true kidney function include: extremes of age and body size, severe malnutrition or obesity, diseases of skeletal muscle, paraplegia or quadriplegia, vegetarian diet, rapidly changing kidney function, and drugs which may interfere with creatinine excretion.

Irrespective of the formula used i.e. Cockcroft-Gault, MDRD (Modified Diet in Renal Disease), or Schwartz formulae, the important concept is that any calculation is a better estimate of kidney function than serum creatinine alone.

STAGING OF CHRONIC KIDNEY DISEASE BY ESTIMATE OF GFR

Although chronic kidney disease is uncommon in children, its prevalence appears to be increasing among adults particularly in the USA. Standardized methods for describing levels of kidney function by using estimates of GFR, allow a categorization of patients into definable groups for clear communication in clinical care and future research. Furthermore, the translation of the raw number of serum creatinine into level of kidney function is critical to increasing awareness of the problem of chronic kidney disease across all age groups.

According to the K/DOQI guidelines, chronic kidney disease (CKD) in both children and adults is defined primarily as an abnormality of kidney function or structure, as determined by a laboratory test, urinalysis or imaging test which has been abnormal for three or more months.[31] Kidney disease is characteristically asymptomatic, and is often not diagnosed until relatively advanced. In children and adults, evidence is accumulating that untreated chronic kidney disease at any level is associated with poor outcomes.[32-36] Importantly, long-term outcomes are impacted by conditions and risk factors that are present long before the need for renal replacement therapy such as dialysis or transplant. Given the modifiable risk factors identified in patients with CKD (anemia, hypertension, dyslipidemia, abnormalities of calcium and phosphate, and nutritional deficien-

cies) it is important to accurately identify CKD populations.[37-39]

ESSENTIAL ASPECTS AND COMPONENTS OF THE NEW CKD CLASSIFICATION SYSTEM

CKD is defined more objectively in the new K/DOQI classification system (Table 1.2) in order to enhance the study and intervention capabilities of the medical community. The proposed new terminology, applicable by patients, clinicians (primary care providers, specialists, and nephrologists) and researchers should ensure both a clear definition of chronic kidney disease and a staging system which is useful in identifying and differentiating groups of patients.

The essential components of the proposed new system are based on a rigorous evidence-based review process, database analysis (population and referred patient groups) and public review process of international and multidisciplinary breadth. The essential components of the guidelines include the following:

1. Kidney function should be estimated using formulae, derived from serum creatinine, given that serum creatinine alone is so imprecise that errors in patient identification and assessment occur using it as a sole assessment of kidney function.

Table 1.2 Stages of CKD defined by ranges of GFR

Chronic Kidney Disease: Stages according to GFR, and Clinical Action Plan – as Defined in Adults

Stage	Description	GFR (ml/min/1.73 m^2)	Action Plan**
1	Kidney damage with normal or increased GFR	> 90	Diagnosis and treatment; treat co-morbid conditions, slow progression, CVD risk reduction
2	Kidney damage with mild decrease in GFR	60–90	Estimate progression
3	Moderate decrease in GFR	30–60	Evaluate and treat complications
4	Severe decrease in GFR	15–30	Preparation for kidney replacement therapy
5	Kidney failure	< 15	Replacement (if uremia present)

** Actions are not confined to specific stages, and should be additive. These descriptions have been identified in adults. Reprinted from NKF, K/DOQI Clinical Practice Guidelines for Chronic Kidney Disease: Evaluation, Classification and Stratification. Am J Kidney Disease 2002; 39: S1–S266[31]

2. Urine abnormalities (such as high protein or albumin:creatinine ratios) are an important component in the evaluation of CKD.

3. The staging of patients with CKD (1 through 5) is based on increasing prevalence of abnormalities associated with kidney disease, and the stages can be described relatively clearly, according to levels based on ranges of estimated GFR.

1) DETAILS OF THE GENERATION OF THE STAGING SYSTEM

The CKD stages are based on an analysis of adult NHANES III data supplemented by data from other large databases including the MDRD study and the Canadian study of patients prior to dialysis.[30,39] Unfortunately, little comparable data are available in children. Using these existing databases, rigorous analyses were conducted to determine the prevalence of abnormalities based on categories of GFR (where GFR was estimated using an abbreviated MDRD formula). This strategy led to a set of proposed stages. The categories appear consistent when applied to independent samples, in that they define different prevalences of co-morbidities associated with chronic kidney disease.[40–42]

The new staging system recommends use of specific formulae; and underscores the need for accurate calibration of serum creatinine assay measurements. Importantly, the formulae have not yet been validated on all the heterogeneous populations in which they will be used. Nonetheless even those debating the specifics of the estimates of GFR, agree that any transformation is more meaningful than using the serum creatinine alone.[43–46]

2) THE STAGES OF CKD: DEFINED BY RANGES OF GFR (TABLE 1.2)

Normal GFR in children from the age of two years into young adulthood is approximately 120–130 ml/min/1.73 m^2. GFR then declines with aging. A GFR level < 60 ml/min/1.73 m^2 represents loss of more then half of normal kidney function in children and young adults. Below this level there is an increasing prevalence of complications of chronic kidney disease. The burden of earlier stages of chronic kidney disease has not yet been systematically studied in children.

The stages of CKD are defined by ranges of estimated GFR, using the best data currently available from large population based cohorts of patients. While it is possible that some refinement in the exact cut points may occur as more data accumulate, the current staging brings some clarity to the description of the progression of CKD. Furthermore the implementation of the staging system permits a common language among people with kidney disease, clinicians, and researchers.

EVIDENCE OF KIDNEY DAMAGE/DYSFUNCTION

According to the analysis of data from the National Health and Nutrition Evaluation Study (NHANES) and corroborated by other database analyses, evidence of kidney dysfunction in adults is obtained by evaluating parameters such as blood pressure, hemoglobin, albumin, calcium, phosphate, and parathyroid hormone levels, as well as assessing functional aspects such as exercise capacity and quality of life. While there is variability of each parameter within each stage, in terms of prevalence and severity, it is clear that worsening kidney function increases the likelihood of more severe derangements of function. Figure 1.2 demonstrates the prevalence of abnormalities at each level of kidney function in adults. Comparable data are not available in children. Most strikingly, at levels of GFR below 60 ml/min/1.73 m^2, there appears to be an increase in all abnormalities.

Kidney damage per se can be determined by imaging techniques, or examination of the urine. The most commonly used imaging modality in children suspected of urologic abnormalities or kidney disease is a renal ultrasound. This can evaluate the structure of the kidneys, urethra, and bladder non-invasively. In children, evaluation for evidence of kidney damage usually begins with a urine dipstick and microscopic urinalysis. In individuals with kidney disease the urine often contains protein (in micro or macro amounts, most commonly albumin), and may contain cellular elements

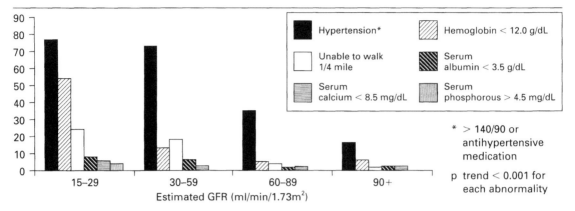

Figure 1.2 Prevalence of abnormalities at each level of kidney function

Reprinted from NKF, K/DOQI Clinical Practice Guidelines for Chronic Kidney Disease: Evaluation, Classification and Stratification. Am J Kidney Disease 2002; 39: S1–S266[31]

such as white cells, epithelial cells, or red cells. Red blood cell casts in the urine are pathognomonic of glomerular diseases. Further evaluation of the child with suspected kidney disease depends largely on the timing and presentation of symptoms, evidence of hematuria, proteinuria, hypertension or evidence of abnormal kidney function.

COMMON KIDNEY PROBLEMS IN PEDIATRICS, AND CHOICE OF LABORATORY STUDIES

ASYMPTOMATIC PROTEINURIA

In children suspected of having kidney damage, a urinalysis should be checked. In non-diabetic children evidence of proteinuria on a dipstick urinalysis should prompt evaluation with a first morning urine protein to creatinine ratio. This should be < 0.2 in children over two years old (Table 1.3). Assessment for chronic kidney disease in post-pubertal patients with diabetes should begin with evaluation for microalbuminuria. An elevation in the urine protein to creatinine ratio or urine albumin to creatinine ratio in diabetic children should prompt further evaluation.[48]

Evaluation of asymptomatic proteinuria in non-diabetic children usually includes evaluation of

Table 1.3 Evaluation for proteinuria in children according to the KDOQI guidelines

	UPr/Cr (mg/mg)	UAlb/Cr (mg/g or µg/mg)
Indication	Assessment of proteinuria in children with positive dipstick	Assess risk of chronic kidney disease in post-pubertal patients with duration of diabetes 5 years
Normal range	< 0.2 (age > 2 yrs) < 0.5 (age 6–24 mos)	< 30 on first am urine specimen
Comments	Also positive in Low Molecular Weight proteinuria	Treat diabetics with microalbuminuria to prevent progressive CKD

Adapted from Hogg et al. National Kidney Foundations' Kidney Disease Outcomes Quality Initiative Clinical Practice Guidelines for Chronic Kidney Disease in Children and Adolescents. Pediatrics 2003; 111:1416–1421, with permission[47]

growth parameters (height and weight), blood pressure, blood chemistries, estimation of GFR using the Schwartz formula and renal imaging studies, most frequently with a renal sonogram.[47] The evaluation of a persistently abnormal first morning urine protein to creatinine ratio in children is outlined in Figure 1.3. It should also include a history and physical with attention to a family history of renal

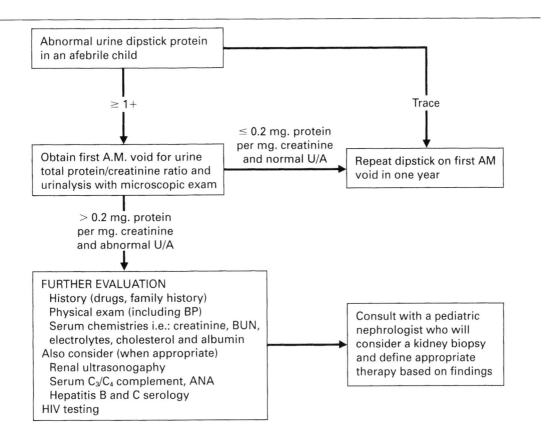

Figure 1.3 Evaluation of persistent proteinuria in children/adolescents

Reprinted from Hogg et al., Evaluation and Management of Proteinuria and Nephrotic Syndrome in Children: Recommendations from a Pediatric Nephrology Panel established at the National Kidney Foundation Conference on Proteinuria, Albuminuria, Risk, Assessment, Detection and Elimination. Pediatrics 2000; 105: p1244, with permission[50]

disease, clues for systemic disease, chronic renal disease, and risk factors for hepatitis or HIV.

In addition to renal sonogram, urinalysis, and assessment of kidney function, blood work should include an electrolyte panel, cholesterol and albumin, a CBC, complement levels (C_3, C_4), and a test for antinuclear antibody and anti-streptolysin O (ASO). Consideration should also be given to testing for HIV, Hepatitis B and C.

HEMATURIA

The presence of microscopic hematuria, i.e. evidence of hemoglobin on a dipstick urinalysis, confirmed by red blood cells in otherwise normal appearing urine on urinalysis on at least two of three occasions, or symptoms of gross hematuria (tea-colored, cola-colored or bloody urine) should also prompt further evaluation. Further history about the timing and onset of hematuria should be obtained: whether it was painful or painless, as well as medications taken, other illness, and family history of hematuria, kidney stones, renal failure, and deafness. Figure 1.4 shows an algorithm for the evaluation of isolated microscopic hematuria. First, the urinalysis should be repeated. A more extensive evaluation should be pursued if the hematuria persists on two or three occasions. There is some

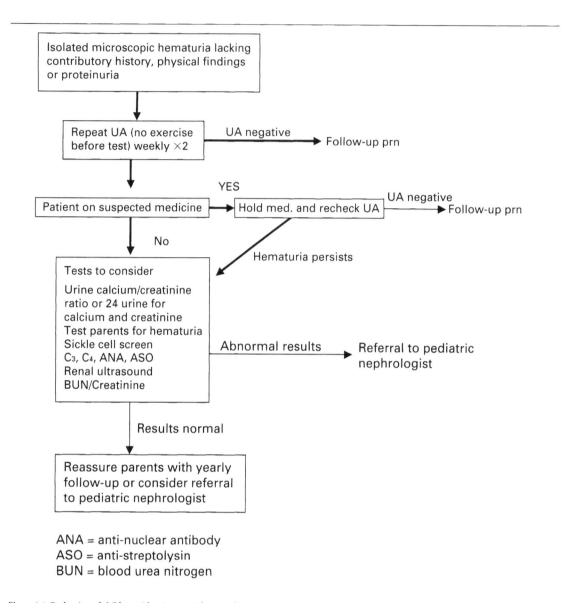

Figure 1.4 Evaluation of children with microscopic hematuria

Modified from Patel et al., Hematuria in children. Pediatr Clin North Am 2001; 48(6): 1528–1529, with permission from Elsevier[51]

debate about the minimal laboratory evaluation for microscopic hematuria, but most pediatric nephrologists would agree that work-up should include evaluation for concurrent significant proteinuria, renal sonogram, evaluation of kidney function (BUN/creatinine), urine calcium to creatinine ratio, complements (C_3,C_4), screen for recent streptococcal infection, and possible autoimmune disease. If history warrants this, an evaluation for stone risk should be considered. Hypercalciuria with elevated urine calcium to creatinine ratio ($>$ 0.2 or $>$ 4 mg/kg/day calcium excretion) is a common cause of hematuria. A positive family history of hematuria may suggest thin basement membrane disease or Alports' nephritis. Sickle cell trait or disease can lead to hematuria, as can structural urologic abnormalities. The presence of significant proteinuria in conjunction with hematuria is much more concerning for an underlying glomerular disease and early referral to a pediatric nephrologist should be considered.

GROSS HEMATURIA

Figure 1.5 shows an algorithm for the evaluation of gross hematuria (urine that looks red, tea-colored or cola-colored). In the absence of a clear history of trauma or suspicion of a urinary tract infection, attention should be directed as to whether the

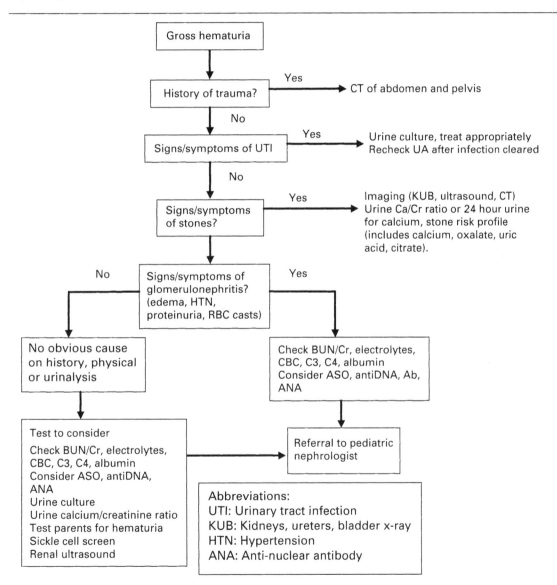

Figure 1.5 Evaluation of children with gross hematuria

Modified from Patel et al., Hematuria in children. Pediatr Clin North Am 2001; 48(6): 1528–1529, with permission from Elsevier[51]

hematuria is painless or painful. Painful hematuria may point to the presence of kidney stones; passage of clots suggests a urologic origin for the blood. A relatively common cause of painless gross hematuria in children is post-streptococcal glomerulonephritis (PSGN), which typically is associated with hypertension and edema, occurring 10–21 days after a strep throat or skin infection. Therapy for PSGN is generally supportive, however, acute renal failure can occur and consultation with a pediatric nephrologists should be considered.

URINARY TRACT INFECTION

The Committee on Quality Improvement of the American Academy of Pediatrics has published an evidence-based guideline summarizing the recommended evaluation of urinary tract infections in febrile infants and young children under 24 months of age. This practice guideline is outlined in Figure 1.6. Once the diagnosis of a urinary tract infection has been confirmed, a renal ultrasound is recommended to evaluate the structure of the kidneys and

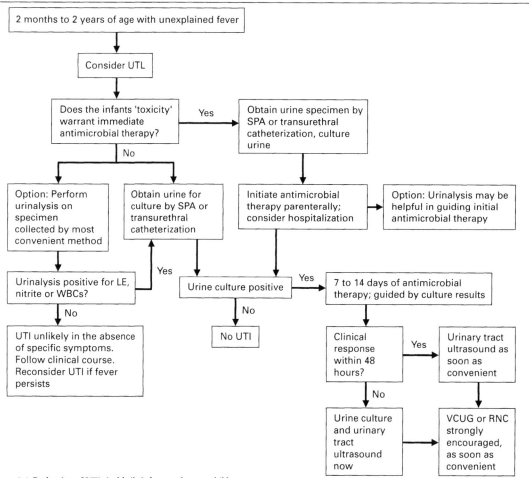

Figure 1.6 Evaluation of UTIs in febrile infants and young children

Abbreviations:

SPA: Suprapubic aspiration, LE: leukocyte esterase, VCUG: voiding cystourethrogram, RNC: renal nuclear cystogram

Reprinted from Committee on Quality Improvement, Subcommittee on Urinary Tract Infection. Practice parameter: the diagnosis, treatment and evaluation of the initial urinary tract infection in febrile infants and young children. Pediatrics 1999; 103:851 with permission[52]

bladder. A voiding cystourethrogram (VCUG) is also strongly encouraged to evaluate for vesico-ureteral reflux. Although current guidelines do not uniformly recommend renal sonography and a VCUG for children more than 24 months of age with a first UTI, these studies are indicated in children with recurrent UTI, or in any child with a first UTI who does not have close medical follow-up.

SUMMARY

There is a clear need for definition, early evaluation, common terminology, and a simple staging system if clinicians are to identify evidence of kidney damage earlier in children and adults. Early evaluation, recognition of kidney disease, and intervention will lead clinicians to screen for risk factors of progressive kidney disease, and ideally to institute appropriate therapies in a timely manner.

Given that the burden of kidney disease in the adult population has increased dramatically over the past decade, the focus has moved to earlier identification and intervention to delay progression and treat comorbidities and complications. Early identification and intervention should begin in childhood and adolescence. A uniform terminology for the definition and staging of CKD such as the NKF K/DOQI system is advantageous in public education, clinical care, observational and interventional research. The proposed system may allow a more accurate assessment of lifetime implications of early kidney damage or abnormal kidney function, identified in early childhood and adolescence. Additionally, strategies which allow efforts to delay progression of kidney damage and treat the co-morbidities associated with abnormalities of kidney function can be implemented.

REFERENCES

1. Vander AJ. Renal Physiology, 4th Edition. McGraw Hill, New York, USA. 1991.
2. Davies JA. How to Build a Kidney. Semin Cell Biol 1993; 4:213–219.
3. Barron CR. Regulatory molecules in kidney development. Pediatr Nephrology 2000; 14:240–283.
4. Gomez RA, Norwood V. Recent advances in renal development. Current Opinion in Pediatrics 1999; 11:135–140.
5. Ingelfinger JR, Woods LL. Perinatal programming, renal development, and adult renal function. Am J Hypertens 2002; 15:46S–49S.
6. Moritz KM, Dodic M, Wintour EM. Kidney development and the fetal programming of adult disease. Bioessays 2003; 25:212–220.
7. Barker DJ, Eriksson JG, Forsen T et al. Fetal origins of adult disease: strength of effects and biological basis. Int J Epidemiol 2002; 31:1235–1239.
8. Schwartz GJ. Does kL/Pcr estimate GFR, or does GFR determine K? Pediatr Nephrol 1992; 6:512–515.
9. Spitzer A. Twenty-one years of developmental nephrology: The kidney then and now. Pediatr Nephrol 2003; 18:165–173.
10. Straues J, Daniel SS, James LS. Postnatal adjustment in renal function. Pediatrics 1981; 68:802.
11. Drukker A, Guignard JP. Renal aspects of the term and preterm infant: a selective update. Curr Opin Pediatr 2002; 14:175–182.
12. Arant BS Jr., Edelmann CM Jr., Spitzer A. The congruence of creatinine and inulin clearances in children: Use of the Technicon Auto Analyzer. J Pediatr 1972; 81:559–561.
13. Dalton RN, Haycock GB. Laboratory investigation. Barratt TM, Avner ED, Harmon WE, editors. Pediatric Nephrology 1999. 343–364.
14. Rahn KH, Heidenreich S, Bruckner D. How to assess glomerular function and damage in humans. J Hypertens 1999; 17:309–317.
15. Silkalns GI, Jeck D, Earon J et al. Simultaneous measurement of glomerular filtration rate and renal plasma flow using plasma disappearance curves. J Pediatr 1973; 83:749–757.
16. U.S. Renal Data System, USRDS 2002 Annual Data Report: Atlas of End-Stage Renal Disease in the United States. National Institutes of Health, National Institute of Diabetes and Digestive and Kidney Disease. 2002.
17. Back SE, Krutzen E, Nilsson-Ehle P. Contrast media as markers for glomerular filtration: a pharmacokinetic comparison of four agents. Scand J Clin Lab Invest 1988; 48:247–253.
18. Olsson B, Aulie A, Sveen K et al. Human pharmacokinetics of iohexol: a new nonionic contrast medium. Investigative Radiology 1983; 18:177–182.
19. Gaspari F, Perico N, Ruggenenti P et al. Plasma clearance of non-radioactive iohexol as a measure of glomerular filtration rate. J Am Soc Nephrol 1995; 6:257–263.
20. Brown SCW, O'Reilly PH. Iohexol clearance for the determination of glomerular filtration rate in clinical practice: evidence for a new gold standard. J Urol 1991; 146:675–679.
21. Erley CM, Bader BD, Berger ED et al. Plasma clearance of iodine contrast media as a measure of glomerular filtration rate in critically ill patients. Crit Care Med 2001; 29:1544–1550.
22. Van Acker BAC, Koomen GCM, Koopman MG et al. Creatinine clearance during cimetidine for measurement of glomerular filtration rate. The Lancet 1992; 340:1326–1329.
23. Hellerstein S, Berenbom M, Alon US et al. Creatinine clearance following cimetidine for estimation of glomerular filtration rate. Pediatr Nephrol 1998; 12:49–54.
24. Schwartz GJ, Feld LG, Langford DJ. A simple estimate of glomerular filtration rate in full-term infants during the first year of life. J Pediatr 1984; 104:849–854.
25. Schwartz GJ, Brion LP, Spitzer A. The use of plasma creatinine concentration for estimating glomerular rate in infants, children and adolescents. Pediatr Clin North Am 1987; 34:571–590.

26. Schwartz GJ, Haycock BG, Chir B et al. Plasma creatinine and urea concentration in children: normal values for age and sex. J Pediatr 1976; 88:828–830.

27. Cockcroft DW, Gault MH. Prediction of creatinine clearance from serum creatinine. Nephron 1976; 16:31–41.

28. Schwartz GJ, Haycock GB, Edelmann CM Jr. et al. A simple estimate of glomerular filtration rate in children derived from body length and plasma creatinine. Pediatrics 1976; 58:259–263.

29. Schwartz GJ, Gauthier B. A simple estimate of glomerular filtration rate in adolescent boys. J Pediatr 1985; 106:522–526.

30. Levey AS, Bosch JP, Lewis JB et al. A more accurate method to estimate glomerular filtration rate from serum creatinine: a new prediction equation. Modification of Diet in Renal Disease Study Group. Ann Intern Med 1999; 130:461–470.

31. NKF, K/DOQI Clinical Practice Guidelines for Chronic Kidney Disease: Evaluation, Classification and Stratification. Am J Kidney Dis 2002; 39:S1–S266.

32. Al-Ahmad A, Rand W, Manjunath G et al. Reduced kidney function and anemia as risk factors for mortality in patients with left ventricular dysfunction. J Am Coll Cardiol 2001; 38:955–962.

33. Herzog CA, Ma JZ, Collins AJ. Poor long-term survival after infarction among patients on long-term dialysis. N Engl J Med 1998; 339:799–805.

34. McCullough PA, Shah SS, Smith ST et al. Risks associated with renal dysfunction in coronary care unit patients. J Am Coll Cardiol 2000; 36:679–684.

35. Mann JF, Gerstein H, Pogue J et al. Renal as a predictor of cardiovascular outcomes and the impact of ramipril: the HOPE randomized trial. Ann Intern Med 2001; 134:629–636.

36. Levin A. Identification of patients and risk factors in chronic kidney disease-evaluating risk factors and therapeutic strategies. Nephrol Dial Transplant 2001; 16:57–60.

37. Levin A. Prevalence of cardiovascular damage in early renal disease. Nephrol Dial Transplant 2001; 16:7–11.

38. Arora P, Obrador GT, Ruthazer R et al. Prevalence, predictors and consequences of late nephrology referral at a tertiary care center. J Am Soc Nephrol 1999; 6:1281–1286.

39. Burt V, Cutler J, Higgins M. Trends in the prevalence, awareness, treatment, and control of hypertension in the adult US population. Data from the Health Examination Surveys, 1960 to 1991. Hypertension 1995; 26:60–69.

40. Levin A, Djurdjev O, Barrett B, et al. Cardiovascular disease in patients with chronic kidney disease: getting to the heart of the matter. Am J Kidney Dis 2001; 8:1398–1407.

41. Levin A, Horl W. for the International Working Group of Kidney Disease. International study of prevalence of kidney disease in high risk populations. JASN 2002; 280.

42. Clase C, Garg A, Kiberd B. Prevalence of low glomerular filtration rate in non diabetic Americans: Third National Health and Nutrition Examination Survey (NHANES III). J Am Soc Nephrol 2002; 13:1338–1349.

43. Clase C, Garg A, Kiberd B. Reply from the authors. Estimating the prevalence of low glomerular filtration rate requires attention to the creatinine calibration assay. J Am Soc Nephrol 2002; 13:2812–2816.

44. McClellan W. As to diseases, make a habit of two things–to help, or at least to do no harm. J Am Soc Nephrol 2002; 13:2817–2819.

45. Jungers P, Zingraff J, Page B et al. Detrimental effects of late referral in patients with chronic renal failure: a case-control study. Kidney Int Suppl 1993; 41:S170–S173.

46. Coresh J, Astor BC, McQuillan G et al. Calibration and random variation of the serum creatinine assay as critical elements of using equations to estimate glomerular filtration rate. Am J Kidney Dis 2002; 39:920–929.

47. Hogg RJ, Furth SL, Lemley KV et al. National Kidney Foundation's Kidney Disease Outcome Quality Initiative Clinical Practice Guidelines for Chronic Kidney Disease in Children and Adolescents: Evaluation, Classification, and Stratification. Pediatrics 2003; 111:1416–1421.

48. Ekblom P. Basement membrane proteins and growth factors in kidney differentiation. In Role of Extracellular Matrix in Development. Edited by Trelstad RL. New York: Alan R Liss; 1984: 173–206.

49. Heilbron DC, Holliday MA, Al-Dahwi A et al. Expressing glomerular filtration rate in children. Pediatr Nephrol 1991; 5:5–11.

50. Hogg RJ, Portman RJ, Millener D et al. Evaluation and management of proteinuria and nephrotic syndrome in children: recommendations from a pediatric nephrology panel established at the National Kidney Foundation conference on proteinuria, albuminuria, risk, assessment, detection, and elimination (PARADE). Pediatrics 2000; 105:1244.

51. Patel HP, Bissler JJ. Hematuria in children. Pediatr Clin North Am. 2001; 48(6):1519–37.

52. Practice parameter: the diagnosis, treatment and evaluation of the initial urinary tract infection in febrile infants and young children. American Academy of Pediatrics. Committee on Quality Improvement. Subcommittee on Urinary Tract Infection. Pediatrics. 1999; 103:851.

2. Radiographic studies in children with kidney disorders: what to do and when

Michael Riccabona and Richard Fotter

INTRODUCTION

Imaging often plays a major role in the diagnostic work up of children with nephro-urologic diseases. In recent years, imaging techniques have undergone significant changes and refinements: these changes have reduced invasiveness and radiation burden by improved resolution. In addition to providing a short anatomic snapshot on an ongoing process, imaging now increasingly focuses on assessment of important functional aspects. Assessment of the impact of these studies on diagnostic, therapeutic, outcome, and life quality efficacy has become a major aspect, as the results of efficacy studies and the growing economic pressure force medicine into evidence-based protocols resulting in new, slimmer, but still comprehensive and reliable imaging algorithms, that are constantly under discussion.[1-9] However, some well-established radiologic studies remain valid; some have undergone major refinements with new, modern techniques that enhance their diagnostic value.[10-12] It is important to note that whereas some new modalities, such as magnetic resonance-urography (MRU), have widened the potential of imaging, some other new methods (e.g. multislice-CT) are used more reluctantly in the pediatric population because of the radiation burden and contrast material risks.

In this chapter, we will provide a description of standard imaging methods that are used to evaluate children with nephro-urologic disorders, as well as try to provide some practical imaging algorithms that the reader may find helpful in typical pediatric clinical presentations. In addition, we will also try to consider the impact of imaging on patient management and prognosis.

IMAGING MODALITIES

ULTRASOUND (US) STUDIES OF THE URINARY TRACT

Renal sonography has evolved into a highly sophisticated imaging modality and is usually the primary imaging tool for examining the urinary tract in children.[3,9-11,13-14] US not only gives reliable information and/or establishes a diagnosis, it may additionally help to direct further imaging studies as needed. Furthermore – as a non-invasive and non-ionizing imaging modality – US allows for repeated investigations that enable close monitoring of the course of many diseases. The US device must be technically suited to neonatal, infant, and pediatric imaging and operators must receive age-specific training and experience in order to produce high quality examinations with consistent results in children. Careful attention to patient preparation is also essential: good hydration and a full urinary bladder are important aspects to avoid missing upper tract dilatation or bladder pathology. A complete pediatric urinary tract US investigation should include evaluation of the following areas of interest:

- The proximal urethra (potentially using a transperineal approach) and entire bladder in longitudinal, transverse and oblique sections.[9,13-16]
- Both ureters – when visible – particularly the uretero-pelvic and uretero-vesical junctions, including the distal ureter and ostial area.
- Both kidneys, in multiple longitudinal and transverse sections supplemented by the use of a high-resolution linear transducer for evaluation of renal parenchyma and the collecting system. It is

also important to measure the dimensions of each kidney and the bladder, with comparison to age, weight, or height-related growth charts.

- The renal collecting system, with accurate measurement of calyceal or pelvic distention and potential pelvic wall thickening.
- Both adrenal glands.

At the end of each study, a post-void evaluation for residual urine, including a re-evaluation of the distal ureters and the renal collecting system (to check for high pressure reflux during voiding), should be conducted. More sophisticated techniques should be integrated into individual studies as dictated by each patient's needs. For example, color Doppler sonography (CDS) or Duplex Doppler US (DDS) evaluation of the renal vessels may be helpful in evaluating renal venous thrombosis and renal artery stenosis in neonates with hypertension, and amplitude coded CDS (aCDS) will allow depiction of focal renal perfusional disturbances such as focal pyelonephritis or infarction (Fig. 2.1).[9–11,13,14,17,18]

Although renal US provides a reliable depiction of most pediatric urinary tract pathology, certain restrictions of US have to be acknowledged, e.g. for excluding vesico-ureteral reflux (VUR), achieving functional information, and in anatomic evaluation of the urethra and the ureters. However, US may depict indirect signs of some disorders, such as thickening of the ureteric and pelvic wall, calyceal distention and/or distortion, dilated ureters, bladder wall thickening and trabeculation, or an increased post-void residual urine volume.[10,11,19] These findings indicate that the next study to be considered should be a VCUG. Further sophisticated refinements of renal US such as extended field of view US, harmonic imaging, three-dimensional US, echo-enhanced voiding cystosonography (ee-CS), as well as the intravenous administration of echo-enhancing agents – the description of which is beyond the scope of this chapter – have and will improve the potential of US and may partially overcome some of the above mentioned restrictions.[9–11,13,20,21] In spite of these advances, US remains equipment and operator

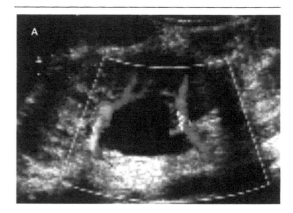

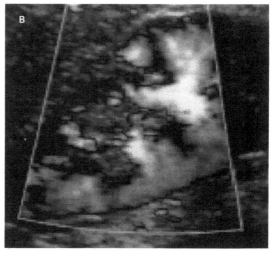

Figure 2.1. Doppler sonography in renal disease

1A) Accessory renal artery depicted by CDS in a hydronephrotic kidney with uretero-pelvic junction obstruction.
1B) Focal renal perfusional disturbance in acute pyelonephritis seen as an area of reduced color signals on amplitude coded color Doppler sonography. (See color plate section)

dependent, and should be regarded as only one component of the pediatric uroradiology imaging options.

PLAIN FILM OF THE KIDNEY, URETERS, AND BLADDER (KUB)

An adapted abdominal plain film, often referred to simply as 'a KUB', may be helpful as a single, relatively low ionizing technique for evaluation or confirmation of certain renal conditions, primarily urolithiasis and spinal malformations that may be associated with abnormal bladder function.[1–3] Important technical aspects include age and size adapted radiation dose, and the use of modern image acquisition systems that permit the lowest possible radiation dose at sufficient resolution.

INTRAVENOUS UROGRAPHY (IVU)

IVU – also called excretory urography or intravenous pyelography (IVP) – is a uroradiologic technique that has largely been replaced by renal US, scintigraphy, and more recently CT and MRI. However, IVU is still one of the most complete diagnostic tools for viewing the upper urinary tract, even though the indications for IVU are in universal decline.[10–12] Certain specific physiologic aspects of the neonatal and infant kidney have to be considered when IVU is utilized, for example, glomerular filtration rate is very low at birth and the tubules are even more immature than the glomeruli. This explains the poor visualization of the kidneys by IVU in the neonate. We therefore recommend that IVU should be delayed at least until the fourth week of life. Dehydration, elevated serum creatinine (with the risk of contrast nephropathy), and allergic reactions to contrast media (though rare in infancy) are relative contraindications to the use of IVU throughout childhood. In the routine IVU, water-soluble, non-ionic contrast agents are used, with the dose adapted to the patients' weight and age. Though today IVU is often tailored to the patients' individual query, the number and timing of films is usually determined at the beginning of the study. In general it consists of a minimum of three films (a baseline KUB, followed by a 3–5 minutes and a 15 minutes view). In patients with obstructive uropathy, delayed films are essential for defining the site and degree of obstruction (Fig. 2.2). In pediatric uroradiology today, IVU is recommended in the child with:

- Hematuria and colic, or other signs or symptoms that suggest a urinary calculus, with indecisive US result.

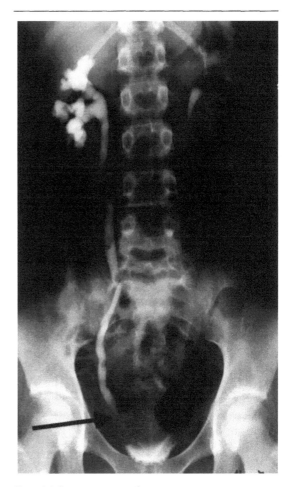

Figure 2.2. Intravenous urography

A delayed KUB – IVU film (1 hour after contrast administration) demonstrates the filling defect in the distal ureter due to a distal ureteral non- (or poorly) calcified ureteric stone

- Certain congenital abnormalities, e.g. urinary incontinence in girls (ectopic ureter?) – if MRI is not available.
- Recent urinary tract surgery, when the urinary tract will be at risk for postoperative deterioration, or for preoperative anatomic assessment.
- Abnormal findings on a renal US that may indicate the need for IVU (e.g. calyceal diverticula, papillary necrosis, medullary sponge kidney).

VOIDING CYSTOUROGRAPHY (VCUG)

The VCUG has assumed significant importance in pediatric uroradiology since it allows for direct visualization of the bladder during filling and emptying. In addition to detection and grading of VUR, the VCUG permits functional assessment of the bladder. The standard VCUG is considered to be the gold standard for urethral evaluation and VUR assessment. However, a significant radiation dose is involved, particularly to the gonads; therefore strict indications must be employed. Follow-up studies of VUR often utilize radionuclide cystography or increasingly ee-CS since these procedures have comparable sensitivity and specificity, with significantly lower or no radiation dose, at the cost of less anatomic detail and less functional information.

To obtain an optimal VCUG in children, the use of modern equipment that is adapted to pediatric needs is of great importance. Transurethral catheterization is utilized under most circumstances. A suprapubic approach may be used for patients with bladder outlet obstruction (e.g. valve, cloacal malformation, trauma), or for psychosocial, cultural and religious reasons. Other important aspects of the VCUG include the following:[10,12,22–26]

- Local anesthesia (Lidocaine jelly) should be used to reduce discomfort. In addition, some pediatric radiologists administer mild sedation (also for amnesia) (e.g. oral, rectal, or nasal midazolam) to reduce distress.
- Antibiotics may be administered prior to the VCUG or added to the contrast infusion to prevent VUR-associated urinary tract infection (UTI).
- The procedure should be performed using warmed contrast material and physiologic filling pressure and speed.
- Cyclic VCUG, usually with three bladder fillings, is advocated to improve VUR detection, particularly in neonates and infants.
- Oblique views of the vesico-ureteral junction should be obtained. Lateral views are helpful for demonstration of low degree VUR and are

essential for anatomic assessment of the (male) urethra (e.g. posterior urethral valve = PUV).
- VCUG must include visualization of the bladder, the ureters, the urethra, and the renal collecting system during voiding.
- A post void evaluation should include assessment of residual volume in the bladder and drainage of refluxed contrast medium from the upper urinary tracts.

There are some variations in methodical details: some centers only image an almost completely filled bladder and during voiding; others use high-pressure contrast infusion to speed up filling. Some centers perform a 'modified VCUG' with intermittent fluoroscopy during bladder filling for evaluation of functional disturbances and early VUR.[10,11,25] The most sophisticated application of VCUG is the combination of fluoroscopy with urodynamics for evaluation of neurogenic bladder dysfunction, a procedure called video-urodynamics.

ISOTOPE STUDIES OF THE URINARY TRACT

Renal isotope scans require the intravenous application of tracers that are marked with a short-lived radiotracer, usually Tc-99m. The activity of the tracer is then monitored by a gamma camera and registered for quantitative assessment. These investigations are focused on various aspects of kidney function including renal perfusion, relative renal function, urine excretion and drainage.[10,11,27] Sedation is only rarely needed, whatever the age of the patient. Most studies use one of four isotopes; the use of each radionuclide will be described in the following sections.

1) A static renogram uses Tc-99m labeled dimercapto-succinic acid (DMSA). This provides an indirect assessment of differential renal function, detection of focal parenchymal defects and a global loss of functioning kidney parenchyma.[27–30] DMSA is extracted from the blood by the proximal tubules and fixed in the tubular cells. Imaging of the kidneys is performed two to four hours post i.v. injection. The main advantage of this 'DMSA renogram' over other scans described below is the

lower background activity, which provides a more reproducible estimation of relative renal function and a clearer depiction of even small renal parenchymal defects (Fig. 2.3).

Accurate determination of glomerular filtration rate can be obtained by measuring the plasma disappearance of an intravenous injection of Tc-99m DTPA or Cr-51 ethylene-diamine tetraacetic acid (EDTA).[25] However, this relatively invasive technique is generally used only for research purposes or in special clinical situations e.g. renal transplant patients.

2) Dynamic 'renograms' use tracers that are taken up by the kidney and excreted into the urine. The isotopes used for this purpose are diethylene-triamine pentaacetic acid (DTPA) or mercapto-acetyl-triglycine (MAG3). The renal extraction of MAG3 is virtually double that of DTPA making MAG3 the isotope of choice for these studies in neonates, infants, and children.[10,11,27] The parameters that can be estimated include renal blood flow, differential renal function, and urine drainage from the kidneys. When dilatation of one or both collecting systems is present and obstruction is suspected, drainage function can be better assessed after administration of a loop diuretic such as furosemide. The quantification of drainage adequacy is accomplished using computer analysis. In order to allow gravity to have its full effect, the bladder should be empty when the MAG3 scan is done.

3) Indirect isotope cystography uses the natural filling of the urinary bladder with a labeled tracer by the kidneys: in the late phase of a dynamic MAG3 study an increase of activity in the area of the ureter and/or the renal collecting system indicates VUR.

4) Direct isotope cystography aims at VUR evaluation. It is carried out very similarly to a VCUG. Instead of instilling radiopaque contrast material into the bladder, a Tc-99m labeled tracer is used, and the gamma camera evaluates the abdomen for any activity in the renal or ureteral area that indicates VUR. With this technique the radiation dose is lower than with a VCUG, at the cost of less anatomic detail, less functional information, and less sensitivity to short-lasting low degree VUR.[10,11,31–33]

Generally accepted indications for renal isotope studies in pediatric patients are:

- Assessment of renal function, particularly for initial diagnosis that can be used as a baseline for follow-up monitoring of therapeutic measures (DMSA).
- Assessment of renal involvement (i.e., acute pyelonephritis or renal scars) in association with VUR and UTI (DMSA).
- Evaluation of renal function and drainage in obstructive uropathy (MAG3).
- Isotope cystography is used for VUR follow-up or screening with direct or indirect isotope cystogram.

COMPUTED TOMOGRAPHY (CT)

Although US continues to be the major imaging modality utilized in pediatric uroradiology, CT has developed a well recognized role for specific pediatric urologic applications.[10,11,34] With the recent advent of spiral and multi-detector CT allowing progressively faster acquisitions without loss of image quality, it has become an easier technique to perform in children with less sedation needs.

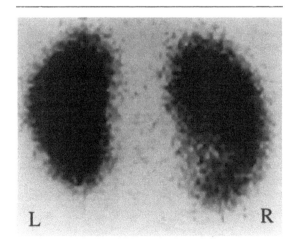

Figure 2.3. Static renal scintigraphy

DMSA scan in a child with aPN. Note the reduced tracer uptake in the lower pole of the right kidney

However, a significant radiation burden persists and needs to be addressed when discussing indications for pediatric uro-CT in spite of the beautiful images and detailed information obtained by modern CT. If a CT is performed, age related protocols at reduced dose (enough to perform a diagnostic investigation, at the cost of some image degradation and noise) are mandatory, and contrast media administration (at weight-adapted dose and age-adapted delay) is necessary for most queries.[10,34] Currently CT is regarded as being particularly valuable in the following nephro-urologic applications:

- Major urinary tract trauma, and acute events such as severe urinary tract hemorrhage (e.g. spontaneous bleeding of an angiomyolipoma).
- Suspected or proven urinary tract malignancy – if no MRI is available.
- As a problem solving tool in atypical chronic urinary tract infections, such as tuberculosis or xanthogranulomatous pyelonephritis (XPN).
- In complicated cases of renal stone disease where US studies and KUB films are unable to provide a definitive answer.
- Investigation of congenital urogenital abnormalities that need simultaneous osseous pelvic anatomy assessment (e.g. for planning treatment) such as in bladder extrophy.
- CT angiography (CTA) in renal vascular disease that potentially involves also smaller vessels which may not be visualized sufficiently by magnetic resonance angiography (MRA).

MAGNETIC RESONANCE IMAGING OF THE URINARY TRACT (MRU)

Modern MRU techniques have improved spatial and temporal resolution and dedicated pediatric coils have improved noise to signal ratio. These new techniques have resulted in MRI studies providing accurate information in both infants and children in the evaluation of renal vessels, assessment of cortico-medullary perfusion and glomerular filtration, as well as visualization of the renal excretory function and urine drainage.[10,11,35–41] Although sedation is often necessary for achieving diagnostic image quality in young children and infants, MRU holds a vast potential for evaluating the child's urogenital tract by a non-ionizing technique that – using intravenous paramagnetic contrast material – offers both anatomic and functional information by a single examination. At present, various conditions, with severe and/or complex pathology, may be studied by MRU (Fig. 2.4). These include:

- Unusual duplex systems, particularly those with poor functioning moieties or dilated ureters, suspected ectopic ureteral orifice or dysplastic renal buds.
- Complex urinary tract and potentially associated genital malformations.
- Renal vascular disease using T1-weighted, gadolinium-enhanced 3d-sequences for MRA.
- Additionally, MRU is increasingly used in patients with impaired renal function, for assessment of kidney or bladder tumors, in complicated urinary tract infection or renal abscess, as well as for postoperative imaging (hemorrhage, urinoma . . .), and in renal transplants.

In all these indications MRU has to a great extent replaced IVU, and appears to be equal or superior to other conventional imaging techniques. In spite of the relatively high cost and its sedation needs, MRU as a 'one stop shop' that reliably assesses anatomy and function, and may help to save costs by replacing inferior diagnostic methods in the individual query. New MRU protocols additionally enable assessment of renal function (relative renal size and function, GFR, renal transit time, renal excretion, and urinary drainage) thus taking over some scintigraphy indications. However, more simple pathology can still be diagnosed and followed with accuracy using the 'old', established imaging techniques.

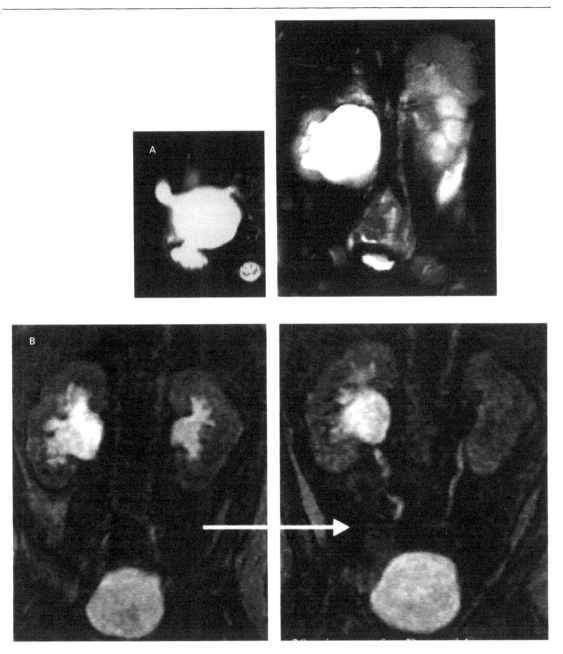

Figure 2.4. MR-urography

4A) Axial and coronal T2 weighted MRU images demonstrate the dilated, fluid-filled renal pelvis, and the anatomy of the uretero-pelvic junction in this infant with severe UPJO and poor function with insufficient contrast excretion on IVU.

4B) Gadolinium enhanced dynamic acquisition during diuretic MRU enables visualization of both anatomy and function (renal perfusion and excretion, as well as urine drainage) in a neonate with equivocal findings for UPJO on diuretic MAG 3 scintigraphy. Left: 15 minutes after Gd; right: 20 minutes after furosemide

ANGIOGRAPHY AND INTERVENTIONAL PROCEDURES

Angiography and interventional radiology represent a small, but important subspecialty of pediatric uroradiology. With the advent of less invasive procedures such as CDS, CTA, and MRA, angiography lost most of its diagnostic importance and is usually employed for confirming suspected pathology, often prior to starting intervention during the same procedure.

Interventional procedures based on modern imaging guidance became safer, thus new approaches were developed and complications have decreased significantly. CT guidance for biopsy and drainage is possible, but rarely used in childhood, as US and fluoroscopy usually suffice and spare radiation. Indeed, many pediatric procedures are performed using US guidance, sometimes complemented by fluoroscopy as a multimodal approach. Modern pulsed fluoroscopy with digital imaging technique has reduced the radiation burden for these procedures. Monitoring of potential complications of any procedure has also become possible by improved resolution of modern equipment, particularly modern US. This new imaging approach detects many peri- and post-interventional conditions.

The most common interventional procedures in the pediatric urinary tract at present are:[10,42]

- Sonographically guided renal biopsy.
- Percutaneous nephrostomy/placement of pigtail/ JJ tubes (combined US + fluoro guidance).
- Puncture/drainage of renal abscess as well as some renal cysts (combined US and fluoroscopy guidance, rarely CT).
- Arteriography of the renal artery and balloon dilatation/stent implantation in renal artery stenosis or aneurysm.
- Intra-arterial embolization, e.g. in severe renal bleeding from posttraumatic injury or renal tumors, for treating arterio-venous malformations, or post-biopsy arterio-venous fistula (AVF).
- Minimal invasive procedures, e.g. percutaneous endopyelotomy or percutaneous nephrolithotomy.

SUGGESTIONS FOR DIAGNOSTIC ALGORITHMS IN PEDIATRIC NEPHRO-UROLOGIC IMAGING

Many nephro-urologic diseases have characteristic and sometimes unique imaging features, while others may be detected but not specified by imaging features. In many conditions, imaging helps to narrow down differential diagnoses or enables safe biopsy for establishing a definite diagnosis. The following suggestions for imaging algorithms are mainly based on the potential of imaging correlated with the clinical presentation, integrating the different imaging techniques, and considering their impact on diagnosis and treatment. Reducing radiation burden and invasiveness in children are most relevant responsibilities for pediatric uroradiology; suggestions for adults may fail in children's nephro-urologic imaging management. Clinical routine and research necessitate close cooperation between all involved disciplines thus creating a consensus on the individual imaging algorithm.

1) CONGENITAL HYDRONEPHROSIS OR UROPATHY

Patients with prenatally diagnosed hydronephrosis need a reliable and economic diagnostic work-up at the lowest possible radiation burden. Subgroups at risk – such as siblings of patients with VUR, children of mothers with VUR, and patients after a febrile/recurrent UTI – will need a more aggressive diagnostic work up; low-risk or screening populations have to follow an even more strict application of the ALARA principle (= 'as low as reasonably achievable'). High grade prenatal hydronephrosis (> 10 mm for third trimester) most probably indicates potential obstruction at the UV or UP junction level or high grade dilating VUR. Low grade (< 7 mm) or moderate (between 7 and 10 mm) prenatal hydronephrosis hold a low potential for relevant obstruction; however, even high grade VUR may be detected in those newborns.[1,2] Planning postnatal imaging management is based on prenatal findings and on the results of the first postnatal US.

Postnatal US should be performed in any case of prenatal hydronephrosis. VCUG is indicated in any case of ureteric dilatation with high grade hydronephrosis, or if postnatal US shows any pathology using 'extended US criteria' (e.g. increased bladder wall thickness, pathologic bladder volume, atypical bladder neck configuration, increased ureteral diameter, increased ureteral and pelvic wall thickness, increased or decreased renal size, altered renal parenchymal structure or parenchymal thinning, and calyceal/pelvic dilatation ...).[1,4,19] In general, postnatal imaging is strategized as follows (Fig. 2.5a, b):

- Fetal low grade hydronephrosis (axial pelvic diameter < 7 mm): postnatal US not earlier than five days after birth (as only by then has renal function matured and allows a reliable evaluation of dilating urinary tract disorders), in a well hydrated baby; if this is normal, no further imaging.
- Fetal moderate grade hydronephrosis (axial diameter of renal pelvis 7–10 mm): postnatal US not earlier than five days after birth, in a well hydrated baby. The need for routine VCUG is under discussion, but should be performed at least in baby boys, and if postnatal US shows any abnormality.

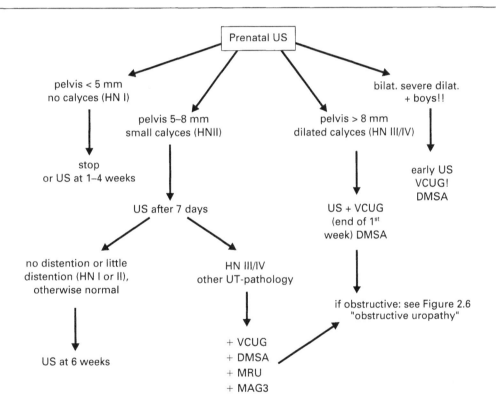

Figure 2.5a. Flowchart: Imaging algorithm in prenatally recognized hydronephrosis

Algorithm for postnatal imaging work up depending on fetal US findings using the HN-classification as established by the Society of Fetal Urology and adapted for postnatal use in infants.

Abbreviations: US = ultrasound, MRU = MR-urograhy, HN I-IV = hydronephrosis grade 1 to 4, DMSA = static renal szintigraphy, MAG3 = dynamic renography, VCUG = voiding cystourethrography.

Adapted from Riccabona M, Fotter R. Reorientation and future trends in paediatric uroradiology: minutes of a symposium. Pediatr Radiol 2004; 34: 295–301[3]

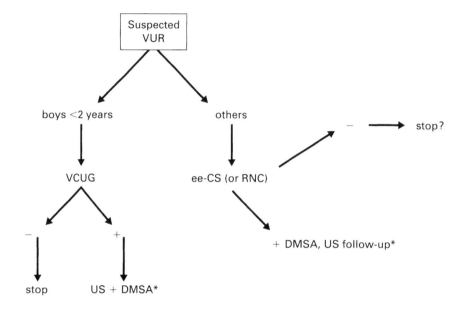

VCUG mandatory in suspected infravesical obstruction

* In case of operation (antireflux procedure): preoperative imaging
that includes VCUG, and sometimes IVU or MRU
(e.g. duplex systems)

In older patients: always think of functional disturbances
with secondary VUR

Figure 2.5b. Flowchart: Imaging algorithm in suspected congenital VUR or PUV

Imaging for VUR depends on cystography: voiding cystourethrography (VCUG) or radionucleid cystograhy (RNC) or echo-enhanced cystosonography (ee-CS).

Abbreviations: VUR = vesicoureteral reflux, PUV = posterior urethral valve, DMSA = static renal scintigraphy

Note: In the future, MRI may partially replace DMSA scintigraphy.

Adapted from Riccabona M, Fotter R. Reorientation and future trends in paediatric uroradiology: minutes of a symposium. Pediatr Radiol 2004; 34: 295–301[3]

- Severe unilateral fetal hydronephrosis (axial diameter of renal pelvis > 10 mm): postnatal US not earlier than five days after birth, and VCUG. The need for routine renal scintigraphy after 8–12 weeks is under discussion.
- Bilateral severe or moderate hydronephrosis, particularly in boys: early US (first or second day of life) and VCUG, followed by renal scintigraphy (timing depends on initial imaging findings, clinical query, and treatment option).
- Prenatal signs of bladder pathology (increased volume, thickened bladder wall, suspected PUV …): early US, and VCUG. Additional imaging depending on these results.

Second step imaging – US follow up at four to six weeks of age, MRU, IVU (not before six weeks), or isotope studies (not before six weeks or three months) – are then based on the prenatal findings and postnatal US and VCUG results.

- In low and moderate grade fetal hydronephrosis without pathology on postnatal US (even using extended US criteria), no additional imaging will be needed in a clinically uneventful child; some perform a late US follow up after three to six months.[3,5,43]
- Neonates with clinically uncomplicated but moderate persisting hydronephrosis may either

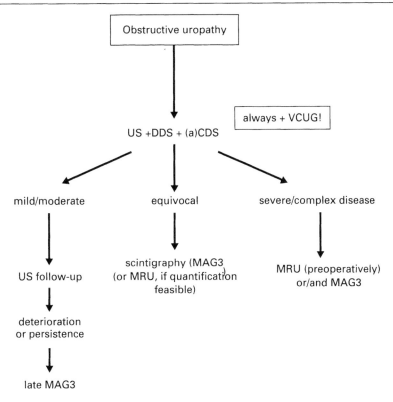

Figure 2.6 Flowchart: Imaging algorithm in obstructive uropathy

US can visualize calicyal, pelvic, or ureteral dilatation. However note, that dilatation does not equal obstruction, and that US is not able to quantify reliably or assess drainage. Therefore, any suspected obstruction needs functional imaging capable of evaluating urine drainage: MAG 3 scinigraphy, IVU, or MRU.

During follow-up, a significant change of dilatation on US, changes in parenchymal echotexture or asymmetric perfusion patterns on DDS/aCDS may indicate deterioration and thus US may serve as a non-invasive and non-ionizing monitoring tool.

Abbreviations: DMSA = static renal scintigraphy, US = ultrasound, MRU = MR-urography, MAG3 = dynamic renography, IVU = intravenous urography, VCUG = voiding cystourethrography.

Adapted from Riccabona M, Fotter R. Reorientation and Future Trends in Paediatric Uroradiology: Minutes of a Symposium. Pediatr Radiol 2004; 34: 295–301[3]

be followed-up solely by US at regular intervals, or may undergo ee-CS/isotope cystography.

- If there is increasing dilatation or any other sonographic pathology such as parenchymal damage, thickened ureteral, or pelvic or bladder wall, a US follow-up and a VCUG are mandatory for differentiation of obstructive versus refluxing uropathy. In general, all neonates and infants with a sonographically abnormal bladder, gross dilatation of the upper collecting system, and renal parenchymal abnormalities should undergo a VCUG, as well as infants with cloacal malformation or spinal cord disorders.

- In obstructive uropathy, a (dynamic) renography at the age of 6–8 weeks is recommended to evaluate renal function and drainage (Fig. 2.6). In some centers, MRU has taken over this indication, particularly in complex cases.[37,38,41] Otherwise IVU may be a useful tool for anatomic preoperative assessment, or differentiation of suspected duplex systems (if there is a clinical impact from that DD). Follow-up in these patients usually consists of regular US examinations, complemented by dynamic MAG3 renal scintigraphy.

2) OTHER CONGENITAL URINARY TRACT MALFORMATIONS

Every suspected congenital urinary tract malformation (multicystic dysplasia = MCD, duplex systems, ectopic ureters, urethral pathology ...) requires postnatal imaging to establish the diagnosis.[3,10,11]

US is the first imaging modality in the postnatal imaging work-up. Neonates with suspected PUV, impaired renal function, severe cloacal malformation, or equivocal bilateral cystic renal abnormalities must be investigated within the first days of life; all other conditions may undergo US after the first week of life. Depending on the initial US result, US follow-up, VCUG (including fistulography or genitography), delayed DMSA or MAG3 scintigraphy, and/or MRI are performed to establish the final diagnosis and monitor the course of the disease.

3) SCREENING

Fetal US is now generally performed under screening conditions. Still, particularly as fetal US is less sensitive towards VUR and unspecific in moderate dilatation, postnatal US screening exams are recommended in high-risk populations:

- Syndromes that bear the risk of associated urinary tract malformation.
- Siblings of patients with VUR.
- Children of mothers with VUR.

Screening is usually complemented by ee-CS (in some centers) or isotope cystography, and by conventional VCUG (particularly in boys with VUR), with additional imaging according to the findings of these initial studies.[1,3,10,11,19]

4) URINARY TRACT INFECTION (UTI)

The imaging protocols in UTI are currently under discussion and are undergoing changes. The reasons for these developments are the growing knowledge, the potential of new modalities, as well as the growing economic pressure, with increasing importance of efficacy-based strategies. At present, imaging is – besides the search for associated or preexisting congenital uropathies – more and more being targeted towards detection of renal involvement, and particularly chronic renal sequelae (scar, reflux nephropathy, hypertension, chronic renal failure). The second goal of modern diagnostic and therapeutic concepts is restoration or preservation of bladder function.[9–11,25,44,45] UTI is diagnosed by clinical symptoms and urine as well as blood analysis. Different queries are important in acute, recurrent, or breakthrough infections. In all these conditions, various therapeutically important information is provided by imaging. In the initial assessment, imaging (= US, DMSA) aids differentiation between upper or lower UTI, evaluates renal involvement, enables detection of associated or preexisting urinary tract malformation, or allows recognition of atypical disease.[7–11,14,17,18,28–30] During follow-up, imaging focuses on monitoring of the acute disease, on evaluation of complications such as abscess formation (initially by US, and complemented by CT or MR), and on long-term evaluation of potential scarring and reflux nephropathy (US + VCUG + DMSA).[9,11,46–48] At present, three major imaging tools are used:

1) US is the first line investigation. US (with aCDS) supports – together with the initial clinical evaluation – differentiation of upper from lower UTI. US additionally evaluates for congenital urinary tract malformations, and helps to screen for possibly complicated disease (e.g. atypical infection, pyonephrosis, abscess, signs for other unusual disease such as bilharziasis ...).
2) Cystography (VCUG, ee-CS, radionuclide cystography) is recommended in every infant with UTI and renal involvement, and patients with recurrent febrile UTI, as these patients have a high VUR incidence that also correlates with renal scarring.
3) DMSA scintigraphy is used to assess both acute renal involvement (= acute pyelonephritis = aPN), and chronic renal lesions, scarring, and

reflux nephropathy. In future this indication may partially be taken over by renal MRI.

We suggest the following imaging algorithm in patients with UTI (Fig. 2.7):

- In first non-febrile UTI, US (including aCDS) may suffice.
- In recurrent or febrile UTI, US (including aCDS) is complemented by early DMSA, at least in all cases with equivocal US findings or mismatch between US results and clinical aspect.
- In patients with recurrent, breakthrough, or febrile UTI a consecutive cystography should

be performed (not earlier than the urine is sterile again, and acute symptoms have disappeared); only in older children may this be postponed.
- In all patients with aPN, a late DMSA at approx. 6–9 months after the UTI is recommended to check for scarring.
- CT or MRI is necessary for evaluation of an atypical or complicated or protracted disease, e.g. DD against tumors, assessment of abscesses, infective stones, renal tuberculosis, or XPN.
- Particularly in girls older than four years, search for functional disturbances such as bladder instability and dysfunctional voiding.

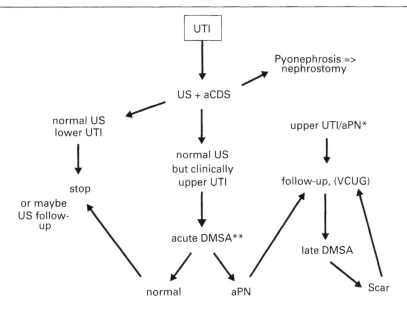

*   or equivocal US => acute DMSA; in future maybe MRI

**   in complicated UTI : MR or CT

    (DD: cyst, abscess, tumor, tbc, XPN, ...)

Figure 2.7. Flowchart: Imaging algorithm for UTI

Imaging in UTI is strategized according to clinical signs of upper UTI, risk factors from patient history, and initial US findings. It aims at detection of renal involvement, prevention of chronic renal scarring, and preservation/restoration of normal urinary bladder function. US and DMSA may suffice if they can achieve these goals, otherwise additional imaging becomes indicated!

Abbreviations: UTI = urinary tract infection, UT = urinary tract, aPN = acute pyelonephritis, DMSA = static renal scintigraphy, (a) CDS = (amplitude coded) color Doppler sonography, Tbc = tuberculosis, VCUG = voiding cystourethrography, XPN = xanthogranulomatous pyelonephritis, US = ultrasound, ee-US = echo-enhanced urosonography, RN-cystography = radionuclide cystography.

Adapted from Riccabona M, Fotter R. Reorientation and future trends in paediatric uroradiology: minutes of a symposium. Pediatr Radiol 2004; 34: 295–301[3]

5) FUNCTIONAL DISORDERS OF THE LOWER URINARY TRACT (bladder-sphincter dysfunction)

A broad spectrum of terms describing bladder sphincter dysfunction without underlying neurologic disease has been published; in general the International Children's Continence Society has distinguished two main types of lower urinary tract dysfunction that now are used as the standard for therapeutic decision making:

- Unstable bladder or bladder instability or urge syndrome (= uninhibited involuntary detrusor contractions during filling), mostly associated with urge or urge incontinence (daytime wetting).
- Dysfunctional voiding (= external sphincter hyperactivity during voiding), eventually leading to a decompensated 'lazy bladder'.

Persisting bladder sphincter dysfunction leads to development of trabeculation, diverticula, and secondary VUR. Bladder sphincter dysfunctions are suspected clinically or are detected by chance. Classification may be achieved using clinical data and the results of functional studies (uroflowmetry, pelvic floor electromyogram, manometry). Based on findings of these functional studies, different imaging algorithms may be applied.[10,11,25,44,45]

- In simple nocturnal enuresis, US may be considered.
- In recurrent or treatment-resistant wetting, protracted disease, secondary voiding disorders, or in complicated disease (e.g. by UTI), modified VCUG[18] may become indicated; a renal DMSA scan should be performed if there is clinical evidence of UTI, or signs of renal damage on US.
- Rare entities such as ectopic ureteral insertion in girls with permanent dribbling have to be considered – the active search for these malformations may necessitate a wider range of studies: in addition to US and cystography, MRU (in some centers IVU), or renal scintigraphy may become necessary.

- In patients with an underlying organic disease (e.g. myelomeningocele, cerebral palsy, cloacal malformations, caudal regression syndromes), US and renal DMSA scan are performed additionally. A 'modified' VCUG[10,11,25] or video-urodynamic studies is advisable.

6) HEMATURIA (AND URINARY TRACT COLIC)

Hematuria is a common finding in children. Besides the finding of, 'dipstick hematuria' some classification can be achieved by presentation and laboratory/microscopy: painful versus painless, macro- versus microhematuria, renal versus postrenal erythrocyte morphology, isolated hematuria or hematuria in conjunction with infection or proteinuria.

There are many conditions that may present with hematuria: among them is nephritis, hemolytic uremic syndrome (HUS), obstructive uropathy, renal or bladder tumor, infection (particularly cystitis), infarction, and renal vein thrombosis. Another condition presenting with abdominal colic and hematuria – though relatively rare in childhood – is urolithiasis. In all these conditions, imaging serves for DD, confirmation of clinically suspected disease, and for management decisions. Imaging in general consists of:[10,11]

- US as the first modality. It may show dilatation of the collecting system (obstructive uropathy), may depict the size and location of an urinary calculus, or demonstrate renal parenchymal disease as well as renal or bladder tumors. US should always be performed with a fully extended bladder, with particular interest in the distal ureter and the uretero-pelvic junction.
- A KUB may be complementary in case of abdominal calcifications or urolithiasis.
- IVU is indicated in suspected urolithiasis with equivocal US results.
- A MAG3 (or a 'quantitative' MRU) study is indicated for grading of obstructive uropathy.
- CT is rarely used in children. It is indicated in complicated stone disease such as an infected

stone, in traumatic (persisting) hematuria for suspected renal infarction, in assessment and staging of tumors (if no MRI is available), as well as for evaluation of tumor complications (e.g. acute severe hemorrhage). In acute renal hemorrhage, percutaneous embolization may offer a treatment option.

- MRI at present is only used for assessment of complex obstructive uropathy or in tumor patients. Indications such as renal infarction or renal vein thrombosis will probably soon also be integrated into the MRI list.
- Advanced US techniques should be applied whenever available, as they increase non-invasive and non-ionizing imaging potential: renal DDS may support grading of obstruction, as acute severe obstruction (even with little distention of the collecting system) may exhibit asymmetrically elevated resistive indices (RI). Elevated RI values can also be observed in other conditions such as HUS or renal vein thrombosis. CDS not only improves diagnosis of renal vein thrombosis or an AVM/AVF; using the twinkling artefact, CDS may support the detection of small calculi. In case of a renal colic, CDS evaluation of the ostial urine inflow jet may clarify ureteral patency (DD partial versus complete obstruction). ACDS may depict renal infarction or segmental infection, and provide information on renal perfusion or tumor vascularization.

The further imaging protocol is then selected depending on the initial information. If US is conclusive, or if other imaging is not likely to enhance the diagnosis (e.g. in nephritic syndrome, suspected HUS . . .), no additional imaging is performed, except for potential preoperative evaluation. In other conditions (e.g. tumor, obstructive uropathy . . .), US offers a definite diagnosis that still needs further assessment or grading by additional imaging (MAG 3, CT, MRI). If there is a suspicion of VUR or urethral pathology, either urethro-cystoscopy or/and a VCUG may become indicated.

7) PROTEINURIA, NEPHRITIC AND NEPHROTIC SYNDROME, RENAL PARENCHYMAL DISEASE, AND OTHER NEPHROPATHIES

The diagnosis of renal parenchymal disease is based partially on laboratory findings; the detection of early disease states as well as of cystic and dysplastic renal parenchymal disease relies on imaging, both in the initial diagnosis as well as for follow-up and DD. Other forms of renal involvement in systemic or immunologic disease (e.g. para- or post-infectious nephritis, nephrotic syndrome, renal involvement with systemic lupus erythematosus, hemolytic-uremic syndrome) are less attractive for imaging: findings may be subtle or even missing and only severe disease exhibits anatomic changes detectable by imaging. Often the diagnosis is established clinically. Usually, an initial imaging assessment is performed for general information and DD hints; during follow-up, imaging may help monitor the course of the disease:

- US is the first and – for most diseases – only imaging tool. It usually allows differentiation of different cystic renal disease entities. In dysplastic or inflammatory renal parenchymal disease US may demonstrate normal findings; sometimes a more or less enlarged kidney with some diffuse alteration of parenchymal echo structure is detected. The most valuable sonographic approach is DDS and aCDS that allow depiction of perfusion alterations. Still, these changes usually are non-specific and relate more to the severity of renal failure than to the type of kidney disease.
- Some specific entities (e.g. calyceal diverticula, medullary sponge kidney) may warrant an IVU, CT or MRI.
- Differentiation of complicated cysts or complex and excessive cystic disease indicates CT or MRI.
- For functional evaluation of particularly dysplastic kidneys (relative renal function), DMSA and MAG3 studies, as well as GFR tests, may be indicated. Otherwise scintigraphy remains non-specific in these queries.

- US guided renal biopsy is performed in certain conditions (e.g. recurrent nephrotic syndrome, progressive/recurrent glomerulonephritis . . .) to histologically establish the diagnosis.

8) RENAL FAILURE (RF)

Acute and chronic renal failure (ARF/CRF) is diagnosed clinically. The role of imaging in these conditions is to aid differentiation of pre-renal from intrinsic or post-renal origin, as well as to monitor the disease process.

- US gives the first information on renal parenchyma, renal size, as well as potential dilatation of the collecting system.
- aCDS/DDS enables assessment of renal perfusion that may be helpful for follow-up during the course of the disease, further for prediction of recurrences or improvement (e.g. DDS in HUS).
- Renal scintigraphy allows assessment of renal perfusion and function.
- CT is practically contraindicated due to the risk of contrast nephropathy.
- MRI at present is not used except for pre-transplant assessment; the future however holds promising applications, particularly for functional MRI in some conditions.
- Interventional procedures (US guided drainage, fluoroscopically guided placement of stents) offer a quick, relatively safe, and reliable relief in post-renal RF.
- During follow-up – particularly of CRF – imaging needs to not only check for the development of renal disease, but also to assess extrarenal complications and sequelae such as osteopathy, growth retardation, cortisol-induced changes (e.g. aseptic necrosis, . . .), or hypertension associated changes. For these queries the entire range of imaging techniques may become necessary.

9) RENAL HYPERTENSION AND OTHER RENOVASCULAR DISEASE

The imaging studies that are often used in the evaluation of renovascular disease are:

- US is usually the first test in a focused search to look for renal origin of systemic hypertension. Gray scale imaging assesses renal size and parenchymal structure. CDS and DDS usually allow a sufficient visualization of the central renal artery and main segmental branches to provide reliable diagnosis of renal artery stenosis. CDS mapping of peripheral renal areas may pick up aliasing in some areas that indicates elevated flow velocity and/or turbulent flow consistent with peripheral stenoses or arterio-venous malformations/AVF. CDS, furthermore, may reliably diagnose conditions such as nutcracker syndrome with a retro-aortal left renal vein, renal artery aneurysm, or renal vein thrombosis.
- Captopril scintigraphy as a screening test is less important in the pediatric setting; however, it may prove helpful in case of indecisive US results before proceeding to more invasive examinations.
- CTA or MRA are indicated for confirmation and detailed assessment, as well as for a reliable 'rule out' test concerning the main renal artery.
- Conventional catheter angiography in children is performed mainly for image guided interventions (e.g. PTA = percutaneous transluminal balloon angioplasty) or for diagnosis of more peripheral or multisegmental disease.[42]

10) PALPABLE OR SUSPECTED TUMOR, AND COMPLICATED RENAL CYSTS

The role of imaging in these entities is detection, confirmation, assessment, and follow-up of renal and bladder tumors:

- Tumors are primarily assessed, confirmed, or detected by US.
- Staging and detailed preoperative assessment indicates sectional imaging such as contrast enhanced spiral CT or MRI. These methods are also indicated if US reveals indecisive findings; histology eventually establishes the definite tumor entity.

Renal cysts in pediatric patients are usually indicative of inherited renal cystic disease (see also Chapter 3 'renal parenchymal disease').

- US is used both for initial diagnosis (often incidentally or in screening conditions) and for follow-up.
- Complicated or atypical and growing cysts, as well as excessive cystic disease, may need additional imaging: for depiction of a calyceal diverticulum or a medullary sponge kidney IVU may be helpful, otherwise MRI or CT (particularly if MRI is unavailable) is used.

11) RENAL TRANSPLANT

Imaging is an important aspect of managing renal transplantation. It starts with the pre-transplant assessment of both donor and recipient, continues with the early postoperative surveillance (renal perfusion and size, obstruction?, vascular anastomosis?, urinoma?, ...), and ends with a continuous evaluation during follow-up as well as of complications such as an infected lymphocele, vascular complications (stenosis, occlusion, thrombosis, AVF ...), rejection, infection, or obstruction:

- US – including US-guided biopsy – is the primary imaging tool that may achieve a lot; equivocal findings or specific queries need additional imaging.
- CTA or MRA complement US for vascular assessment.
- Nuclear medicine studies (MAG 3) and increasingly MRI provide information on transplant function or failure.
- If the native kidneys are left in situ, they also need regular imaging (usually by US and MRI) for cystic transformation or secondary malignancy.

12) NEONATAL IMAGING

Owing to the immaturity of the neonatal and especially preterm kidney, contrast enhanced studies are not only non-diagnostic, but also risk the development of contrast nephropathy and should therefore be avoided. As a result, US is the main imaging tool, particularly as it can be applied at the patient's bedside.

- US including ee-CS and aCDS is the main imaging tool. In general this allows us to answer all common and relevant queries (renal vein thrombosis, DD of ARF, congenital hypodysplasia or cystic renal disease, congenital renal tumor, dilating uropathy, PUV ...), to establish the most important and common diagnoses, or to direct additional imaging.
- VCUG is the modality of choice in suspected VUR and PUV.
- Percutaneous nephrostomy is only indicated in case of severe bilateral hydronephrosis with compromised overall renal function or in (untreatable) pyo-hydronephrosis with urosepsis.
- Static scintigraphic renal scans are useful for global information, but have less accuracy than in the older child.
- CT is rarely indicated; complicated cases are usually imaged by MRU if available.

CONCLUSION

All the accumulated new data on the natural history and the causes of many urinary tract diseases have significantly influenced the ongoing discussion on diagnostic and therapeutic management; thus they also brought up new imaging concepts. A conservative approach with medical treatment is now considered the general first line strategy in many conditions that still required surgery only a decade ago, except for patients with severe anatomic malformations. Operative strategies themselves are being re-evaluated. Finally, it is essential to assess the potential impact of any new investigation or algorithm on patient management or therapeutic concepts. Old and new imaging protocols have to be validated in randomized, efficacy oriented, and prospective studies. These results may then provide sufficient evidence-based data to justify altering the established imaging algorithms, which up to then should not be dropped light mindedly.

At present, imaging will remain essential in many diseases based on well approved imaging algorithms. Mostly they start with US and are complemented by scintigraphy, VCUG, and MRU (or IVU) depending on the clinical query and the underlying disease. To assure the utmost quality at lowest possible invasiveness, these examinations should preferably be performed by well trained personnel in a properly equipped environment that usually is guaranteed in a pediatric radiology department. The definition of imaging algorithms and indication for additional – particularly invasive – imaging should not only rely on international standards, but needs to be adapted to the local circumstances and facilities as well as to the individual patient, thus heavily relying on a good and intensive, regular communication between pediatric uroradiologists and all physicians/clinicians involved.

REFERENCES

1. Avni EF, Hall M, Schulman CC. Congenital uro-nephropathies: is routine voiding cysto-urethrography always warranted? Clin Radiol 1988; 53:247–250.

2. Morin L, Cendron M, Crombleholme M et al. Minimal hydronephrosis in the fetus: clinical significance and implications for management. J Urol 1996; 155:2047–2049.

3. Riccabona M, Fotter R. Reorientation and future trends in paediatric uroradiology: minutes of a symposium. Pediatr Radiol 2004; 34:295–301.

4. Garin EH, Campos A, Homsy Y. Primary vesicoureteral reflux: review of current concepts. Pediatr Nephrol 1998; 12:249–256.

5. Noe NH. The current status of screening for vesicoureteral reflux. Pediatr Nephrol 1995; 9:638–641.

6. Fanos V, Cataldi L. Antibiotics or surgery for vesico-ureteric reflux in children. Lancet 2004; 364:1720–1722.

7. Stark H. Urinary tract infection in girls: the cost-effectiveness of currently recommended investigative routines. Pediatr Nephrol 1997; 11:174–177.

8. Ring E, Zobel G. Urinary infection and malformations of urinary tract in infancy. Arch Dis Child 1988; 63:818–820.

9. Riccabona M, Fotter R. Urinary tract infection in infants and children: an update with special regard to the changing role of reflux. Eur Radiol 2004; 14:L78–L88.

10. Fotter R. (ed). Pediatric Uroradiology. 2002. Springer, Berlin–Heidelberg–New York.

11. Riccabona M, Lindbichler F, Sinzig M. Conventional imaging in paediatric uroradiology. Eur J Radiol 2002; 43:100–109.

12. Carty H, Brunelle F, Stringer D, Kao SC (eds). Imaging Children, 2nd edition, Elsevier Science, Volume I. 2005. The Urinary Tract 537–882.

13. Riccabona M. Potential of modern sonographic techniques in paediatric uroradiology. Eur J Radiol 2002; 43:110–121.

14. Riccabona M, Schwinger W, Ring E, Aigner R. Amplitude coded colour Doppler sonography in paediatric renal disease. Europ Radiol 2001; 11:861–866.

15. Good CD, Vinnicombe SJ, Minty IL et al. Posterior urethral valves in male infants and newborns: detection with US of the urethra before and during voiding. Radiology 1993; 198:387–391.

16. Schöllnast H, Lindbichler F, Riccabona M. Ultrasound (US) of the urethra in infants: comparison US versus VCUG. JUM 2004; 23:769–776.

17. Dacher JN, Pfister C, Monroc M, Eurin D, LeDoneur P. Power Doppler sonographic pattern of acute pyelonephritis in children: comparison with CT. Am J Roentgenol 1996; 166:1451–1455.

18. Winter DW. Power Doppler sonographic evaluation of acute pyelonephritis in children. J Ultrasound Med 1996; 15:91–96.

19. Avni FE, Ayadi K, Rypens F, Hall M, Schulman CC. Can careful ultrasound examination of the urinary tract exclude vesicoureteral reflux in the neonate? Br J Radiol 1997; 70:977–982.

20. Darge K, Tröger J, Duetting T et al. Reflux in young patients: Comparison of voiding ultrasound of the bladder and the retrovesical space with echo-enhancement versus voiding cystourethrography for diagnosis. Radiology 1999; 210:201–207.

21. Kenda RB, Novljan G, Kenig A, Hojker S, Fettich JJ. Echo-enhanced ultrasound voiding cystography in children: a new approach. Pediatr Nephrol 2000; 14:297–300.

22. Fernbach SK, Feinstein KA, Schmidt MB. Pediatric voiding cystourethrography: a pictorial guide. Radiographics 2000; 20:155–168.

23. Paltiel HJ, Rupich RC, Kiruluta HG. Enhanced detection of vesicoureteral reflux in infants and children with use of cyclic voiding cystourethrography. Radiology 1992; 184:753–755.

24. Lebowitz RL, Olbing H, Parkkulainen KV, Smellie JM, Tamminen-Moebius TE. International system of radiographic grading of vesicoureteral reflux. Pediatr Radiol 1985; 15:105–109.

25. Fotter R, Kopp W, Klein E, Höllwart M, Uray E. Unstable bladder in children: functional evaluation by modified voiding cystourethrography. Radiology 1986; 161:811–813.

26. Lebowitz RL. The detection and characterisation of vesicoureteral reflux in the child. J Urol 1992; 148:1640–1642.

27. Piepsz A. Radionuclide studies in paediatric nephro-urology. Eur J Radiol 2002; 43:146–153.

28. Biggi A, Dardanelli L, Pomero G et al. Acute renal cortical scintigraphy in children with a first urinary tract infection. Pediatr Nephrol 2001; 16:733–738.

29. Benador D, Benador N, Slosman DO, Nussle D, Mermillod B, Girardin E. Cortical scintigraphy in the evaluation of renal paraenchymal changes in children with pyelonephritis. J Pediatr 1994; 124:17–20.

30. Jakobsson B, Nolstedt L, Svensson L, Söderlundh S, Berg U. 99mTc-dimercaptosuccinic acid (DMSA) in the diagnosis of acute pyelonephritis in children: relation to clinical and radiological findings. Pediatr Nephrol 1992; 6:328–334.

31. Chapman SJ, Chandler C, Haycock GB et al. Radionuclide cystography in vesicoureteral reflux. Arch Dis Child 1988; 63:650–671.

32. Godley ML, Ransley PG, Parkhouse HF et al. Quantitation of vesicoureteral reflux by radionuclide cystography and urodynamics. Pediatr Nephrol Sem 1990; 4:485–490.

33. Mandel GA, Ehggli DF, Gilday DL et al. Procedure guideline for radionuclide cystography in children. Society of Nuclear Medicine. J Nucl Med 1997; 38:1650–1654.

34. Maudgil DD, McHugh K. The role of CT in modern pediatric uroradiology. Eur J Radiol 2002; 43:129–138.

35. Borthne A, Nordshus T, Reiseter T et al. MR urography: the future gold standard in pediatric urogenital imaging? Pediatr Radiol 1999; 29:694–701.

36. Avni F, Bali MA, Regnault M et al. MR urography in children. Eur J Radiol 2002; 43:154–166.

37. Riccabona M, Simbrunner J, Ring E, Ebner F, Fotter R. Feasibility of MR-urography in neonates and infants with abnormalities of the upper urinary tract. Eur Radiol 2002; 12:1442–1450.

38. Rohrschneider WK, Haufe S, Wiesel M, Tonshoff B, Wunsch R, Darge K, Clorius JH, Tröger J. Functional and morphologic evaluation of congenital urinary tract dilatation by using combined static-dynamic MR urography: findings in kidneys with a single collecting system. Radiology 2002; 224:683–694.

39. Lonergan GJ, Pennington DJ, Morrison JC, Haws RM, Grimley MS, Kao TC. Childhood pyelonephritis: comparison of gadolinium-enhanced MR imaging and renal cortical scintigraphy for diagnosis. Radiology 1998; 207:377–384.

40. Rodriguez LV, Spiekman D, Heifkens RJ, Shortliffe LD. MR imaging for the evaluation of hydronephrosis, reflux and renal scaring in children. J Urol 2001; 166:1023–1027.

41. Riccabona M. Pediatric MRU – its potential and its role in the diagnostic work-up of upper urinary tract dilatation in infants and children. World J Urol 2004; 22:79–87.

42. Riccabona M, Sorantin E, Hausegger K. Imaging guided interventional procedures in paediatric uroradiology – a case based overview. Eur J Radiol 2002; 43:167–179.

43. Wennerström M, Hansson S, Jodal U et al. Disappearance of vesicoureteral reflux in children. Arch Pediatr Adolesc Med 1998; 152:879–883.

44. Sillen U. Bladder dysfunction in children with vesicoureteric reflux. Acta Paediatr 1999; 431S:40–47.

45. Snodgrass W. The impact of treated dysfunctional voiding on the non-surgical management of vesicoureteral reflux. J Urol 1998; 160:1823–1825.

46. Olbing H, Claësson I, Ebel K et al. Renal scars and parenchymal thinning in children with vesicoureteral reflux. J Urol 1992; 148:1653–1656.

47. Merrick M, Notghi A, Chalmers N et al. Long term follow-up to determine the prognostic value of imaging after urinary tract infection: Part 1: Reflux. Arch Dis Child 1995; 72:388–392.

48. Goldman M, Lahat E, Strauss S et al. Imaging after urinary tract infection in male neonates. Pediatrics 2000; 195:1232–1235.

3. Congenital abnormalities of the kidney and urinary tract

Alan R Watson

INTRODUCTION

Congenital abnormalities of the urinary tract are an important cause of morbidity and occasionally mortality in children. Many patients require a joint nephrouroradiology approach and such an example would be a male infant presenting with urosepsis and acute renal failure due to posterior urethral valves.

Ever since the advent of antenatal obstetric ultrasound, abnormalities of the urinary tract have been increasingly recognized in children, the majority of whom will remain asymptomatic. We are still defining the natural history of many conditions detected as a result of antenatal ultrasound, hence pediatricians and nephrologists will have an increasing role to play in the monitoring process.[1]

It has also become apparent that many causes of chronic renal failure in childhood are due to kidney maldevelopments. Databases from around the world confirm that renal dysplasia, obstructive uropathy, and reflux nephropathy account for almost 60% of established renal failure in childhood.[2] As a result of antenatal ultrasound many infants with gross vesicoureteric reflux have been shown to have globally 'scarred' kidneys due to presumed associated dysplasia before infection has occurred.

DEVELOPMENT OF THE RENAL TRACT

There is a lot of current interest in nephron formation which involves:

- Ureteric bud induction.
- Collecting system development with branching tubulogenesis.
- Metanephric mesenchyme conversion to epithelium.
- Glomerulogenesis.

New nephrons continue to form in the human kidney until the 34th week of gestation. Thereafter, increase in nephron mass is by increase in tubular length and glomerular size. Nephron mass is a critical issue with respect to long-term kidney function. There are some concerns that infants who survive extreme prematurity have reduced nephron numbers in the long term. Part of the spectrum of twin-to-twin transfusion in utero can include renal dysplasia in one twin with chronic renal failure from birth.[3]

Most congenital abnormalities of the kidneys and urinary tract (CAKUT) occur spontaneously and are understandable in terms of maldevelopments of the embryonic processes. Genetic influences are evident in conditions such as autosomal dominant or autosomal recessive polycystic kidney disease, and abnormalities in association with recognized syndromes. Research efforts are currently being concentrated on the genetic basis for abnormalities such as vesicoureteric reflux and duplex kidneys.

CAKUT problems are more prevalent in parts of the world where there are high consanguinity rates. Rather than describing abnormalities according to morphologic criteria, it is hoped that basic cellular and molecular biology studies will enable future classifications of CAKUT to be based upon correlations of morphology with pathogenic mechanisms.[4]

ANTENATALLY DETECTED URINARY TRACT ABNORMALITIES (AUTAs)

The incidence of AUTAs has increased considerably over the past two decades, rising from one in 964 births between 1984 and 1988 to one in 364 total births in the years 1989 to 1993, due in a large part to the routine introduction of detailed fetal scanning at 18–20 weeks gestation.[5] The number of conditions observed in Nottingham in this 10 year period are shown in Table 3.1.

In a later cohort of patients studied in our unit between 1999 and 2002 the incidence was one in 155 total births (Table 3.1). One immediately notes that the increased detection rate is attributable to 'non-specific dilatation' of the renal pelvis, a diagnosis that is only arrived at after postnatal investigations. It is generally accepted in obstetric ultrasound departments that a renal pelvic diameter of 5 mm at 18–20 weeks will require rescanning in the third trimester, and a renal pelvic diameter equal or greater than 7 mm at that stage would lead to postnatal referral. This has clearly resulted in an increased number of asymptomatic infants being investigated for minor degrees of pelvic dilatation with the priority being to minimize invasive investigations (see later).

ANTENATAL INTERVENTION

It was thought initially that antenatal ultrasound would reveal dilated urinary tracts with problems such as posterior urethral valves, which would then be amenable to intrauterine intervention in fetal medicine units (Fig. 3.1). In the initial enthusiastic phase, fetuses had vesicoamniotic shunts placed for conditions that were not truly obstructive such as prune belly syndrome and gross vesicoureteric reflux. Many shunts became displaced and had to be reinserted (Fig. 3.2). The criteria for intervening remain debatable. This may be contemplated in a situation with a male infant with obstructive uropathy due to post urethral valves where there is evidence of bilateral renal involvement and falling amniotic fluid volume.[6] Such situations require detailed assessment in a fetal medicine unit with joint counselling including a pediatric nephrologist and/or urologist. The neonatal staff should also be fully informed so that if the pregnancy proceeds successfully, delivery should take place in a regional center where immediate nephrourology

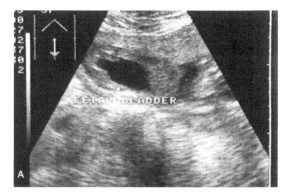

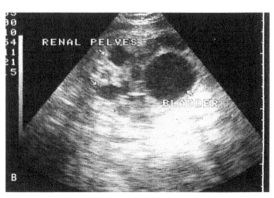

Figure 3.1 (A) Antenatal ultrasound at 28 weeks showing enlarged 'beaked' bladder in male fetus suggesting posterior urethral valves. (B) Ultrasound in same fetus at 32 weeks showing progressive calyceal dilatation and large bladder

Table 3.1 Antenatally detected urinary tract abnormalities – spectrum of conditions in Nottingham (a) 1984–1993[1] and (b) 1999–2002

	a %	b %
Pelviureteric junction obstruction	26	7
Multicystic dysplastic kidney	18	11
Vesicoureteric junction obstruction	8	2
Vesicoureteric reflux	7	10
Duplex systems	6	2
Posterior urethral valves	5	1
Others, e.g. renal agenesis, single kidney	16	12
Non-specific dilatation	14	55

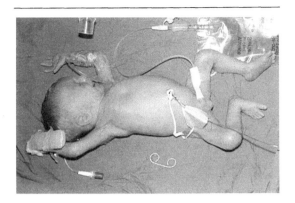

Figure 3.2 Newborn male infant with posterior urethral valves and antenatally inserted vesicoamniotic shunt which was floating free and not draining. (See color plate section)

support is available as well as neonatal intensive care.

Counseling for AUTAs is an imprecise art. Experience has taught us that one always has to be cautious about making an exact diagnosis antenatally, especially when prognosticating on the appearance of echogenic kidneys. Amniotic fluid volume is usually the most reliable indicator of renal outcome as severe early oligohydramnios is usually fatal in association with pulmonary hypoplasia.

Management points for AUTAs include:

- Joint counseling with obstetric staff when an intervention such as a vesicoamniotic shunt is contemplated.
- Dialogue with obstetric staff so that they are aware of outcomes for many of the suspected AUTAs.
- Counseling of parents when requested.
- Information materials in the form of leaflets or booklets to supplement the counseling.
- Liaison with pediatric urologist (if not already involved) especially if true obstructive uropathy expected.
- Neonatal staff should have clear protocol of postnatal management for those with unilateral and/or minor abnormalities.
- After initial ultrasound, it is often helpful to

discuss further investigations at joint nephrouro-radiology meetings.

INVESTIGATIONS

For infants with a AUTA a suggested scheme of postnatal investigations is shown in Figure 3.3. There is a wide spectrum of mainly unilateral conditions in asymptomatic infants and it is our usual practice to allow infants home if there are no other neonatal problems and the child is passing urine well. In the rare situation where there is a palpable mass at birth or bilateral obstruction has been identified suggesting posturethral valves or gross reflux, then the infant would be detained and an early ultrasound obtained. Very rarely is intervention such as a nephrostomy required for an obstructed system. Early urethral catheterization would be advocated in post urethral valves. For the majority of infants the appropriate practice points include:

- Discharge home with parents as long as outpatient arrangements have been made to perform the ultrasound during the first few weeks of life.
- Some units commence all children on prophylactic antibiotics. An alternative view that we have followed is to prescribe prophylactic antibiotics only when there is major dilatation of the ureters or bladder on the antenatal scan and vesicoureteric reflux is a strong possibility.
- If postnatal ultrasound shows kidneys of equal size with renal pelvic dilatation of less than 10 mm, no ureteric dilatation, and no calyceal dilatation or cortical thinning then the child is not brought back for routine review. We would term this non-specific dilatation (Table 3.1). The parents and primary care physician/general practitioner are informed and referral suggested only if any clinical symptoms or urinary tract infection occurs.
- The contrary view is that mild dilatation of the renal pelvis can be associated with significant vesicoureteric reflux. However, in the absence of other kidney abnormalities and no ureteric dilatation when performed by a competent radiologist, VUR is unlikely to be high-grade. In the

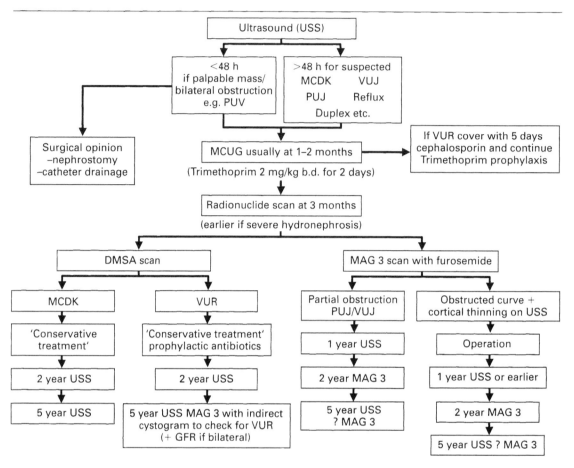

Figure 3.3 Scheme for postnatal investigations of AUTAs

author's experience this approach to discharging infants with non-specific dilatation has not resulted in any problems over 10 years of observation.

- If a micturating cystourethrogram (MCUG) is performed then this is usually delayed to 1–2 months. Antibiotic coverage of trimethoprim for 48 hours is prescribed.

- However, if gross (grade IV–V) VUR is detected on MCUG then a five-day course of a cephalosporin antibiotic is prescribed before the infant returns to regular prophylaxis. Cases of septicemia have arisen from early MCUG investigation with inadequate antibiotic cover.

- The radionuclide scan is usually deferred to three months unless there is severe hydronephrosis

(greater than 30 mm renal pelvic diameter) on the initial USS, in which case the scan is performed earlier.

- DMSA scans usually define non-function in a unilateral multicystic dysplastic kidney, and are also used to document differential function in the presence of severe VUR. Suspected obstruction due to pelviureteric junction or vesicoureteric junction obstruction is quantified using a radionuclide scan and furosemide injection.

- Since invasive tests in an asymptomatic infant can generate considerable anxiety for the parents, it is appropriate to provide them with information materials if they haven't already received them. A liaison nurse is invaluable to support prospective parents in the antenatal clinic and coordinate follow-up with the maternity unit and family after birth.

RENAL AGENESIS

Bilateral renal agenesis is incompatible with prolonged life, due to the associated pulmonary hypoplasia and oligohydramnios sequence with Potter's facies, low set ears, and rocker bottom feet (Fig. 3.4).

Unilateral renal agenesis occurs in about 0.1% of the infant population, is more common in males, and has been described in association with abnormalities of the external ear on the ipsilateral side.

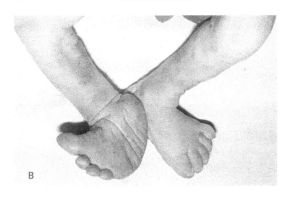

Figure 3.4 (A) Oligohydramnios sequence with low set ears, micrognathia, small chest. (B) Rocker bottom feet and equinovarus deformity. (See color plate section)

Atresia of the corresponding ureter is frequent and supports the view that unilateral renal agenesis is commonly the result of failure of formation of the ureteric bud, or its inability to stimulate differentiation of the nephrogenic mesoderm. The commonest abnormality in the general population is a single kidney (1 in 1000 approximately), but it is possible most of these are due to an involuted multicystic dysplastic kidney (see below).

Ultrasound and dimercaptosuccinic acid (DMSA) scan, including views of the whole abdomen and pelvis to exclude ectopic location, should be undertaken. The presence of a normal hypertrophied kidney on the contralateral side should lead to reassurance, and there is no need for long-term follow-up unless there are associated problems.

RENAL FUSION AND ECTOPIA

The metanephric blastema is originally situated in the pelvis and ascends to its subdiaphragmatic position during early fetal life. During the ascent some rotation occurs so that the renal pelvis, which originally lies anterior to the disk-shaped pelvic metanephros, comes to lie medial to the lumbar kidney. Moreover, the kidney assumes its reniform shape by virtue of its lumbar position and the rotation it undergoes. An ectopic non-ascended kidney is therefore likely to be non-reniform in shape, being usually diskoid, and to have a pelvis and ureter arising anteriorly. The ureter may have a normal vesical opening but may also open in an ectopic position in the bladder, bladder neck, urethra, or vaginal vault. The blood supply is derived from nearby arteries such as the common iliac.

- Ectopic kidney is frequently found in the pelvis and may be higher up the posterior wall or crossed to the opposite side.
- Such crossed ectopia is often fused with a normal kidney – crossed fused ectopia.
- Fusion of normally placed kidneys may occur at the lower poles and give rise to horseshoe kidney (Fig. 3.5). The fusion of such kidneys prevents normal medial rotation, and the ureters arise

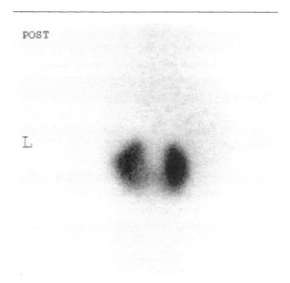

POST

L

Figure 3.5 DMSA scan showing typical picture of horseshoe kidney with bridge at lower pole

from an anterior or lateral, rather than medial, position relative to the renal parenchyma.

POTENTIAL PROBLEMS

- Ectopic kidney can be more vulnerable to trauma and cause obstruction at the time of delivery.
- Ureteric drainage may be impeded with stasis and infection.
- Ectopic ureteric orifice in the bladder is often associated with VUR and prone to infection.
- Horseshoe kidney may be associated with Turner's syndrome in particular.

MANAGEMENT

- Investigation with ultrasound and radionuclide imaging, usually with DMSA, but Mag 3 preferred if obstruction is suspected.
- MCUG if ureteric or pelvic dilatation or UTI.
- Most children who are asymptomatic do not need long-term follow-up if the family are fully informed.

DUPLEX SYSTEMS

Varying degrees of duplication occur. Double and completely separate pelves may occur (on one or both sides), draining via separate ureters to separate ureteric orifices in the bladder. There may be two pelves and one ureter or the two ureters may unite in Y fashion during the descent to the bladder. Such duplication is sometimes associated with vesico-ureteric reflux or other abnormalities and this gives rise to problems such as recurrent infection.

CLINICAL FEATURES

- Duplex kidneys is one of the commonest abnormalities detected on imaging of the urinary tract, with a strong familial tendency.
- Commonly, one of the ureters is associated with a ureterocele (cystic dilation of the intra-vesical portion of the ureter) which can lead to obstruction and hydronephrosis (Fig. 3.6).
- The ureter leading from the lower pelvis to the upper ureteric orifice is most often the abnormal one. Cystography might reveal unilateral or bilateral VUR.
- Either ureteric orifice in the duplex kidney may open ectopically into the bladder, the urethra, or the vagina. The important clinical clue is continued wetting during the day. Suspect if child apparently never had a dry day, but may be dry at night if small dysplastic upper pole. This abnormal pole of the kidney may be hard to define on ultrasound but may require DMSA or intravenous pyelogram.

MANAGEMENT

- No treatment if patient is asymptomatic ± one episode of UTI that is uncomplicated.

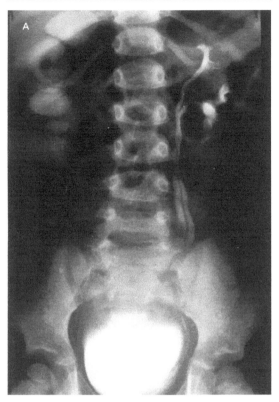

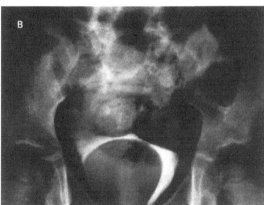

Figure 3.6 IVU in a three-year old girl investigated for urinary tract infection showing (A) duplex system on left side and hydronephrosis in duplex system on right side with hydronephrosis being associated with (B) ureterocele, showing as filling defect in bladder

- Surgical decompression ('pinging') of ureterocele if obstruction in newborn period.
- Antibiotic prophylaxis for VUR and surgical correction if breakthrough infections (VUR into duplex less likely to resolve).
- Surgical correction of ectopic ureter can be most rewarding for patient and surgeon as it can dramatically make a child 'dry' after years of 'wetting'.

RENAL DYSPLASIA AND HYPOPLASIA

It is difficult to know whether these two conditions should be separated. True hypoplasia (i.e. a normally developed but unduly small kidney) is rare. It is best identified by its small size and diminution of the number of papillae and calyces present. Most cases are associated with some degree of dysplasia as well (Fig. 3.7). Renal dysplasia may produce diminution or increase in total renal size, but its characteristic feature is the presence of pluripotent undifferentiated mesenchyme, which may give rise to aberrant tissue such as cartilage and smooth muscle within the kidney. Cyst formation is common and has been attributed to premature cessation of branching by the ureteric bud which, being unable to induce nephron formation, degenerates and becomes cystic. Obstruction to the ureter in fetal life is also a factor in pathogenesis, and causes well marked dilatation of Bowman's capsule in some cases. The dysplasia may be unilateral in which case the opposite kidney functions normally, or may be bilateral. Oligomeganephronia is one form of bilateral dysplastic kidney that is characterized by a reduced number of very large nephrons, which undergo progressive focal sclerosis.

CLINICAL PRESENTATION

- Maldevelopment of the kidney may be recognized antenatally with abnormally echogenic kidneys.

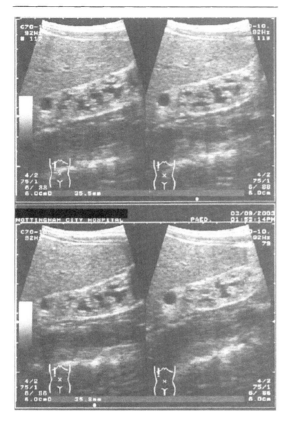

Figure 3.7 Postnatal ultrasound in infant with chronic renal failure associated with bilateral small abnormally echogenic kidneys with small cysts suggesting dysplasia

- Echogenic kidneys have many causes and prognostication is difficult until serial measurements of kidney growth and renal function have been undertaken.
- Children with renal dysplasia may present with acute on chronic renal failure with incidental acute illnesses such as gastroenteritis.
- Many children with renal dysplasia may go undetected but children who fail to thrive should always have urinalysis and creatinine measured.
- Children with renal dysplasia may be polyuric and progress into chronic renal failure in adolescence when they outgrow their kidney reserve.

MULTICYSTIC DYSPLASTIC KIDNEY

The most common cystic lesion recognized antenatally is multicystic dysplastic kidney (MCDK). In this disorder, renal dysplasia associated with a number of cysts is believed to result from failed coordination between the developing metanephros and the branching ureteric bud. The condition may be bilateral in association with other lethal abnormalities or syndromes, and such fetuses die from the oligohydramnios sequence.[7] Most cases are unilateral with an occasional infant having a palpable abdominal mass.[8]

CLINICAL PRESENTATION AND MANAGEMENT

- Usually asymptomatic and detected antenatally.
- Postnatal ultrasound confirms cystic features (Fig. 3.8A) and DMSA scan confirms nonfunction in the MCDK kidney (Fig. 3.8B).
- Approximately 20% have VUR into the contralateral kidney, and other abnormalities can also occur such as pelviureteric junction obstruction.
- Most VUR is mild to moderate; follow-up in our unit has shown no cases of pyelonephritis and no difference in UTIs between those with or without VUR. MCUG is therefore no longer *routine* in our unit unless ureteric dilatation (implying gross VUR) on first ultrasound.
- Occasional reports of hypertension, sepsis, and, extremely rarely, malignancy have been used to justify nephrectomy, but long-term follow-up has confirmed that most MCDK kidneys involute with time (47% at five years and 60% at 10 years).[8]
- An involuted MCDK may be a major contributor to the commonest abnormality in general population, i.e. single kidney.

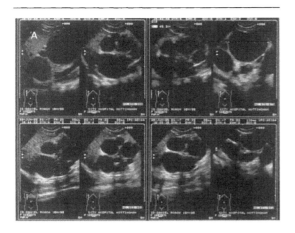

Figure 3.8 (A) Postnatal USS of infant with unilateral right MCDK (left normal). (B) Confirmation of non-functioning right MCDK on DMSA

PELVIURETERIC JUNCTION (PUJ) OBSTRUCTION

PUJ obstruction is identified by renal pelvic, but no ureteric, dilatation. It is obviously a spectrum condition with children presenting from the neonatal period into adulthood with symptoms such as intermittent abdominal pain, flank mass, haematuria, and urinary tract infection associated with a classical dilated pelvis on ultrasound or IVU. The symptoms above are usually surgical indications for a pyeloplasty (Fig. 3.9).

However, the findings of variable degrees of renal pelvic dilatation on antenatal ultrasound have provided one of the biggest dilemmas with respect to postnatal management. The surgical adage that 'dilatation does not equal obstruction' is particularly pertinent in infants with antenatally detected PUJ holdup.[9] On the other hand, the kidney is growing and maturing rapidly in the first two years of life and sustained high pelvic pressures may impede normal development.

MANAGEMENT

- Radiologic assessment of the PUJ consists of ultrasound with attention to the renal pelvic diameter, calyceal dilatation, cortical thickness, and overall kidney size.
- Radionuclide investigation of choice is a Mag 3 (^{99m}Tc-labeled mercaptoacetyl triglycine) scan combined with furosemide to determine differential function, response to diuretic, and degree of holdup on delayed films (Fig. 3.10).
- MCUG under trimethoprim cover is also performed in young infants as pseudo PUJ holdup can occur with gross vesicoureteric reflux.
- Symptomatic patients usually proceed to pyeloplasty.
- Asymptomatic infants with antenatally detected PUJ holdup are usually operated upon only if there is a tense distended kidney in the newborn period, or if serial scans show significant calyceal dilatation with thinning of the cortex and reduction of differential function below 40% on radionuclide scan, combined with delayed excretion on late films.
- There is little in the way of controlled data, and a consensus view is best arrived at with a combined meeting between urologists, nephrologists, and radiologists.

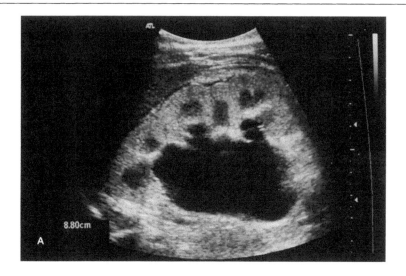

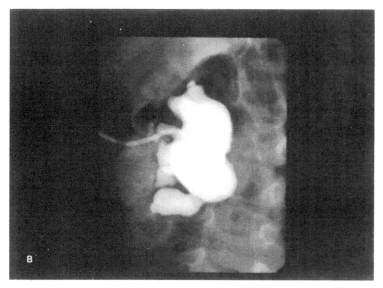

Figure 3.9 (A) USS in infant with acute renal failure due to PUJ obstruction in single kidney with marked pelvic and calyceal dilation. (B) Nephrostogram in same patient confirming PUJ obstruction

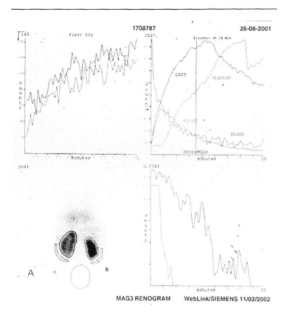

MAG3 RENOGRAM   WebLink/SIEMENS 11/02/2002

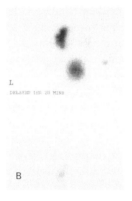

Figure 3.10 (A) MAG 3 renogram in asymptomatic infant being evaluated for PUJ obstruction. Delayed excretion L side. (B) Delayed film at 1hr 20mins in same patient (lower image) shows clearing of dye. Patient followed with serial ultrasound

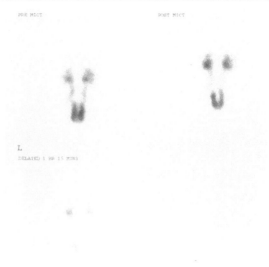

Figure 3.11 MAG 3 images in infant being evaluated for VUJ obstruction. Filling of ureters noted on both sides but clearing on delayed image

As with PUJ obstruction, some infants may present at a later stage with urinary tract infection, pyonephrosis, hematuria, or loin pain.

- Radiologic investigations include ultrasound scan and MAG 3 scan with furosemide (Fig. 3.11).
- MCUG under trimethoprim cover is performed as some megaureters that result from VUJ holdup are associated with VUR.
- Symptomatic VUJ obstruction is usually operated on with a tapered reimplant operation.
- Most infants with antenatally detected VUJ holdup remain asymptomatic, and are observed with serial ultrasound studies.

VESICOURETERIC JUNCTION (VUJ) OBSTRUCTION

This condition may be recognized antenatally by renal pelvic and ureteric dilatation. Children with antenatally detected VUJ holdup are asymptomatic.

VESICOURETERIC REFLUX (VUR)

Asymptomatic infants investigated for VUR as a result of antenatal ultrasound have shown that some already have very poorly functioning

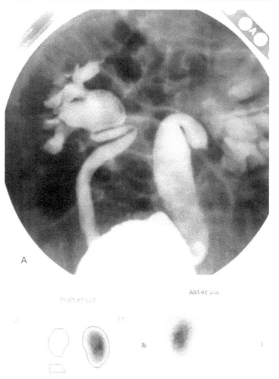

A

B

Figure 3.12 (A) Gross bilateral vesicoureteric reflux in asymptomatic newborn evaluated for antenatal hydronephrosis. (B) DMSA scan in same patient showing little function on left side. (See color plate section)

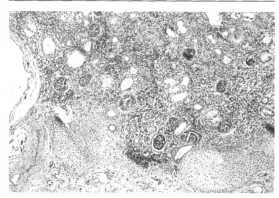

Figure 3.13 Features of renal dysplasia in kidney removed from asyptomatic infant with non-functioning kidney and gross VUR. (See color plate section)

MANAGEMENT

- Ultrasound to document renal length in relation to patient length as baseline for kidney growth.
- Initial MCUG performed under trimethoprim prophylaxis. If gross VUR is found then a five day course of cephalosporin is advocated, and the parents warned to return if the child is unwell. Cases of severe urosepsis have occurred in the newborn period following catheterization.
- DMSA scan to document differential function.
- Conservative medical management generally advocated for even gross VUR. The degree of reflux can dramatically improve in the first two years of life.
- Trials of medical vs surgical treatment have shown no benefit from routine surgery although few infants were included.[11]
- Further management of VUR will be discussed in Chapter 12.
- A strong familial tendency for VUR can occur in up to 30% of siblings,[12] but we only advocate ultrasound screening of siblings if gross VUR in index case. If further pregnancies ensue, then mother is cautioned to have sonography in both early and late pregnancy.

kidneys at the outset, even in the absence of infection[10] (Fig. 3.12). Many of these kidneys with so-called congenital reflux nephropathy are already probably severely dysplastic kidneys (Fig. 3.13).

POSTERIOR URETHRAL VALVES (PUV)

PUV affects male infants with an incidence of approximately 1 in 12,000 pregnancies.[1] Even with antenatal detection and, occasionally, intervention with vesicoamniotic shunts in utero, many fetuses do not survive to term or die in the neonatal period because of the associated oligohydramnios and the severe lung abnormalities. However, posterior urethral valves represent a spectrum of disorders, with some neonates presenting with bladder outflow obstruction, infection, and acute renal failure (ARF) in the newborn period in association with urosepsis (Fig. 3.14), whereas other children present later with apparently minor symptoms.

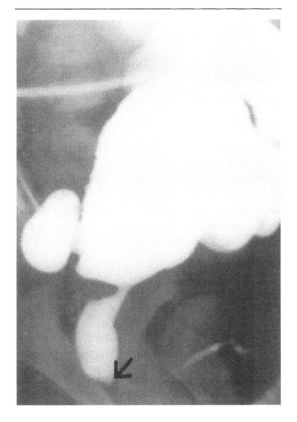

Figure 3.14 Cystogram showing posterior urethral valves (arrow), large bladder, bladder diverticulum (on right side), and reflux in a three-month-old male infant presenting with urosepsis

PRESENTATION AND MANAGEMENT

- PUV is usually managed in association with pediatric urology colleagues in a regional center.
- Fulguration of the valves is undertaken when infection has been eradicated and the child's urethra is big enough to accept the smallest resectoscope.
- Diversion of the urinary tract with procedures such as ureterostomy is no longer routine and intermittent catheterization may be initiated for large bladder residuals and recurrent infection.
- Prognosis will depend upon the degree of associated renal dysplasia and bladder abnormality requiring joint management between nephrology and urology staff.
- Children usually have prolonged daytime and night-time wetting and urodynamic assessment may be necessary.

NEUROPATHIC BLADDER

Myelomeningocele is the main cause of neuropathic bladder in the pediatric population. The number of children born with this condition has diminished with neonatal screening programs. The child with prolonged day and nighttime wetting needs to have a full spinal and neurologic examination to exclude the possibility of a neuropathic bladder from other causes such as spinal dysraphism.

Children with myelomeningocele are usually born with normal kidneys. Damage can ensue if the bladder is not drained adequately (Fig. 3.15).

- Neuropathic bladder sphincter dysfunction is complex, and these children require careful assessment in specialist centers with expertise in urodynamics.
- Clean intermittent catheterization has dramatically improved the prognosis for children with neuropathic bladder. It can provide a means of both improving continence as well as safeguarding kidney function.

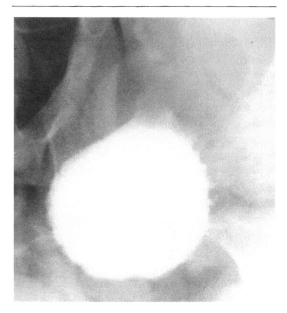

Figure 3.15 Cystogram showing small capacity highly trabeculated bladder in a child with myelomeningocele

Table 3.2 Renal cystic disorders

Genetic disorders

Autosomal recessive
Autosomal recessive polycystic kidney disease (ARPKD)
Juvenile-onset nephronophthisis
Other rare syndromes associated with multiple malformations

Autosomal dominant
Autosomal dominant polycystic kidney disease (ADPKD)
Von Hippel-Lindau disease (VHL)
Tuberous sclerosis complex (TSC)
Adult-onset medullary cystic disease

X-linked
Orofaciodigital syndrome type 1

Non-genetic disorders

Developmental
Medullary sponge kidney
Renal cystic dysplasia; multicystic dysplasia; cystic dysplasia associated with lower urinary tract obstruction; diffuse cystic dysplasia (syndromal and non-syndromal)

Acquired
Simple cysts
Hypokalemic cystic disease
Acquired cystic disease (in advanced renal failure)

- Oxybutynin to inhibit detrusor overactivity is often combined with intermittent catheterization.
- Small capacity bladders may require augmentation procedures using the patient's own bladder or bowel.
- The appendix can be used to fashion a Mitrofanoff channel between the bladder and the umbilicus, or laterally, for intermittent catheterization.
- Patients and families derive great benefit from close support by a specialist nurse.

RENAL CYSTIC DISEASE

There are a number of disorders that share renal cysts as a common feature (Table 3.2).

These disorders may be inherited or acquired. Consideration of the clinical context and associated systemic manifestations may help distinguish cystic disorders one from another. A solitary cyst in a young child may indicate a calyceal diverticulum rather than a simple cyst, which is more common in adult life. Bilateral enlarged kidneys in a neonate should raise the suspicion of autosomal recessive polycystic kidney disease, which is more likely in this context than autosomal dominant polycystic kidney disease or tuberous sclerosis complex. Renal insufficiency in an adolescent might suggest juvenile nephronophthisis or autosomal recessive polycystic kidney disease as possible etiologies.

AUTOSOMAL RECESSIVE POLYCYSTIC KIDNEY DISEASE (ARPKD)

ARPKD is an inherited malformation complex with varying degrees of renal collecting duct dilatation and biliary ectasia.[13] There is an estimated incidence of 1 in 20,000 live births and it appears to occur more frequently in Caucasians than in other ethnic populations.

The ARPKD locus has now been mapped to the short arm of chromosome 6 (6p21–12), and to date all phenotypic variants appear to result from mutations in the single gene.[14]

Late in the 1970s, ARPKD was subdivided into four distinct phenotypes according to the age of presentation and the proportion of dilated renal collecting ducts. However, the process typically begins in utero and the renal cystic lesions appear to be superimposed on a normal developmental sequence. The renal abnormality primarily involves fusiform dilatation of the collecting ducts. The early liver lesion appears to involve defective remodeling of the ductal plate in utero such that primitive bile duct configurations persist and progressive portal fibrosis evolves.

CLINICAL FEATURES

- The clinical spectrum of ARPKD is variable and depends on the age at presentation.[15] Most patients are identified either in utero or at birth.
- The most severely affected fetuses present in pregnancies with oligohydramnios and have enlarged echogenic kidneys. They may die at birth because of pulmonary hypoplasia.
- Those infants who survive the perinatal period have hypertension, renal failure, and portal hypertension.
- Renal hypertension usually develops in the first few months and ultimately affects 70–80% of patients.

- There is also an increase in the incidence of urinary tract infections.
- Portal hypertension can be the predominant clinical abnormality in older children and adolescents with ARPKD. These children typically present with hepatosplenomegaly and bleeding esophageal or gastric varices as well as hypersplenism. Hepatocellular function is usually preserved, but ascending suppurative cholangitis is a serious complication and can cause hepatic failure.

DIAGNOSIS

In the antenatal period, oligohydramnios or enlarged echogenic kidneys suggest ARPKD. Postnatally, ultrasound can reveal symmetrically enlarged diffusely echogenic kidneys with poor demarcation from surrounding tissues, as well as cortex, medulla, and renal sinus. With high resolution ultrasound, the regular ray of dilated collecting ducts may be imaged, and intravenous urography and computed tomography scanning will show similar features. In older children, the development of scattered small cysts and progressive fibrosis can alter the reniform character, and ARPKD in older children can be mistaken for autosomal dominant polycystic kidney disease (ADPKD). The liver may be normal in size or enlarged and is usually less

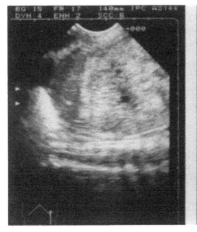 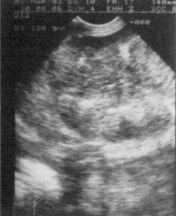

Figure 3.16 Ultrasound of newborn infant with Tuberous Sclerosis Complex showing enlarged bilateral echogenic kidneys

echogenic than the kidneys. Prominent intra-hepatic bile duct dilatation suggests associated Caroli's disease. With age, the portal fibrosis tends to progress, and there may be hepatosplenomegaly and a patchy increase in hepatic echogenicity.

OUTCOME

The estimated perinatal mortality is 30–50%. For those who survive the first month of life, the reported mean five-year patient survival rate is 80–95%.[16] The prognosis outside the perinatal period is improved, because of the availability of aggressive interventions such as unilateral or bilateral nephrectomy, and the availability of dialysis and transplantation for this group of children. For those with end-stage renal failure and severe portal hypertension, combined liver and kidney transplantation may be indicated.

AUTOSOMAL DOMINANT POLYCYSTIC KIDNEY DISEASE (ADPKD)

ADPKD is a multisystem disorder characterized by multiple bilateral renal cysts and is associated with cysts in other organs, such as liver, pancreas, and arachnoid membranes. It is one of the most common hereditary diseases affecting approximately 1 in 400 to 1 in 1000 individuals.

The genes responsible for ADPKD have provided a major breakthrough in the study of the disease. PKD1 is the gene on chromosome 16 and is responsible for 85% of clinically detected cases. PKD2 has been identified in the long arm of chromosome 4, and there is likely to be a third gene. Proteins encoded by PDK1 and PKD2 have been named polycystin 1 and polycystin 2 respectively. Molecular genetic work has stimulated a great deal of research into variation in disease progression between patients, and this appears to depend upon underlying mutations, modifying genes, somatic mutations, and environmental factors.[17]

CLINICAL FEATURES

- It is rare for ADPKD to manifest clinically in childhood, but an occasional child may have

significant renal enlargement with hypertension. Urinary tract infections are also known to exacerbate kidney disease in adults with ADPKD.
- Although ADPKD may be recognized incidentally on renal ultrasound scans done for urinary tract infection investigation etc., there is a general consensus that asymptomatic children from affected families should not be routinely screened for this condition either by ultrasound or genetic studies. They should be free to make their own autonomous decision as to whether they want to be investigated when they reach adulthood.

FAMILIAL NEPHRONOPHTHISIS (NPH) AND MEDULLARY CYSTIC DISEASE COMPLEX

Familial (juvenile) nephronophthisis (NPH) and medullary cystic disease complex are histologically similar diseases, differing in their mode of transmission and age of onset.

PATHOGENESIS

Recent studies have mapped a gene (NPHP1) for juvenile NPH to the chromosome region 2q13. Approximately 85% of renal NPH involves defects in NPHP1, which involves a novel protein product called nephrocystine.[18] Large homozygous deletions have been detected in 80% of affected members of NPH and in 65% of sporadic cases.

Pathologically, the disease is characterized by a chronic sclerosing tubulo-interstitial nephropathy with sparse inflammatory cell infiltration, and the development of medullary cysts late in the disease course. There is an irregular thickening of the tubular basement membrane (TBM) with the absence of certain TBM components and the novel expression of alpha-5 integrin in tubular epithelial cells.

CLINICAL FEATURES

- Reduced urinary concentrating capacity is common in patients with NPH and this usually precedes a decline in glomerular filtration rate. The mean age of onset is four years.

- Polyuria and polydipsia are common symptoms and the patients may be anemic, even before the onset of renal insufficiency.
- Growth retardation, out of proportion with the degree of renal insufficiency, is a common finding.[19]
- A gradual decline in renal function is typical and end-stage renal failure usually develops by adolescence.
- The disease is not known to recur in renal allografts.
- In 10–15% of NPH there is an association with retinitis pigmentosa caused by retinal degeneration (Senior-Loken syndrome) and presents with coarse nystagmus and early blindness. NPH associated with ocular motor apraxia and co-existing retinal degeneration (Cogan's syndrome) has been reported in several kindreds, and a subset of these patients have also had mental retardation. Congenital hepatic fibrosis occurs occasionally in patients with NPH.

AUTOSOMAL DOMINANT MEDULLARY CYSTIC KIDNEY DISEASE

This nephropathy is histologically undistinguishable from recessive NPH, and has been reported with male to male transmission in successive generations, suggesting an autosomal dominant mode of inheritance. Progression to end-stage renal failure occurs in the third to fourth decade of life.

MEDULLARY SPONGE KIDNEY

Again, this condition more commonly comes to light in adult life, when calcification in the renal pyramids may give rise to calculi, abdominal pain, and hematuria. It is occasionally identified in childhood for the same reasons, but more often because of the urographic appearance of streaky opacification in the renal pyramids.

TUBEROUS SCLEROSIS COMPLEX (TSC)

TSC is an autosomal dominant disorder in which tumor-like malformations, called hamartomas, develop in multiple organ systems. This affects 1 in 1000 individuals but spontaneous mutations appear to occur at high frequency and are estimated to account for 60% of new cases.

Renal cystic disease is the earliest finding in TSC (Fig. 3.16) and may be the presenting manifestation in infants and children before even the seizures and mental retardation have become manifest alongside the facial angiofibromas, hypomelanotic macules and periungual fibromas.

Angiomyolipomas are the principal hamartomas in TSC. They rarely occur before five years of age, but increase in frequency and size and give rise to hemorrhage or mass effects leading to severe hypertension and progressive decrease in renal function. Malignant tumors, found in TSC patients, were originally thought to be a renal cell carcinoma, but are now regarded as malignant epitheloid angiomyolipomas.[20]

SUMMARY AND THOUGHTS FOR THE FUTURE

- Antenatal ultrasound has resulted in increasing numbers of asymptomatic infants being referred for postnatal investigations, and has changed our perceptions of the natural history of many conditions. Many long-term outcomes still need to be defined. In the meantime we need to avoid over-investigation and needless exposure to radiation of infants with largely benign conditions.
- As currently performed, antenatal ultrasound does not pick up all congenital abnormalities as most fetuses only have one detailed scan at 18–20 weeks.
- Dysplasia/hypoplasia is a major cause of established renal failure in childhood and we can do little to alter the prognosis in childhood.
- Multicystic dysplastic kidney is usually a benign unilateral condition with serial follow-ups

showing involution of the kidney with time. MCDK may be a major contributor to the single commonest urinary tract abnormality in the general population, i.e. a single kidney. Removal of the MCDK kidney does not appear justified.

- Antenatally detected hydronephrosis due to PUJ holdup has provided the greatest postnatal dilemmas. There are no randomized control data on which to base firm recommendations as to which infants require surgery. The number being operated on appears to be falling with time as a more conservative approach is adopted; the same applies to infants with VUJ obstruction.

- Randomized controlled trials have shown a comparable outcome for VUR managed conservatively or by operative intervention. Infants born with VUR recognized antenatally have demonstrated that the kidneys may be very severely damaged in association with gross VUR in the antenatal period. Congenital reflux nephropathy does question the value of intensive investigations for UTI in later childhood.

- Autosomal recessive polycystic kidney disease remains a very rare condition. It is not invariably fatal in the newborn period and again is part of a spectrum disorder.

- Autosomal dominant polycystic kidney disease may be recognized even in utero with cysts. There does not appear to be significant benefit from screening asymptomatic children for this condition. Tests can be carried out in adulthood with their full consent.

REFERENCES

1. James CA, Watson AR, Twining P, Rance CH. Antenatally detected urinary tract abnormalities: changing incidence and management. Eur J Pediatr 1998; 157:508–511.
2. Lewis M, Watson AR, Clark G. Report of the paediatric renal registry 1999. London: Renal Association; 1999.
3. Abdelraheem M, Watson AR. Chronic renal failure due to twin-to-twin transfusion. Brit J Ren Med 2003; 8(3):19–20.
4. Pohl M, Bhatnagar V, Mendoza SA, et al. Toward an etiological classification of developmental disorders of the kidney and upper urinary tract. Kidney Int 2002; 61:10–19.
5. Watson AR. Management of antenatally detected urinary tract abnormalities. Curr Paeds 1999; 9:232–236.
6. Quintero RA, Arias F, Cotton DB, et al. In-utero percutaneous cystoscopy in the management of fetal lower obstructive uropathy. Lancet 1995; 346:537–540.
7. Al-Khaldi N, Watson AR, Zuccollo J, Twining P, Rose DH. Outcome of antenatally detected cystic dysplastic kidney disease. Arch Dis Child 1994; 70:520–522.
8. Sukthankar S, Watson AR, on behalf of the Trent & Anglia Paediatric Nephrourology Group. Unilateral multicystic dysplastic kidney disease: defining the natural history. Acta Paediatr 2000; 89:811–813.
9. Ulman I, Jayanthi VR, Koff S. The long-term follow up of newborns with severe unilateral hydronephrosis initially treated nonoperatively. J Urol 2000; 164(3 Pt 2):1101–1105.
10. Anderson PAM, Rickwood AMK. Features of primary vesicoureteric reflux detected by prenatal sonography. Br J Urol 1991; 67(3):267–271.
11. World Health Organization. International Society of Hypertension guidelines for the management of hypertension. Guidelines subcommittee. J Hypertens 1999; 17:151–183.
12. Aggarwal VH, Verrier Jones K. Vesicoureteric reflux – screening of the first degree relatives. Arch Dis Child 1989; 64:1538–1541.
13. Guay-Woodford LM. Autosomal recessive disease: clinical and genetic profiles. In: Torres V, Watson M, editors. Polycystic kidney disease. Oxford: Oxford University Press; 1996. 237–267.
14. Guay-Woodford LM, Muecher G, Hopkins SD, et al. The severe perinatal form of autosomal recessive polycystic kidney disease (ARPKD) maps to chromosome 6p21.1–p12: implications for genetic counselling. Am J Hum Genet 1995; 56:1101–1107.
15. Jamil B, McMahon LP, Savige JA, et al. A study of long-term morbidity associated with autosomal recessive polycystic kidney disease. Nephrol Dial Transplant 1999; 14:205–209.
16. Roy S, Dillon M, Trompeter R, Barratt T. Autosomal recessive polycystic kidney disease: long-term outcome of neonatal survivors. Pediatr Nephrol 1997; 11:302–306.
17. Peters DJM, Breuning MH. Autosomal dominant polycystic kidney disease: modification of disease progression. Lancet 2001; 358:1439–1444.
18. Konrad M, Saunier S, Heidet L, et al. Large homozygous deletions of the 2q13 region are a major cause of juvenile nephronophthisis. Hum Mol Genet 1996; 5:367–371.
19. Ala-Mello S, Kivivuori S, Ronnholm KAR, Koskimies O, Siimes M. Mechanism underlying early anemia in children with familial juvenile nephronophthisis. Pediatr Nephrol 1996; 10:578–581.
20. Torres V. Tuberous sclerosis complex. In: Torres V, Watson M, editors. Polycystic kidney disease. Oxford: Oxford University Press; 1996. 283–308.

FURTHER READING

Web Based
www.merck.com/mrkshared/mmanual/section19/chapter261
(Merck Manuals)

www.urologyhealth.org/pediatric/index
(American Urological Association)

www.centrus.com.br/DiplomatFMF/SeriesFMF/18-23-weeks/chapter08/renalfmf.htm
(Sylabus from fetal medicine sepcialists)

Text Books
O'Donnell B, Koff SA (eds). Pediatric Urology (3rd Edn) Butterworth-Heinemann, Oxford, 1997

Thomas DFM, Rickwood MC, Duffy PG (eds). Essentials of Paediatric Urology. Martin Dunitz, London, 2002

Webb N, Postlethwaite R (eds). Clinical Paediatric Nephrology. Oxford University Press, Oxford, 2003

4. Neonatal kidney problems

Jean-Pierre Guignard

MATURATION

1) MATURATION DURING FETAL LIFE

Urine formation by the fetal kidney starts at approximately 9–12 weeks of gestation, increases to 12 ml per hour by the 32nd week of gestation and reaches 28 ml per hour shortly before birth. Urine formation is not essential for fetal survival, the homeostasis being maintained by the placenta. Increase in the weight of the kidneys during the last 20 weeks of gestation bears a linear relationship to gestational age, body weight, and body surface area.[1]

2) POSTNATAL MATURATION

GLOMERULAR FUNCTION (FIGS. 4.1 and 4.2)

Birth is the signal for a striking increase in glomerular filtration rate (GFR). From a value of 15–20 ml per minute per 1.73 m^2 at birth in term neonates, GFR doubles in the first two weeks of life. GFR reaches mature levels between 6 and 12 months (Fig. 4.2).

TUBULAR FUNCTION

Tubular function is relatively immature at birth but then matures rapidly after birth.

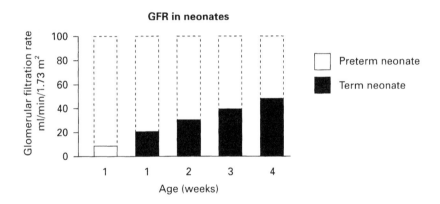

Figure 4.1 Maturation of GFR during the first month of life. The dark columns represent values found in neonates. The 100 ml/min/1.73 m^2 level represents normal mature levels of GFR. (See color plate section)

(Adapted from refs 1 and 2)

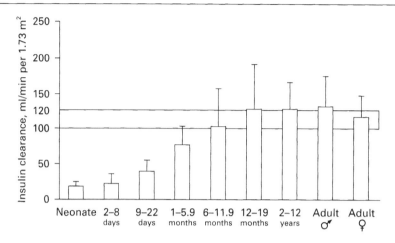

Figure 4.2 Maturation of GFR, as measured by inulin clearance and corrected for BSA, in infants and children

Diluting ability: Neonates can decrease urine osmolality to 40 mosm/kg/H_2O. Because of their low GFR, prematures may have limited capacity to excrete large amounts of free-water.

Concentrating ability: The renal concentrating mechanism is not fully efficient in newborn infants. Term neonates can increase the urine osmolality to 700–800 mosm/kg/H_2O and premature infants to 500–700 mosm/kg/H_2O.

SYMPTOMS AND SIGNS OF RENAL DISEASE IN THE NEONATE

Oligohydramnios: Deficient urine production in utero is the most common cause for deficient amniotic fluid. This condition may be associated with renal agenesis, renal hypoplasia, renal dysplasia, or severe obstruction of the urinary tract. The lack of amniotic fluid around the fetus is responsible for the non-renal features of the 'Potter's syndrome', which includes altered facies (Fig. 4.3), aberrant hand and foot positioning, pulmonary hypoplasia, and late fetal growth deficiency.

Polyhydramnios: Excess amniotic fluid (more than two liters) indicates severe swallowing difficulties due to either neurologic disturbances or upper obstructive disorders of the GI tract. Polyhydramnios may also result from nephrogenic diabetes insipidus, or from severe congenital Bartter's syndrome.

Placenta: In normal term newborns, the placenta weight represents 13–16% of the newborn weight. Nodular formations on the fetal side of the placenta suggest renal anomalies. Anomalies of the umbilical cord are associated with a high incidence of various congenital malformations, including some in the urinary tract. This usually takes the form of a '2-vessel cord' which contains only one umbilical artery.

Perinatal problems: Fetal distress in utero, difficult delivery, and perinatal asphyxia may result in acute tubular necrosis, acute papillary necrosis, renal venous thrombosis, and acute renal failure.[3,4]

3) MICTURITION

Ninety-two percent of newborn infants pass urine during the first 24 hours of life, and 99 percent within the first 48 hours. Urologic and/or renal disorders should be ruled out if no diuresis has occurred by 48 hours of life.

4) URINE VOLUMES

A healthy infant excretes 15–30 ml/kg per 24 hours of urine during the first two days of life and 25–120 ml/kg per 24 hours during the next four weeks.[1]

5) PHYSICAL EXAMINATION

General configuration: In patients with deficient urine production in utero, the face may show the classic Potter's facies with wide-set eyes, beaked nose, low-set ears, and a prominent fold arising from the inner canthus (Fig. 4.3). Potter's facies is often associated with renal agenesis. Isolated anomalies of the external ear, the genitalia, the anus, the lumbosacral area, and the thoracic spine may also be associated with abnormalities of the urinary tract.

Abdominal palpation: Careful examination of the abdomen reveals renal masses in 0.5 to 0.8 percent of infants.[5] A renal mass must be evaluated by ultrasonography and by other imaging techniques, as needed. Possible causes of abdominal masses in the neonate are listed in Table 4.1.

Edema: The main causes of edema in neonates are listed in Table 4.2. Edema is observed in congenital forms of nephrotic syndrome secondary to microcystic disease, congenital syphilis, toxoplasmosis, cytomegalovirus, nephroblastoma, renal venous thrombosis, and mercury intoxication.

Ascites in the newborn: The main causes leading to or associated with neonatal ascites include: abnormalities of the gastrointestinal, of the portohepatic, or the genitourinary tract. About 25% of cases of neonatal ascites are caused by urinary tract disease.

Hydrops fetalis: Renal causes of hydrops include congenital anomalies of the urinary tract and congenital nephrotic syndromes such as seen with syphilis, toxoplasmosis, and cytomegalic inclusion disease.

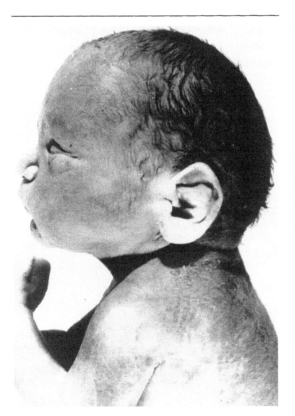

Figure 4.3 Potter's facies

Table 4.1 Abdominal masses in the neonate

Type of mass	Percentage of total
Renal	55
Hydronephrosis	
Multicystic dysplastic kidney	
Polycystic kidney disease	
Mesoblastic nephroma	
Renal ectopia	
Renal vein thrombosis	
Nephroblastomatosis	
Wilms' tumor	
Genital	15
Hydrometrocolpos	
Ovarian cyst	
Gastrointestinal	15
Nonrenal retroperitoneal	10
Hepato-spleno-biliary	5

6) GROSS HEMATURIA

Significant hematuria, which is rare in the neonate, may be the consequence of a variety of disorders at different levels of the urinary system.[6] These are listed in Table 4.3.

Table 4.2 Main causes of edema in the newborn

Physiologic
Cardiac
Renal
Miscellaneous
  Asphyxia
  Hyaline membrane disease
  Erythroblastosis
  Umbilical venous thrombosis
  Lymphedema
  Congenital ascites (chylous ascites, cirrhosis, peritonitis)
  Vitamin E deficiency
  Hypomagnesemia and hypocalcemia
  Cystic fibrosis
  Hypoparathyroidism
  Turner syndrome

Table 4.3. Main causes of hematuria in the newborn

Bleeding tendency	
Vascular disorders	Acute tubular necrosis
	Corticomedullary necrosis
	Renal venous thrombosis
	Adrenal hemorrhage
Cystic diseases	ARPKD/ADPKD
	Cystic dysplasia
	Multicystic kidney
Tumors	Wilms' tumor
	Mesoblastic nephroma and fetal hamartoma
	Angioma
Trauma	
Obstructive/refluxing uropathy	
Nephritides	Pyelonephritis
	Interstitial nephritis (drugs)
	Glomerulonephritis

7) MALFORMATION SYNDROMES

Malformations of the urogenital tract have been found in as many as 10 percent of newborn infants.[7] They may be isolated or part of a complex syndrome. Isolated renal malformations may be sporadic or inherited as a single gene mutation. They include renal agenesis, renal hypoplasia, renal ectopia, ureteral anomalies, horseshoe kidneys, multicystic-dysplastic disease, and infantile or adult polycystic disease.

Renal malformations or dysfunction may be part of a complex malformation syndrome in association with chromosomal abnormalities such as trisomy syndromes (Table 4.4), single gene mutation syndromes, and sporadic malformation syndromes, or may result from teratogenic causes.

Cystic disease of the kidney: Multicystic-dysplasia and infantile polycystic disease are the cystic malformations most commonly seen in newborn infants.

Table 4.4 Renal anomalies in trisomy syndromes

Trisomy	Renal anomaly
11	Dysplastic multicystic kidneys
13–15	Bilateral hydronephrosis
	Renal cysts
16–18	Horseshoe kidneys
	Hydronephrosis
	Dysplastic multicystic kidneys
	Renal cortical cysts
	Abnormal nodule of renal blastema
21	Agenesis/hypoplasia

INVESTIGATION

1) URINALYSIS

Hematuria: Microscopic hematuria may be secondary to vascular disorders, malformative uropathies, interstitial nephritis, cystic and dysplastic disorders, and tumors (Table 4.3).

Proteinuria: Transient proteinuria is often present during the first weeks of life. After the seventh day of life, proteinuria is usually below 0.15 mg per kg per hour. The amount of albumin and/or protein in the urine decreases over time during the first six weeks of life and can be measured most conveniently in random urine specimens (Table 4.5). The main causes of proteinuria in the neonate are listed in Table 4.6.

Glucosuria: In low birth-weight infants, significant glucosuria may be observed at a plasma glucose concentration below 150 mg/dl (8.3 mmol/l).

Bacteriuria: Significant bacteriuria is found in 0.7–3.4 percent of neonates and is more frequent in pre and post-mature infants. Male infants are more frequently affected than girls by 5 to 1.

2) BLOOD TESTS

Creatinine: The level of plasma creatinine at birth reflects the maternal plasma creatinine level since creatinine passes freely across the placenta. Hence the level bears no reflection on the neonate's renal function at that time. The plasma creatinine rises transiently after birth in very low birth-weight infants (Table 4.7).[8,9] This is probably due to the

---

Table 4.6 Main causes of proteinuria in the newborn

Physiologic proteinuria
Vascular disorders
   Renal venous thrombosis
   Corticomedullary necrosis
Congenital nephrotic syndrome
   Hereditary diseases
   Finnish type
   Onycho-osteodysplasia (nail-patella syndrome)
   Severe infantile sialidosis
Infectious diseases
   Syphilis
   Toxoplasmosis
   Cytomegalovirus
   AIDS
Drugs
   Mercury compounds
   Other nephrotoxic compounds

Table 4.5 Albumin and protein to creatinine concentration ratio in neonates

Age (days)	Albumin/creatinine g/mol	Protein/creatinine g/mol
1	35	120
15	12	110
43	8	92

Table 4.7 Changes in plasma creatinine over time for different gestation groups

Group gestation age (wk)	Birth creatinine (μmol/l)*	Peak plasma creatinine (μmol/1)*	Time to peak plasma creatinine (h)*
23–26	67–92	195–247	40–78
27–29	65–89	158–200	28–51
30–32	60–69	120–158	25–40
33–45	67–79	99–140	8–23

*Mean ± 95% confidence intervals. Adapted from Miall LS, et al. Pediatrics 1999; 104:b

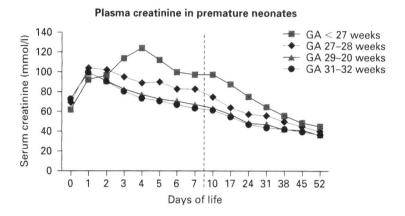

Plasma creatinine in premature neonates

Figure 4.4 Plasma (serum) creatinine concentrations during the first 52 days of life of premature infants. (See color plate section)
(Adapted from ref. 8)

tubular reabsorption of creatinine, as a consequence of the back-diffusion of creatinine across leaky immature tubules.[10] The level subsequently falls over the next few weeks (Fig. 4.4). Once the plasma creatinine stabilizes, GFR can be estimated by the Schwartz formula: GFR (ml/min/1.73 m²) = k × length (cm)/creatinine (μmol/1). (Factor K = 33 in full term infants and 24 in LBW infants.)

Sodium: Hyponatremia is a common finding in the newborn. It may be secondary to impaired excretion of free water or to sodium wasting.

Late hyponatremia may be observed in very low birth-weight infants given less than 1.3 mmol/kg per 24 h of sodium, and can be prevented by giving additional sodium (3–4 mol/kg per 24 h).

Bicarbonate: The bicarbonate threshold is low in newborns, with values of 21–23 mmol/l in the term neonate, and 19–22 mmol/l in the preterm infant.

BLOOD PRESSURE AND HYPERTENSION

Measurement of blood pressure by the Doppler technique has largely replaced older techniques.

The Doppler ultrasonic device is incorporated underneath a 4–5 cm cuff assembly. It gives an accurate estimate of systolic blood pressure, but overestimates direct intra-arterial measurement by approximately 5 mmHg. Blood pressure is low at birth. It varies according to both gestational and postnatal age, and increases steadily during the first months of life (Table 4.8).[11,12] When arterial hypertension occurs in the neonate it causes a high-risk of cardiorespiratory failure, cerebral distress, and growth failure. Aggressive control of hypertension may improve the diagnosis.[11,13]

Table 4.8 Normal mean arterial blood pressure in the newborn infant*

Age	< 1.0 kg	1.0–1.5 kg	> 2.5 kg
Birth	33 ± 15	39 ± 18	49 ± 19
1 week	41 ± 15	47 ± 18	60 ± 19
2 weeks	45 ± 15	50 ± 18	64 ± 19
4 weeks	48 ± 15	53 ± 18	68 ± 19

* Mean ± 95% confidence limits for single measurements; measurement via umbilical artery catheterization or by Dynamap[11]

1) ETIOLOGY OF ARTERIAL HYPERTENSION

Neonatal hypertension is either secondary to congenital malformations or to acquired diseases. The main causes are listed in Table 4.9.

Renal artery thrombosis is an important, and potentially severe, cause of hypertension which usually occurs in patients who have had umbilical artery catheters for a number of days. An intrinsic stenosis or an extrinsic compression of a renal artery can also induce renin-dependent hypertension. Hypertension has also been observed in newborn infants following closure of abdominal wall defects, after intra-nasal use of 10 percent phenylephrine, in neonates from heroin- or methadone-addicted mothers. Tight coarctation of the aorta, proximal to the ductus arteriosus, may produce severe hypertension. High blood pressure has been associated with endogenous or exogenous excess of mineralo- or gluco-corticoids, and after rupture of an adrenal hematoma.

Table 4.9 Main causes of hypertension in the newborn

Vascular	Renal artery hypoplasia, stenosis, thrombus
	Coarctation of the aorta
	Aortic thrombus
Renal	Polycystic kidney disease
	Multicystic dysplasia, hypoplastic kidney
	Obstructive uropathy
	Acute and chronic renal failure
Tumors	Neuroblastoma
	Mesoblastoma
	Pheochromocytoma
Endocrine	Congenital adrenal hyperplasia
	Cushing's syndrome
	Thyrotoxicosis
Central nervous system	Raised intracranial pressure
	Meningitis
	Convulsions
Respiratory	Bronchopulmonary dysplasia
Miscellaneous	Drugs: phenylephrine eyedrops (10% solution)
	Infants of drug-taking mothers
	Adrenal hemorrhage with renal artery compression
	Closure of abdominal wall defects
	Idiopathic (prematures)?

---

2) CLINICAL MANIFESTATIONS

Hypertension may be asymptomatic, produce non-specific symptoms such as proteinuria, hematuria and failure to thrive, or cause significant cardio-respiratory and neurologic disturbances. The risk of intra-ventricular hemorrhage is present in premature infants. Renal enlargement associated with hypertension suggests polycystic kidney disease, multicystic dysplasia, obstructive uropathy, renal tumor, or an adrenal hematoma compressing the renal artery.

3) TREATMENT

The approach to a neonate with hypertension should be tailored to the individual patient and based on the severity of the problem and the presence of complicating factors. Hypertensive crises must be treated vigorously because of the risk of intracranial hemorrhage and heart failure. Potent vasodilators such as sodium nitroprusside can be life saving. In most instances the initial therapy should be given intravenously with subsequent conversion to oral medications when appropriate. Some of the medications that are used in the treatment of hypertension in neonates are listed in Table 4.10.

RENAL FUNCTION DURING NEONATAL RESPIRATORY DISORDERS

Perinatal asphyxia or hypoxemia, as seen in severe idiopathic respiratory distress syndrome or in secondary respiratory distress syndrome after complicated or traumatic deliveries, can profoundly affect renal function.[3,4] Hypovolemia, hypotension, metabolic acidosis, and respiratory acidosis are often present and may result in the renal functional changes observed in these conditions (Fig. 4.5). Severe or prolonged hypoxemia causes oliguria. The prerenal failure may, however, lead to parenchymal injury, with consequent acute tubular necrosis or, in very severe forms, acute cortical necrosis, if the prerenal factors are not corrected.[14,15]

Table 4.10 Antihypertensive drugs in the neonate

Agent	Starting dosage	Intervals	Maximum recommended	Route of administration
Furosemide	1 mg/kg	q 4–6 h	5 mg/kg/dose	PO/IV
Hydrochlorothiazide	1 mg/kg	q 8 h	3 mg/kg/dose	PO
Propranolol	0.25 mg/kg/dose	q 6–8 h	5 mg/kg/dose	PO/IV
Atenolol	0.5 mg/kg/dose	q 12–24 h	4 mg/kg/dose	PO
Labetalol	0.5 mg/kg/dose	q 1–4 h	2 mg/kg/dose	IV
Sodium nitroprusside	0.5 µg/kg/min	–	6 µg/kg/min	IV
Captopril	0.1 mg/kg/dose	q 8–12 h	0.5 mg/kg/dose	PO
Enalapril	5 µg/kg/dose	q 8–24 h	20 µg/kg/dose	IV
Nifedipine	0.5 mg/kg/dose	q 4–6 h	2 mg/kg/dose	PO

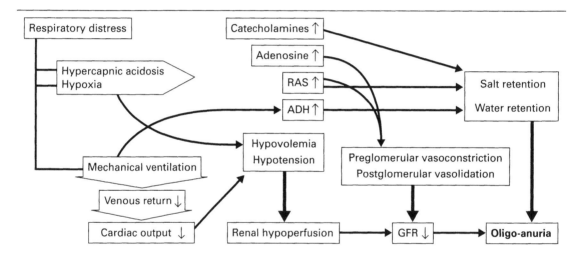

Figure 4.5 Pathophysiology of the oliguric renal insufficiency secondary to severe respiratory distress

ACUTE RENAL FAILURE

ARF is characterized by a sudden decrease in glomerular filtration rate, which leads to disturbances in water, electrolytes, and acid-base homeostasis, and to accumulation of nitrogen end products. Renal failure may have a prerenal, an intrinsic or a postrenal etiology (Table 4.11). Prerenal insufficiency is the most frequent form

of ARF.[3,4] It is preventable if treated early and adequately.

1) ETIOLOGY

The major causes of acute renal failure in the neonatal period are listed in Table 4.11. They are divided into pre-renal, renal, and post-renal causes, but it must be remembered that some infants may

Table 4.11 Causes of acute renal failure in neonates

Prerenal

Hypovolemia or renal hypoperfusion
Asphyxia
Respiratory distress syndrome (RDS)
Dehydration
Hemorrhage (maternal antepartum, twin-to-twin transfusion, intraventricular bleeding, hemolytic disease)
Sepsis
Cardiac disease (patent ductus arteriosus, aortic coarctation)
Polycythemia (hyperviscosity)

Renal

Acute tubular necrosis (ATN)
Persistent prerenal disturbances
Nephrotoxins (nephrotoxic antibiotics, e.g. aminoglycosides, contrast agents, angiotensin-converting enzyme [ACE] inhibitors)
Myoglobinuria, hemoglobinuria, hyperuricemia
Vascular disorders (renal vein thrombosis, renal artery thrombosis, aortic thrombosis, disseminated intravascular coagulation)
Congenital renal anomaly (dysplasia, hypoplasia, polycystic kidney, agenesis)
Pyelonephritis
Transient acute renal failure of the neonate
Maternal etiology (gentamicin, indomethacin, ACE inhibitors, paraproteinemia)

Postrenal

Congenital anomaly (ureteral or urethral obstruction, neurogenic bladder, megacystis-megaureter)
Obstruction secondary to circumcision
Renal candidiasis
Calculi
Neurogenic bladder

---

have more than one of these components leading to acute renal failure.

2) DIAGNOSIS

Oliguria is defined as a urine output of less than 1.0 ml/kg per hour in preterm infants and 0.5 ml/kg per hour in term neonates.

Laboratory studies: Renal failure can be defined as a plasma creatinine concentration above 90 μmol/l after the fifth postnatal day and a daily increase of 20 μmol/l per day. Urinary indices can help to dis-

tinguish prerenal from renal failure. A U/P osmolality ratio above 2, and a sodium of fractional excretion below 2 are in favor of a prerenal insufficiency. These criteria do not apply to very low birth-weight infants. Additional details regarding the interpretation of normal and abnormal renal function indices are provided in Chapters 1 and 15.

Imaging studies: Ultrasonography is useful in evaluating poorly or non-functioning kidneys. Radioisotopic scanning and renograms may be useful in evaluating the size, position, and function of poorly functioning kidneys, and for providing more specific information about renal perfusion and possible abnormalities in the renal arteries and renal veins.

3) TREATMENT OF ACUTE RENAL FAILURE

The cause of ARF in the neonate should be precisely defined and prerenal factors such as hypovolemia, hypotension, and hypoxemia should be rapidly corrected (Fig. 4.6). Subsequent management will usually require medical (conservative) measures alone although dialysis is sometimes needed.

CAREFUL TREATMENT OF FLUID AND ELECTROLYTES DISTURBANCES IS OF FOREMOST IMPORTANCE

Accurate and frequent monitoring of the patient's fluid (volume) status is critical and measures should be taken to maintain the patient in normal fluid balance. This includes frequent measurements of body weight whenever possible.

Hyponatremia is most often a dilutional disturbance, which must be corrected by fluid restriction rather than sodium chloride administration.

Hyperkalemia: This disturbance is life threatening and must be rapidly corrected.

Convulsions: These are usually secondary to electrolyte imbalance. Symptomatic therapy consists of

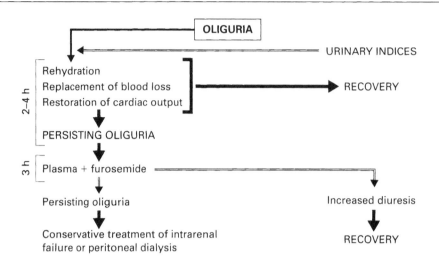

Figure 4.6 Management of acute oliguric renal failure. (See color plate section)

giving iv phenobarbital, 6 mg/kg, or diazepam, iv or rectally, 0.3 mg/kg.

Other aspects of the conservative management of acute renal failure are described in Chapter 15.

4) ACUTE RENAL REPLACEMENT THERAPY

Peritoneal dialysis has been the method of choice in most neonatal units for infants with fluid overload associated with pulmonary edema, congestive heart failure, water intoxication, or persistent renal failure that is not responding to more conservative measures. In more recent years, a number of units have also adopted hemo(dia)filtration as an alternative approach to these infants,[16] especially those who have contraindications to peritoneal dialysis.

5) PROGNOSIS OF ARF

Prerenal failure has a good prognosis if the predisposing factors can be rapidly corrected. Intrinsic renal failure may have a poor outcome, the degree of recovery of renal function being dependent on the nature of the parenchymal lesion and the presence and severity of associated conditions.

ACQUIRED DISEASES

1) URINARY TRACT INFECTION (UTI)

The clinical manifestations of urinary tract infections in neonates are highly variable, from asymptomatic bacteriuria to severe shock secondary to septicemia (Table 4.12). Gastrointestinal symptoms are frequent and include poor feeding and failure to thrive, vomiting, and diarrhea. Other symptoms are fever, lethargy, irritability, and dehydration. Cyanosis, convulsions, and jaundice are sometimes observed. Malformations of the urinary tract, including vesicoureteral reflux, hydronephrosis, ureterocele, ureteropelvic obstruction, or urethral valves are present in 42–55% of infected neonates.[17] To exclude the presence of urinary tract malformations, imaging studies should be obtained in any neonate with proven UTI.

Diagnosis of UTI: When urine is collected from a bag, which may be the method selected in a neonate that shows only mild symptoms/signs, infection can be diagnosed when the specimen contains more than 100,000 colonies/ml of a single bacterium. Any

Table 4.12 Symptoms of neonatal urinary tract infection

	Total number	%
Total number of neonates	1762	100
Infected neonates	43	2.4
Symptomatic infections	34	1.9
Asymptomatic infections	9	0.5
Incidence of symptoms in infected neonates		
Vomiting	16	37
Weight loss, dehydration	13	30
Fever	9	21
Diarrhea	6	14
Palpable kidneys	6	14
Poor feeding	5	12
Jaundice	16	37
Metabolic acidosis	9	21
Miscellaneous	15	35

Adapted from Maherzi M, Guignard JP, Torrado A. Urinary tract infection in high-risk newborn infants. Pediatrics 1978; 62:521[24]

count above 10^4 colonies/ml is suspect and should be confirmed by suprapubic puncture. When a neonate shows signs of severe illness, it is appropriate to obtain the initial specimen by suprapubic aspiration or bladder catheter.

Bacteriology: *E. coli* is the organism most frequently encountered in UTI of the newborn infant, followed by *Klebsiella pneumoniae* and *Proteus mirabilis*. The presence of two bacterial organisms in the urine, a sign of contamination in older children, is occasionally observed in neonates with UTI.[18,19]

TREATMENT OF ACUTE INFECTIONS

When confirmed, UTI must be treated without delay.[19] The choice of antibiotic(s) must be based on the knowledge of the most common locally invading organisms and their antibiotic sensitivities. Initial treatment usually includes iv amoxicillin (30 mg/kg q 8 hours) in association with an aminoglycoside such as gentamycin (2.5 mg/kg q 8–12 hours) or amikacin (7.5 mg/kg q 8–12 hours) for 10 days, with careful monitoring of blood aminoglycosides and creatinine levels. Treatment is adjusted according to the sensitivity of the cultured organisms. Neonatal UTI may also respond to a third generation cephalosporin such as ceftriaxone (50–100 mg q 24 hours). Doses and intervals of administration are given in Table 4.13.

Oral therapy: After the acute phase, treatment can be switched to oral drugs according to the sensitivity of the bacterium that is identified (Table 4.13).

Prophylaxis: Long-term prophylactic therapy must be administered to patients in whom the UTI is associated with vesicoureteral reflux, while an obstructive malformation should be relieved as soon as possible. Chemoprophylaxis is best achieved with amoxicillin, 10 mg/kg q 12 hours for the first 2 months of life, with cotrimoxazole 1–2 mg/kg q 12 hours for the subsequent four months and with nitrofurantoin, 1 mg/kg q 12 hours later (Table 4.13).

2) RENAL VENOUS THROMBOSIS (RVT)

RVT is frequently secondary to perinatal stress, and is more frequent in infants of diabetic mothers or in infants with cyanotic congenital heart disease. RVT is characterized by large hemorrhagic kidneys, oliguric renal insufficiency, thrombocytopenia, and anemia. Proteinuria may be minimal. Ultrasonography demonstrates a large non-functioning, non-cystic kidney. The treatment includes correction of the underlying disorders and symptomatic management of renal insufficiency. The use of heparin has been recommended when there is evidence of continuing intravascular coagulation. Recent evidence suggests that recombinant human tissue plasminogen activator may be a good alternative.[15] The outcome is often fatal. Secondary hypertension is an occasional late complication.

Table 4.13 Antimicrobial agents for the treatment of acute urinary tract infection

Agent	Dose mg/kg	Intervals q h	Warnings
Parenteral (iv/im)			
Amikacin	7.5	8–12	Adapt to GFR, ototoxicity, nephrotoxicity
Amoxicillin	15	8–12	Adapt to GFR, neutropenia
Co-amoxiclavulanic	15 (amox)	12	Diarrhea
Cefotaxime	50	8–12	Adapt to GFR, thrombocytopenia, leucopenia
Ceftazidime	50	8–12	Idem cefotaxime
Ceftriaxone	50–100	24	Displacement of bilirubin, thrombocytopenia, leucopenia
Gentamicin	2.5	8–12	Adapt to GFR, ototoxicity, nephrotoxicity
Oral			
Amoxicillin	20–40	8	Adapt to GFR, neutropenia
Cefixime	8	12	Adapt to GFR, leucopenia, thrombocytopenia
Cotrimoxazole	3	12	Adapt to GFR, not before 1 month of age, Stevens-Johnson syndrome
Prophylaxis			
Amoxicillin	10	2	First 2 months of life
Cotrimoxazole	2 (TMP)	12	Not before 2 weeks of age
Trimethoprim	2	12	Not before 2 weeks of age
Nitrofurantoine	1	12	Not before 4 months of age

3) CORTICAL, MEDULLARY, AND PAPILLARY NECROSIS

Cortical, medullary, and papillary necrosis occur after severe prolonged episodes of ischemia. Major causes include perinatal asphyxia, septic shock, severe hemorrhage, gastroenteritis, erythroblastosis fetalis, severe hyperbilirubinemia, hyperosmolar states, and angiography with hypertonic contrast agents. Treatment is symptomatic and the prognosis is poor.

CONGENITAL NEPHROPATHIES

1) CONGENITAL NEPHROTIC SYNDROME

Congenital nephrotic syndrome of the Finnish type is often associated with placental hypertrophy, prematurity, and fetal distress.[20] Prerenal diagnosis is suggested by an elevation of alpha-fetoprotein in maternal blood and amniotic fluid. The disease is resistant to corticosteroids and immunosuppressive drugs and often fatal in the first year of life. Other conditions, such as congenital syphilis, congenital toxoplasmosis, and possibly congenital cytomegalovirus infection may induce congenital nephrosis (Table 4.14).

2) BARTTER'S SYNDROME

Bartter's syndrome is characterized by polyuria, hyposthenuria, hypokalemia, metabolic alkalosis,

Table 4.14 Etiology of the nephrotic syndrome in the newborn

1. Idiopathic: Finnish type (microcystic disease)
2. Secondary:
   - infectious: syphilis, toxoplasmosis, cytomegalic inclusion disease
   - vascular: renal vein thrombosis
   - toxic: heavy metals

hyperreninemia, and normal blood pressure; it may cause severe dehydration in the neonate.[21] Symptomatic treatment along with the use of inhibitors of prostaglandin synthesis is recommended.

3) NEPHROGENIC DIABETES INSIPIDUS

Nephrogenic diabetes insipidus is characterized by polyhydramnios, unexplained fever, and hypernatremic dehydration secondary to unrecognized polyuria. A postnatal loss of birth-weight greater than 10 percent in a normally fed infant whose urine osmolality is below 200 mosm per kg H_2O (specific gravity, 1.005) should suggest the possibility of this disorder. Administration of vasopressin fails to increase the urine concentration or decrease the polyuria. Treatment consists of the administration of adequate quantities of fluids with a low osmotic load (such as breast milk) and possible use of thiazide diuretics along with amiloride.[21]

4) OLIGONEPHROPATHY

Various pathologic conditions and diseases associated with a low birth weight and a deficit in the number of nephrons (Table 4.15) are major causes of morbidity and mortality in adulthood, such as hypertension, diabetes, and chronic renal failure[22].

DRUGS AND THE NEONATAL KIDNEY

1) FUROSEMIDE

Furosemide, a very efficient natriuretic agent, also promotes calcium excretion. Prolonged administration of furosemide has been associated with renal calcification. Secondary hyperparathyroidism and bone disease have been described after long-term administration of furosemide to preterm infants. By stimulating prostaglandin synthesis, furosemide may increase the incidence of patent ductus arteriosus.

2) DOPAMINE

Doses of 0.5–2.0 µg/kg per min have been claimed to improve urine flow, sodium excretion, and possibly GFR in preterm stressed infants. The usefulness and safety of dopamine in neonates is, however, debated.

3) ANTIBIOTICS

The nephrotoxicity of gentamicin and the cephalosporins is not well documented in newborns. Drugs eliminated mainly by glomerular filtration must be adapted to both gestational and postnatal age (Table 4.16).

Table 4.15 Causes of reduced nephron number

Development factors
    Renal maldevelopment, including obstructive nephropathy
    Intrauterine growth retardation
    Maternal diabetes
Nutritional factors
    Reduced maternal protein intake
    Reduced maternal vitamin A intake
    Reduced fetal potassium intake
Toxic/iatrogenic influences
    Maternal glucocorticoids
    Maternal aminoglycosides
    Maternal β-lactam antibiotics

Table 4.16 Drugs requiring dose adjustment when GFR is compromised

Antibiotics
Aminoglycoides (amikacin, gentamicin, totramycin)
Amoxicillin, amoxicillin-clavulanic acid
Cephalosporins (cefixime, cefotaxime, ceftazidime)
Cotrimoxazole
Ticarcillin
Vancomycin

Antifungal agents
Fluconazole

Cardiac drugs
Digoxin

4) INDOMETHACIN

Inhibition of prostaglandin synthesis has been recommended for the pharmacologic closure of the ductus arteriosus in premature infants. A significant transient decrease in glomerular filtration rate has been reported in some infants treated with indomethacin. The same risks are present when using other COX-non selective or COX2 selective inhibitors.[23]

5) ANGIOTENSIN CONVERTING ENZYME INHIBITORS (ACEI)

When used in neonates and infants, ACEI may decrease the renal perfusion pressure and lead to acute renal insufficiency. The risk is increased by the concomitant use of loop diuretics.[2] The same risk occurs with angiotensin AT-1 receptor antagonists.

6) CONTRAST AGENTS

The following major side effects have been described after the use of hypertonic angiographic contrast agents: renal venous thrombosis, medullary necrosis, hypoperfusion, ischemia, and renal insufficiency. The use of non-ionic contrast agents reduces the risk of toxicity in neonates.

7) DRUGS ADMINISTERED TO THE MOTHER

Angiotensin converting enzyme inhibitors: Persistent fatal anuria has been described in neonates whose mother had been given ACEI. Renal dysgenesis and increased neonatal morbidity has also been reported.[4]

Indomethacin: When given to the pregnant mother to prevent premature onset of labor, indomethacin (like all non-selective or selective NSAIDs) may impair renal function in the fetus and in the neonate. This postnatal effect is usually transient.[4,14]

REFERENCES

1. Guignard JP. Renal function in the newborn infant. Pediatr Clin North Am 1982; 29:777–790.
2. Guignard JP, John EG. Renal function in the tiny, premature infant. Clin Perinatol 1986; 13:377–401.
3. Karlowitz MG, Adelman RD. Nonoliguric and oliguric acute renal failure in asphyxiated term neonates. Pediatr Nephrol 1995; 9:718–722.
4. Toth-Heynh P, Drukker A, Guignard JP. The stressed neonatal kidney: from pathophysiology to clinical management of neonatal vasomotor nephropathy. Pediatr Nephrol 2000; 14:227–239.
5. Pinto E, Guignard JP. Renal masses in the neonate. Biol Neonate 1995; 68:175–184.
6. Brem AS. Neonatal hematuria and proteinuria. Clin Perinatol 1981; 8:321–332.
7. Becker N, Avner ED. Congenital nephropathies and uropathies. Pediatr Clin North Am 1995; 42:1319–1341.
8. Gallini F, Maggio L, Romagnoli C et al. Progression of renal function in preterm neonates with gestational age < or = 32 weeks. Pediatr Nephrol 2000; 15:119–124.
9. Miall LS, Henderson MJ, Turner AJ et al. Plasma creatinine rises dramatically in the first 48 hours of life in preterm infants. Pediatrics 1999; 104(6):e76.
10. Guignard JP, Drukker A. Why do newborn infants have a high plasma creatinine? Pediatrics 1999; 103:4/e49.
11. Ong WH, Guignard JP, Sharma A, Aranda JV. Pharmacological approach to the treatment of neonatal hypertension. Sem Neonatal 1998; 3:149–163.
12. Flynn JT. Neonatal hypertension: Diagnosis and management. Pediatr Nephrol 2000; 14:322–341.
13. Guignard JP, Gouyon JB, Adelman RD. Arterial hypertension in the newborn infant. Biol Neonate 1989; 55:77–83.
14. Guignard JP, Matos V. Protection of the immature kidney. Nephrology Dialysis Transplantation 1995; 10:71–79.
15. Gouyon JB, Guignard JP. Management of acute renal failure in newborns. Pediatr Nephrol 2000; 14:1037–1044.
16. Zobel G, Rodl S, Urlesberger B et al. Continuous renal replacement therapy in critically ill patients. Kidney Int 1998; 66:S169–S173.
17. El-Dahr SS, Lewy JE. Urinary tract obstruction and infection in the neonate. Clin Perinatol 1992; 19:213–222.
18. Shaw KN, Gorelick MH. Urinary tract obstruction and infection in the neonate. Pediatr Clin North Am 1999; 46:1111–1124.
19. Hellerstein S. Urinary tract infections. Old and new concepts. Pediatr Clin North Am 1995; 42:1433–1457.
20. Holmberg C, Antikainen M, Ronnholm K et al. Management of congenital nephrotic syndrome of the Finnish type. Pediatr Nephrol 1995; 9:87–93.
21. Zelikovic I. Molecular pathophysiology of tubular transport disorders. Pediatr Nephrol 2001; 16:919–935.
22. Merlet-Benichou C, Gilbert T, Vilar J. Nephron number: variability is the rule. Causes and consequences. Lab Invest 1999; 79:515–527.
23. Guignard JP. The adverse renal effects of prostaglandin-synthesis inhibitors in the newborn rabbit. Sem Perinatol 2002; 26:398–405.
24. Maherzi M, Guignard JP, Torrado A. Urinary tract infection in high-risk newborn infants. Pediatrics 1978; 62:521.

5. Mass screening for kidney disease in children – should it be done? If so, when?

Pyung-Kil Kim, Young-Mock Lee and Kyo Sun Kim

BACKGROUND

Many forms of chronic kidney disease (CKD) are believed to start in childhood. Children and adolescents are frequently asymptomatic for many years, resulting in their diagnosis and treatment being delayed and consequently a poor prognosis may ensure. The patients often develop symptoms and signs only after the disease has progressed considerably.

In order to recognize such patients earlier in their disease course, mass screening for chronic renal diseases, such as chronic nephritis, has long been suggested. It is possible that renal diseases might be detected at a very early stage and progressive CKD may be delayed or prevented in these patients if screening programs lead to earlier treatment.[1]

Screening of asymptomatic school children is currently employed for the early detection of chronic renal diseases in a number of countries around the world, although this is certainly not universal. Urinalysis is known as the simplest and the least expensive method. Urine testing is well suited for children, because urine specimens are usually readily available and are obtained noninvasively. Thus urinalysis is the most common screening test for asymptomatic children.

In order to perform screening successfully, it is important to understand the natural course and treatment of diseases detectable with those tests. An ideal screening test should screen for conditions that can be diagnosed with certainty, benefit from early diagnosis, be subject to appropriate follow-up, and be cost-effective. Detection of urinary abnormalities in asymptomatic patients results in significant parental and patient concern and may lead to an extended medical evaluation. The question as to whether mass screening of children detects

sufficient treatable pathology to justify the tangible and intangible costs is an important issue.

INTERNATIONAL ATTITUDES

Urinary mass screening is performed in several countries on a national basis. In Korea, since 1981, screening tests started with small numbers of children. Since 1998, all primary, middle, and high school students in Korea have been obligated to participate in the screening. Since the start of a school-screening program for the detection of urinary abnormalities, asymptomatic children with hematuria and/or proteinuria have been encountered with increasing frequency. However, little information regarding the underlying renal histologic changes and clinical findings in these children is available.

Most reports on urinary mass screening have been focused on the efficiency of the test detecting hematuria and proteinuria without providing details about the prognosis of children with abnormal findings. Not many systematic studies have been reported on that issue throughout the world. Most authors have tried to evaluate the distribution of the final diagnosis made on children with positive school urinary screening and follow-up tests. Diagnoses were made based on pathologic findings observed in renal biopsies performed on children satisfying certain conditions.[2]

Several studies have helped define the value of screening urinalysis in school-aged children. Dodge et al.[3] screened more than 12,000 school children in the United States for proteinuria and hematuria over a five-year period. They defined proteinuria as 10 mg/dl or more, and hematuria as five or more red blood cells (RBC) per high powered field (HPF) in the urine sediment in two or three of three specimens. They found proteinuria in 0.942% of the females and 0.33% of the males, and hematuria in 0.34% and 0.12%, respectively. Cumulative occurrence of proteinuria and hematuria was found to be high (>6%). Five hundred and twelve children with proteinuria and 78 with hematuria were followed for one to five years after initial detection and referred to their physician or clinic for additional evaluation and management. Significant renal disease was identified in eight of the children.

Vehaskari et al. conducted a study in 8,954 Finnish school children. They defined hematuria as six or more RBC/0.9 mm^3 in uncentrifuged urine.[4] Based on the results in one urine sample, 364 children (4.1%) had hematuria. However, only 83 of the children had hematuria in two or more samples, with 59 of them having both hematuria and proteinuria. Of the 83 children with hematuria in two or more samples, repeat testing after a further six months showed the abnormality to be persistent in only 33. Biopsies performed on 28 of the children showed two cases of IgA nephropathy, one of focal segmental glomerulosclerosis, one of extracapillary glomerulonephritis, and one of hereditary nephritis. Eleven biopsies showed nondiagnostic changes and 12 were normal. Although renal biopsies provided diagnoses in many of the cases, none of the lesions was subsequently treated.

Annual school screening in Japan was used to follow about 560,000 children (6–14 years of age) for 13 years.[5] When hematuria was defined as six or more RBC/HPF in a centrifuged sample, the prevalence of proteinuria and hematuria was 0.17% and 0.67% of the study population. The detection rates of urinary abnormality were approximately 2% at the first screening, 0.2% after two screenings, and 0.1% after three screenings. A definite diagnosis of renal disease was made in about 0.02%. This school urinary screening program was responsible for the detection of 70–80% of the children diagnosed with IgA nephropathy and non-IgA mesangial proliferative glomerulonephritis, and 65–80% of children diagnosed with membranoproliferative glomerulonephritis.[6]

Benbassat et al.[7] reviewed published data on the frequency of underlying disorders in school children with microscopic or gross hematuria. They found five reports of microscopic hematuria in screened asymptomatic school children, three reports of microscopic hematuria detected by case finding, and five surveys of kidney biopsies in referred children with microscopic and gross hematuria. They listed the reported underlying disorders, and estimated the benefit from their early detection and treatment. Some children had disorders that may benefit from early treatment (membranoproliferative glomerulonephritis, obstructive uropathy, urolithiasis), or counseling (hereditary nephropathy, renal cystic disease). The combined prevalence of these five diseases was 0–7.2% in children with microscopic hematuria detected by screening, and 3.3–13.6% in those with microscopic hematuria detected by case finding. The combined prevalence of membranoproliferative glomerulonephritis and hereditary nephropathy among kidney biopsies was 11.6–31.6% in children with microscopic hematuria, and 3.6–42.1% in children with gross hematuria. They suggested that isolated hematuria, once detected, justified investigation.

These several studies do not appear to warrant mass screening for hematuria or proteinura in asymptomatic school children, since most of the children with microscopic hematuria had no significant underlying diseases and there was no evidence that detection of hematuria prevented renal function impairment. However, most of the reports that have been made throughout the world have not provided data concerning the final diagnosis of children with abnormal screening results, and most of the analyses done concerning renal biopsy results have lacked sufficient subjects and data.

In order to obtain additional information regarding this issue, we conducted a retrospective study of school children who had renal biopsies performed after they were referred to us for the evaluation of an abnormal urinalysis that was detected in a school screening program between 1985 and 2001.[2] The screening program was carried out in three steps. First, an early morning urine specimen was examined by a simple dipstick method for the detection of hematuria, proteinuria, and sugar. If the urine test was positive, a second test was performed in the same manner two weeks later. Patients having hematuria and/or proteinuria in both tests were referred to our hospital for further evaluation. Renal biopsies were subsequently performed in 461 children who had continuous abnormal urinalysis lasting longer than six months, but had no specific abnormal findings in additional laboratory or imaging studies (Table 5.1). The mean age at the time of the renal biopsy was 10.0 ± 2.7 years.

We observed abnormal pathologic findings in 285 of the 461 children (61.8%) (Table 5.2). IgA nephropathy was seen in 121 cases (26.2%), and thin glomerular basement membrane disease in 127 (27.5%). Poststreptococcal glomerulonephritis occurred in eight (1.8%), minimal change

Table 5.1 Types of abnormal findings in urinary mass screening (n=461)

Results of urinalysis	Number of patients (%)
Isolated microscopic hematuria	289 (62.7)
Microscopic hematuria with proteinuria	163 (35.3)
Isolated proteinuria	9 (2.0)
Total	461 (100)

Table 5.2 Final pathologic diagnosis (n=461)

Pathologic diagnosis	Number of patients (%)
No histologic abnormality	176 (38.2)
Abnormal pathology	285 (61.8)
Thin GBM disease	127 (27.5)
IgA nephropathy	121 (26.2)
Poststreptococcal GN	8 (1.8)
Minimal change NS	8 (1.8)
Mesangial proliferative GN	7 (1.5)
Alport syndrome	4 (0.9)
FSGS	3 (0.7)
Membranous glomerulopathy	3 (0.7)
Membranoproliferative GN	2 (0.4)
Lupus nephritis	1 (0.2)
Oligomeganephronia	1 (0.2)
Total	461 (100)

Abbreviations: GBM, glomerular basement membrane; GN, glomerulonephritis; NS, nephrotic syndrome; FSGS, focal segmental glomerulosclerosis

nephrotic syndrome in eight (1.8%), and mesangial proliferative glomerulonephritis in seven (1.5%). Other conditions such as Alport syndrome, focal segmental glomerulosclerosis, and membranous glomerulonephropathy were found in less than 1% of the cases. Our data suggest the need for a more aggressive method of diagnosis, since no positive laboratory findings, or specific symptoms, but abnormal urinalysis only was noted, even in those rare diseases.

CLINICAL PICTURE

Our study showed several pathologic abnormalities in children who had only isolated microscopic hematuria (Table 5.3). Among the 289 cases of isolated hematuria, 97 (33.6%) had thin glomerular basement membrane disease, 46 (15.9%) IgA nephropathy, and 136 (47.1%) normal pathology. Of the 163 patients who had co-existing microscopic hematuria and proteinuria, 75 cases (46%) were found to have IgA nephropathy. Thirty cases (18.4%) had thin glomerular basement membrane disease, and 40 cases (24.5%) had normal pathology. Different studies, including ours, have cited IgA nephropathy and thin glomerular basement membrane disease as the main causes of asymptomatic hematuria in childhood. The significance of an early diagnosis of IgA nephropathy is uncertain and its treatment in the absence of any symptoms is controversial.[10] This is discussed in more detail in Chapter 9. In the future, development of new therapies for kidney diseases such as IgA nephropathy and hereditary nephritis, may increase the value of mass urinary screening. Our study revealed that 52.9% of 289 children, with isolated microscopic hematuria, showed abnormal pathologic findings while 75.5% of the 163 children with co-existing microscopic hematuria and proteinuria, showed them as well.

Classifying the degree of microscopic hematuria by the number of RBCs seen under a microscopic high power field, it was found that the worse the hematuria, the worse the pathologic findings that were observed. A statistically positive correlation between the severity of microscopic hematuria and

Table 5.3 Pathologic diagnosis in three groups: isolated microscopic hematuria (Group I), microscopic hematuria with proteinuria (Group II), isolated proteinuria (Group III)

Pathologic diagnosis	Group I (%)	Group II (%)	Group III (%)
No histologic abnormality	136 (47.1)	40 (24.5)	0
Abnormal pathology	153 (52.9)	123 (75.5)	
Thin GBM disease	97 (33.6)	30 (18.4)	0
IgA nephropathy	46 (15.9)	75 (46.0)	0
Poststreptococcal GN	4 (1.4)	4 (2.5)	0
Minimal change NS	0	1 (0.6)	7 (77.8)
Mesangial proliferative GN	1 (0.3)	5 (3.1)	1 (11.1)
Alport syndrome	1 (0.3)	3 (1.8)	0
FSGS	0	3 (1.8)	0
Membranous glomerulopathy	2 (0.7)	0	1 (11.1)
Membranoproliferative GN	0	2 (1.2)	0
Lupus nephritis	1 (0.3)	0	0
Oligomeganephronia	1 (0.3)	0	0
Total	289 (100)	163 (100)	9 (100)

Abbreviations: GBM, glomerular basement membrane; GN, glomerulonephritis; NS, nephrotic syndrome; FSGS, focal segmental glomerulosclerosis

Table 5.4 Final pathologic diagnosis depending on the severity of hematuria in groups of isolated microscopic hematuria

Microscopic hematuria	Normal histology (%)	Abnormal pathology (%)	Total (%)
6–10 RBC/HPF	62 (58.5)	44 (41.5)	106 (100)
10–20 RBC/HPF	58 (50.4)	57 (49.6)	115 (100)
Many RBC/HPF	16 (23.5)	52 (76.5)*	68 (100)

* : $P<0.01$
Abbreviation: HPF, high power field

the incidence of renal disease was noted. In cases of persistent microscopic hematuria with more than 10 RBCs seen under high power field, further evaluation is strongly recommended, since the rate of abnormal pathologic findings in this group was higher than 50% (Table 5.4).

Our observations agree with those of Vehaskari et al.,[4] who reported that in patients with co-existing hematuria and proteinuria, the degree of hematuria correlated well with the severity of the morphologic alterations in glomeruli in asymptomatic hematuria and proteinuria of the school-age population.

In our study, only 2% of the biopsied patients had isolated proteinuria. This was due to the fact

that most children with asymptomatic proteinuria are often later found to have transient or orthostatic proteinuria, which does not require renal biopsy. Other studies have also emphasized the importance of making the diagnosis of transient or orthostatic proteinuria in order to avoid unnecessary procedures in mass screening programs.

In a second mass screening-based study, conducted in Korea by Cho et al,[8] 452 children with urinary abnormalities were evaluated: 173 of these patients had renal biopsies. Among the biopsy cases, 51 cases (29.4%) had IgA nephropathy, 99 cases (57.2%) had mesangial proliferative glomerulo-nephritis, and 17 cases (9.8%) had other abnormalities similar to the ones that we had observed in our study.

Hisano and Ueda[9] reported that 54 children with hematuria and proteinuria were detected by a mass screening program and evaluated by clinical findings and renal histology. IgA nephropathy was found in 29 patients, diffuse mesangial proliferative glomerulonephritis in 16, membranous glomerulopathy in four, membranoproliferative glomerulonephritis in three, and focal segmental glomerulosclerosis in two. The incidence of renal insufficiency in IgA nephropathy in the children detected in this mass screening program was 3%.

In another Korean study, Lee et al.[11] reviewed the findings of urinary mass screening in 550,000 school children from 1987 to 1994 to evaluate the prevalence of proteinuria, and to estimate the risk of incipient renal diseases. The prevalence of asymptomatic proteinuria was 0.2–0.36%. Of those, the percentage of patients with transient proteinuria was 17%, orthostatic proteinuria 55%, persistent proteinuria 6%, proteinuria with hematuria 20% and isolated proteinuria 2%. Renal biopsy was performed on 80 children with proteinuria and hematuria or persistent proteinuria lasting longer than six months. Of these, IgA nephropathy was diagnosed in 38.9%, membranoproliferative glomerulonephritis 10.0%, membranous glomerulopathy 7.5%, reflux nephropathy 7.5%, focal segmental glomerulosclerosis 6.2%, and hepatitis B associated glomerulonephritis 7.5%.

Lin et al.[12] evaluated the prevalence of heavy proteinuria and chronic renal insufficiency and progression risk factors in children undergoing urinary screening. They concluded that early detection of children with heavy proteinuria by mass urinary screening, followed by early appropriate treatment, and monitoring of significant risk factors, might help to decrease or delay the progression of renal disease.

In a Japanese study, a total of 52 patients, who had been diagnosed with membranoproliferative glomerulonephritis type I, were studied. Thirty-five patients were identified on screening, and clinical symptoms were identified in 17 patients. There were more patients with hypertension and/or proteinuria in the symptomatic group than in the screening group. The renal survival rate in the screening group was 100% over 15 years, while the rate in the symptomatic group was 56%. They suggested that early identification by school urinary screening might enable early management and so improve the prognosis of membranoproliferative glomerulonephritis.[13]

Sakai and Kitagawa[14] also studied 113 cases of chronic progressive renal disease based on renal biopsy. Thirty-one of these 113 patients were found by routine urinalysis at area schools. Many of the asymptomatic children were found to have renal diseases, such as membranoproliferative glomerulonephritis, focal segmental glomerulosclerosis, and IgA nephropathy. Although it is difficult to decide whether or not medical management is required for asymptomatic children, the histologic findings may provide guidance for planning an appropriate therapeutic program in the early stages of various types of renal disease. This early detection may enable us to observe these potentially progressive renal diseases from an early phase, and to provide clues for the investigation of the pathogenesis of these renal diseases.

On the other hand, Ito et al.[15] evaluated the incidence of chronic renal failure in children with asymptomatic proteinuria and/or hematuria detected by a mass screening program in school and kindergarten. They reviewed 403 children who were referred due to urinary abnormalities. Of them, 4 cases were diagnosed with acute glomerulonephritis, 8 Alport syndrome, 7 focal glomerulonephritis, 7 focal segmental glomerulo-sclerosis, 3 Henoch-Schönlein purpura nephritis, 148 IgA nephropathy, 12 membranous glomerulopathy, 24 membranoproliferative glomerulonephritis (including seven cases of focal membranoproliferative glomerulonephritis), and 1 with lupus nephritis. Of these children, 2 of the 8 cases of Alport syndrome, 1 of the 7 cases of focal segmental glomerulosclerosis, 6 of the 148 cases of IgA nephropathy and none of the 24 cases of membranoproliferative glomerulonephritis, developed chronic renal failure. They concluded that the incidence of chronic renal failure in children, with various kinds of renal disease detected by a mass screening program, is lower than that of symptomatic children.

ARGUMENTS IN FAVOUR OF SCREENING

The theoretical merits of mass screening programs for the detection of renal disease include the detection of glomerulonephritis with the possibility of early therapeutic intervention. Renal histopathology in children with asymptomatic urinary abnormalities revealed less severe changes than those found in children diagnosed following clinical manifestations of nephritis.[6] These observations suggested that children with asymptomatic glomerular disease and chronic renal disease should have a better prognosis than those with clinical symptoms, especially if specific treatment is available.

Asymptomatic urinary abnormalities in childhood rarely became aggravated. A small proportion of the subjects who showed exacerbations were those with IgA nephropathy; these patients had considerable glomerular damage on the first biopsy, non-IgA nephropathy with severely damaged glomeruli, focal segmental glomerulosclerosis, membranoproliferative glomerulonephritis or Alport syndrome. Further study is needed in the future to establish an effective screening program and treatment of children who show persistent abnormal urinary findings, especially those with combined hematuria and proteinuria, or isolated proteinuria that is fixed and persistent.

These studies suggest that annual urinary mass screening has greatly facilitated the discovery of chronic kidney diseases in asymptomatic children, and is useful for early intervention and prevention of the occurrence of chronic, progressive renal failure. With routine annual urinalysis screening, chronic renal disease can be diagnosed early, before progression to chronic renal failure. As a result of providing earlier detection, the apparent prevalence of chronic renal glomerular disease has increased. Also, studies on the natural course of some renal diseases are continually being carried out. However,

in order to carry on the mass screening tests successfully, further studies on the natural course of renal diseases and more effective treatment have to be done.

CONCLUSION

We conclude that screening urinalysis can be recommended. We propose that screening dipstick urinalysis be obtained at preschool entry age (between five and six years of age) and annual dipstick urinalysis from school entry age till adolescence. This will provide invaluable epidemiologic information, and the opportunity for setting up clinical trials in the early stages of disease. Continuous follow-up studies will be made in cases of abnormal urinalysis. More aggressive medical approaches, such as renal biopsy, should also be considered, if necessary, as a method of making diagnosis with more systematic analysis. Further systematic studies and analysis according to their results are strongly recommended.

REFERENCES

1. Roberts KB. A synopsis of the American Academy of Pediatrics' practice parameter on the diagnosis, treatment, and evaluation of the initial urinary tract infection in febrile infants and young children. Pediatr Rev 1999; 20:344–347.
2. Lee YM, Kim JH, Lee JS et al. Analysis of renal biopsies performed in children with abnormal findings in urinary mass screening. Korean J Nephrol 2002; 2:349–355.
3. Dodge WF, West EF, Smith EH et al. Proteinuria and hematuria in school children: epidemiology and early natural history. J Pediatr 1976; 88:327–347.
4. Vehaskari VM, Rapola J, Koskimies O et al. Microscopic hematuria in school children. Epidemiology and clinicopathologic evaluation. J Pediatr 1979; 95:676–684.
5. Murakami M, Yamamoto H, Ueda Y et al. Urinary screening of elementary and junior-school children over a 13-year period in Tokyo. Pediatr Nephrol (1991) 5:50–53.
6. Kitagawa T. Lessons learned from the Japanese nephritis screening study. Pediatr Nephrol 1988; 2:256–263.
7. Benbassat J, Gergawi M, Offringa M et al. Symptomless microhematuria in school children: causes for variable management strategies. QJM 1996; 89:845–854.
8. Cho BS, Kim SD, Choi YM et al. School urinalysis screening in Korea: prevalence of chronic renal disease. Pediatr Nephrol 2001; 16:1126–1128.
9. Hisano S, Ueda K. Asymptomatic hematuria and proteinuria: renal pathology and clinical outcome in 54 children. Pediatr Nephrol 1989; 3:229–234.

10. Nolin L, Courteau M. Management of IgA nephropathy: Evidence-based recommendations. Kidney Int Suppl 1999; 70:s56–62

11. Lee CG, Lee DW, Yang SW et al. Analysis of urinary mass screening for elementary, junior and high school children over an 8-year period in Seoul. J Korean Pediatr Soc 1997; 40:1347–1359.

12. Lin CY, Sheng CC, Chen CH et al. The prevalence of heavy protein-uria and progression risk factors in children undergoing urinary screening. Pediatr Nephrol 2000; 14:953–959.

13. Kawakaki Y, Suzuki J, Nozawa R et al. Efficiency of school urinary screening for membranoproliferative glomerulonephritis type I. Arch Dis Child 2002; 86:21–25.

14. Sakai T, Kitagawa T. Screening system for asymptomatic renal disease in children in Japan. Acta Paediatr Jpn 1990; 32:677–681.

15. Ito K, Kawaguchi H, Hattori M. Screening for proteinuria and hema-turia in school children – Is it possible to reduce the incidence of chronic renal failure in children and adolescents? Acta Paediatr Jpn 1990; 32:710–715.

6. Hematuria and proteinuria

Juan Rodríguez-Soriano

Hematuria and proteinuria are among the most important signs by which a child is identified as having possible renal disease. Pediatricians must be able to orient the clinical investigations of children with these signs in an orderly way to make a correct differential diagnosis, and thus identify possible causes which justify the referral of the patient to a specialized center of pediatric nephrology.[1]

In general, children presenting with hematuria and/or proteinuria may be separated into different clinical categories: a) children with hematuria without or with minimal proteinuria; b) children with hematuria associated with significant proteinuria; and c) children with proteinuria without accompanying hematuria. Each one of these clinical settings suggests different etiologies and often has a different prognosis.

HEMATURIA

DEFINITION

A small number of red blood cells (RBC) may be normally excreted in the urine. Microscopic hematuria is defined by the presence in freshly voided urine of more than 3 RBC / hpf or more than 5 RBC/mm^3. Nowadays, microscopic hematuria is generally discovered by the use of dipsticks. The zone of the paper strip impregnated with orthotoluidine recognizes the presence of hemoglobin or myoglobin because the peroxidase-like activity of these substances catalyzes the oxidation of orthotoluidine. It should be recognized, however, that this test is more sensitive to detect free hemoglobin and myoglobin than intact RBC. Nevertheless, a positive test (1 + or more) is generally equivalent to at least five intact RBC / hpf. Sensitivity reaches almost 100%, and

sensitivity lies between 65 and 99%. False negative results may be due to urines with a pH below five, while false positive results may be due to the presence of reducing substances in the urine, such as contaminants or peroxidases of bacterial origin.

Macrosopic hematuria is easily recognized by the presence of red or brown urine. It is important to distinguish between urines having a reddish-brown color, similar to coca-cola or dark tea, which point out to a renal parenchymal origin, and urines having a rutilant red color, with or without blood clots, which point to bleeding from the mucosa along the urinary tract.

HEMOGLOBINURIA AND MYOGLOBINURIA

The absence of RBCs in the urinary sediment despite the presence of a positive orthotoluidine test, suggests the possible diagnosis of hemoglobinuria or myoglobinuria. The most frequent cause for this is the hemolysis of RBCs in a dilute urine specimen that has been allowed to stand for a long time. More rarely, hemoglobinuria is associated with intravascular hemolysis and is accompanied by a pinkish color of serum, and a fall in blood haptoglobin levels. Myoglobinuria is relatively rare. Unlike hemoglobinuria, the serum of patients with this condition maintains its clear color. The diagnosis should be suspected when antecedants of rabdomyolysis (secondary to generalized trauma, excessive burns, physical exercise, heat stroke, grand mal seizures, status asthmaticus, polymyositis, snake bites, etc.) are present. Increased plasma levels of muscle enzymes such as creatine phosphokinase support the diagnosis.

COLORANTS IN URINE

Not all red urine is due to the presence of blood, hemoglobin or myoglobin. Many substances may cause a reddish or brown color when present in the urine. These include: antipyrine, azathioprine, bile pigments, desferroxamine, diphenylhydantoin, lead, phenolphthalein, phenothiazines, pyridium, rifampicin, and urates. Ingestion of beets, blackberries, sweets containing rhodamine B, or urinary infection by *Serratia marcescens* (red diaper syndrome) may also be followed by the passage of a red urine.

RED BLOOD CELL MORPHOLOGY

A simple method to localize the source of hematuria in most patients involves an examination of the morphology of urinary RBCs by phase-contrast microscopy.[2] A sample of fresh urine is centrifuged for approximately 10 min at 1500 rpm. The urinary sediment is resuspended in 0.5 ml of the supernatant urine, and a few drops of the urine are placed on a glass slide and examined with a phase contrast microscope. A glomerular origin of the hematuria is suspected when at least 10% of the RBCs examined are dysmorphic or distorted in shape. Characteristically, small blebs of cytoplasm are seen to extend from the cell membrane (acantocytes or G1 cells) (Figs 6.1 and 6.2). A non-

glomerular origin of the hematuria is associated with urinary RBCs, which almost all are intact and uniform, without distortion of the cell membrane (Fig. 6.1). The same findings may be observed in Wright stains of urine sediments studied by regular microscopy, although it is more difficult to define the dysmorphic features using this last method. Also, the mean corpuscular volume distribution curves of RBCs obtained in a semi-automated cell counter show differences between glomerular and non-glomerular hematuria. RBCs of glomerular origin are smaller and with a volume distribution curve which is irregular and asymmetric, whereas RBCs of non-glomerular origin have size and volume distribution curves identical to those of RBCs obtained directly from venous blood. The quotient of mean corpuscular volume of urinary RBCs/ mean corpuscular volume of blood RBCs is always below one in glomerular hematuria and at about one in non-glomerular hematuria.[3]

URINARY SEDIMENT

Detection and quantification of proteinuria, and careful study of the urinary sediment, are important aspects of the work-up of patients with

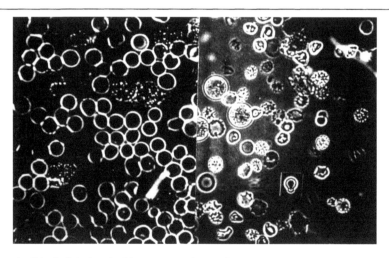

Figure 6.1 Morphology of red blood cells in the urine (phase-contrast microscopy)

Left: Normal red blood cells from the urinary sediment of a patient with non-glomerular hematuria. *Right*: Dysmorphic red blood cells from the urinary sediment of a patient with glomerular hematuria

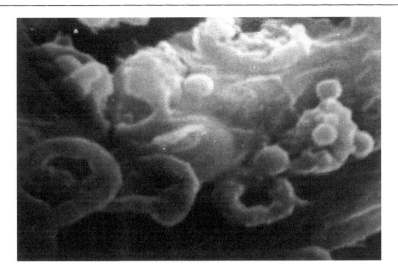

Figure 6.2 Morphology of red blood cells in the urine of a patient with glomerular hematuria (scanning electron microscopy)

hematuria. The presence of leukocytes, casts, or bacteria should be documented by microscopy. The presence of RBC casts strongly supports a glomerular origin of the hematuria. As stated previously, it should be remembered that RBCs may be lysed in urines which either are very dilute or are strongly alkaline, especially if some time has elapsed since the specimen was obtained.

DIFFERENTIAL DIAGNOSIS OF HEMATURIA

1) HEMATURIA OF GLOMERULAR ORIGIN

As mentioned, this type of hematuia is usually accompanied by dysmorphic RBCs in the urine. Table 6.1 lists many glomerular disorders, both primary or secondary, to systemic and hereditary diseases, that may cause glomerular hematuria. Common diagnoses in children include post-streptococcal glomerulonephritis, IgA nephropathy, Henoch-Schönlein purpura, hereditary nephritis (Alport's syndrome), and recurrent benign hema-

turia. More details of some of these disorders can be found elsewhere in this text.

Glomerular hematuria may be microscopic or macroscopic (gross), and may occur as an acute clinical episode, or persist over time either as chronic microscopic hematuria or in the form of recurrent relapses of gross hematuria. It may be accompanied by minimal proteinuria or, more significantly, severe proteinuria.

2) HEMATURIA OF NON-GLOMERULAR ORIGIN

This type of hematuria is usually associated with intact RBCs in the urine. Table 6.1 lists various conditions that may produce this abnormality, such as hemorrhagic cystitis, renal calculi, idiopathic hypercalciuria, renal trauma, congenital renal anomalies, obstructive uropathy, renal tumors, and drugs. Hematuria following strenuous exercise may be observed in older children and adolescents performing sport activities. In general, post-exercise hematuria disappears after a period of 24–72 h.

Table 6.1 Differential diagnosis of hematuria

Glomerular hematuria	Non-glomerular hematuria
Familial	**Congenital**
Hereditary nephritis or Alport's syndrome	Polycystic kidney disease
Recurrent benign hematuria	Sickle-cell anemia
	Coagulation disorders
Acquired	**Acquired**
Poststreptococcal glomerulonephritis	Drug-induced
IgA nephropathy	Contrast media
Membranoproliferative glomerulonephritis	
Membranous glomerulonephritis	**Urinary tract disorders**
Focal segmental glomerulosclerosis	Hemorrhagic cystitis
Bacterial endocarditis	Renal calculi
Shunt nephritis	Idiopathic hypercalciuria
Interstitial nephritis	Renal trauma
	Obstructive uropathy
Systemic	Tumors of the kidney
Systemic lupus erythematosus	Schistosomiasis
Henoch-Schönlein purpura	Vascular abnormalities
Hemolytic-uremic syndrome	Exercise
	Other (idiopathic)

In contrast to glomerular hematuria, non-glomerular hematuria may be accompanied by symptoms such as flank pain in cases of urolithiasis, or of dysuria, frequency and urgency in cases of hemorrhagic cystitis.

3) HEMATURIA OF UNDETERMINED ORIGIN

Occasionally, all investigations, including ultrasonographic and radiologic studies, fail to demonstrate the cause of the hematuria. The hematuria is then classified as *essential* or *idiopathic*. Some of these apparently idiopathic cases may present the so-called 'nutcracker phenomenon', that is, the compression of the left renal vein between aorta and superior mesenteric artery.[4] This diagnosis may be suspected by Doppler ultrasonography and confirmed by direct study of renal vessels, either by selective arteriography or by gadolinium-enhanced magnetic resonance angiography. Nevertheless, it is not completely clear that the 'nutcracker phenomenon' is the direct cause of the hematuria since it may also be observed in normal children, or in children without hematuria who are investigated

because of the presence of orthostatic proteinuria or chronic fatigue syndrome.

WORKUP OF HEMATURIA

Any child presenting with red or brown urine should be evaluated. Some of the studies that may be incorporated into the diagnostic approach are presented in Figure 6.3.[5] Careful assessment of the patient's history, physical examination, and laboratory findings may allow the physician to classify the hematuria as glomerular or non-glomerular, and thus proceed along the different lines of diagnostic studies shown in the figure.

The evaluation should investigate the characteristics of the gross hematuria: color, presence of blood clots, duration, relationship to micturition, etc. as well as the accompanying circumstances: renal trauma, abdominal or flank pain, dysuria, fever, weight loss, and antecedents of exercise, respiratory or cutaneous infection, and administration of nephrotoxic drugs. Personal history should exclude the presence of known renal diseases, congenital heart disease, or antecedents of renal vein

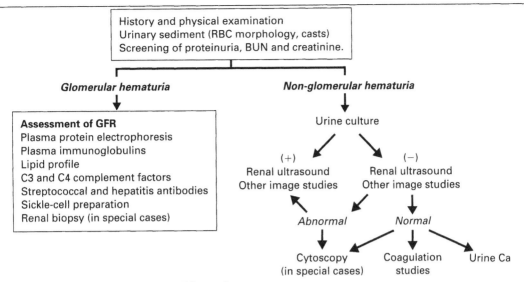

Figure 6.3 Diagnostic workup of a child presenting with hematuria

thrombosis. Family history is extremely important and questions should be posed not only with regards to the existence of family members with known hematuria, but also with renal calculi, hereditary nephropathies, neurosensorial deafness, and coagulation disorders. It is also important to examine the urines of parents and siblings in the search for undetected microhematuria. This is a relatively frequent finding and usually implies that the patient has benign familial hematuria, although more serious diagnoses may also be present.

Physical examination must look for the presence of edema, purpura or exanthema, renal masses, and flank tenderness. Presence of megacystis will point to urinary obstruction. Examination of the urethra may reveal meatal stenosis. Eyes should be carefully examined looking for corneal or lens abnormalities. Measurement of blood pressure with age and size appropriate equipment is mandatory.

Laboratory studies that should be included in the evaluation of children with hematuria begin with a careful urinalysis to search for dysmorphic RBCs. If the initial workup reveals significant proteinuria and/or dysmorphic RBCs, the physician should be favoring a diagnosis of glomerular hematuria, and further investigations should be oriented in this direction. In this way, the child can be spared from

undergoing many radiology studies. Quantification and electrophoresis of blood proteins and immunoglobulins, lipid profile, determination of C3 and C4 fractions of complement, presence of antinuclear antibodies, streptococcal and hepatitis serology, sickle-cell preparation in black children, etc. may help to delineate the diagnosis, but the determination as to which tests are relevant for an individual patient is best approached in collaboration with a pediatric nephrologist. Performance of a percutaneous renal biopsy is not always necessary if the diagnosis is clinically established. However, it may be indicated if a suspected diagnosis must be confirmed before initiating aggressive therapeutic procedures such as corticosteroid therapy, or the administration of immunosuppressive drugs.

If the initial workup points to the diagnosis of non-glomerular hematuria (absence of proteinuria and of dysmorphic RBCs in the urine), one should consider obtaining a urine culture. If it is positive, the diagnosis of cystitis or acute pyelonephritis is established. Specific imaging studies (renal ultrasonography, isotopic studies, voiding cystourethrography, intravenous urography, etc.) may then be indicated. If the urine culture is negative, renal ultrasonography may detect calculi, cysts, dilation of urinary tract, renal masses, etc. If renal ultrasonography and plain X-ray of the abdomen are normal or detect the presence of calculi, a urinary calcium/urinary creatinine (UCa/UCr) ratio should be measured to establish the diagnosis of hypercalciuria. Idiopathic hypercalciuria represents the most frequent cause of non-glomerular hematuria in children, and is thought to be a forerunner of renal calculi in some patients. If a coagulation disorder is suspected, specific blood tests must be performed. Cystoscopy is an aggressive procedure in children and has very limited indications. It may be carried out to determine which kidney is bleeding in cases of persisting non-glomerular hematuria of undetermined origin, but this is not often helpful.

Asymptomatic microscopic hematuria is a frequent abnormality on urinary screening of schoolchildren.[6,7] Its prevalence is 0.56% among screened children of 6–11 years of age, and 0.94% among screened children of 11–13 years of age. Its cumulative incidence rises with repeated examinations, so that by 12 years of age, 3.2% of girls and 1.4% of boys may present >5 RBC/hpf on at least one of five consecutive annual examinations.[8] This is discussed in greater detail in Chapter 4. In many children, microscopic hematuria is transient in nature and never reappears on successive examinations. When microhematuria persists and is associated with significant proteinuria, a complete study, which may include a renal biopsy, is warranted. There is more uncertainty about the outcome of cases of isolated microscopic hematuria, without proteinuria: it is generally believed that most children do not have a serious disease. However, some authors have claimed that a high percentage of children should be referred because microscopic hematuria may later be associated with proteinuria, and have a bad long-term prognosis. In my opinion, this is not the case when microscopic hematuria has been detected by screening. If the urine culture is negative, UCa/UCr ratio is not elevated, and renal ultrasonography is normal, the parents should be informed that there is probably no serious renal disease in their child but that annual examinations are recommended. If proteinuria remains absent, and blood pressure stays within the normal range, the parents may be reassured about the benignity of the outcome. However, without performing a renal biopsy the possibility of a renal disease such as IgA nephropathy or thin basement membrane disease cannot be completely excluded.

PROTEINURIA

DEFINITION

Normal urinary protein excretion in an afebrile individual at rest is below 100 mg/m^2/24 hr (4 mg/m^2/hr). There are age and sex differences as well as diurnal variations; for example, protein excretion is higher during the day while the child is not recumbent. Normally, about 2–4 g of proteins are filtered through the glomeruli in adults, and are almost completely reabsorbed in the proximal tubule by a complex process of endocytosis. Two-thirds of the normally excreted proteins represent a mixture of albumin and other small proteins which escape reabsorption in the proximal tubule: immunoglobulins, transferrin, β2 microglobulin, etc. The remaining one-third represents Tamm-Horsfall protein and other glycoproteins which are directly secreted in the distal nephron.

The detection of proteinuria is generally established by the use of dipsticks containing tetrabromosulfonephthalein (Labstix, Albustix, etc). This method may only detect proteinuria when the concentration is above 15 mg/dl. Different intensities of green color indicate the presence of trace (about 15 mg/dl), *1+* (about 30 mg/dl), *2+* (about 100 mg/dl), *3+* (about 300 mg/dl) and *4+* (above 1000 mg/dl) proteinuria. It should be noted that a false negative result is possible when the urine is very dilute. False positive results are also possible when the urine is alkaline, very concentrated, or contains antiseptics (chlorhexidine), or contrast media. In these circumstances, the diagnosis of proteinuria should be confirmed by the turbidometric method using sulfosalicylic acid.

Quantification of the urinary protein excretion is usually performed in a 24-hr timed collection by the turbidometric method. Proteinuria is considered significant when the protein excretion is above 4 mg/m^2/hr, and in the 'nephrotic range' when it exceeds 40 mg/m^2/hr. However, collection of timed urine specimens is difficult in infants and children. For this reason, the use of a spot urine protein/urine creatinine ratio[5] (UPr/UCr) has been proposed as a surrogate for 24-hr urine protein excretion.[9] The best screening method is to perform the study in a first morning urine sample obtained immediately after the child gets out of bed. A UPr/UCr ratio below 0.2 represents physiologic proteinuria or orthostatic proteinuria, whereas ratios above 0.2 indicate significant degrees of proteinuria. It is important to make sure that the child empties his/her bladder prior to going to bed. 'Nephrotic' proteinuria is manifested by ratios above two. In children under two years of age the cut-off point for normalcy is 0.5. There is a paper strip (Clinitek) which simultaneously quantifies protein and creatinine in the urine using a reflectance meter. When values for the UPr/UCr ratio above 0.30 are considered, sensitivity and specificity are 76% and 89%, respectively, thus making this method a reliable one to screen for proteinuria.[10]

In some circumstances it may be important to carry out qualitative studies to separate different types of proteinuria. Glomerular proteinuria is the result of an increased filtered load of protein, generally due to altered glomerular permeability. Normal tubular reabsorptive mechanisms are overwhelmed, and albumin and other proteins will appear in increased amounts in the urine. Glomerular proteinuria may be more or less selective depending on the size of the proteins present in the urine. It is selective when it is formed by proteins of small molecular weight such as albumin or transferrin, and non-selective when it is formed by large proteins such as IgG. The protein selectivity index is calculated by measuring the clearance ratio of IgG to that of transferrin. When greater than 0.2, proteinuria is termed non-selective, and when it is less than 0.1 is termed selective. 'Selective proteinuria' usually indicates minimal change nephrotic syndrome responsive to steroids, whereas non-selectivie proteinuria is observed in complex forms of glomerulonephritis resistant to steroids.

Microalbuminuria refers to albumin excretion rates below those conventionally accepted as significant proteinuria (i.e. a level that would not show up as positive on a standard dipstick). Among insulin-dependent diabetics, this type of proteinuria may strongly predict the appearance of persistent clinical proteinuria and diabetic nephropathy.

Tubular proteinuria is the consequence of defective proximal tubular endocytosis and is generally manifested by the presence in the urine of proteins of low molecular weight such as β2-microglobulin, lysozyme, retinol-binding protein, immunoglobulin light chains, etc.

DIFFERENTIAL DIAGNOSIS OF PROTEINURIA

The finding of proteinuria in an isolated urine sample occurs with relative frequency; a prevalence of 2.5% has been estimated in schoolchildren between 8–15 years of age. However, the finding of persistent proteinuria (at least in four different urine samples) is much more uncommon, and its prevalence drops to 0.1%.[11] The causes of isolated, asymptomatic proteinuria are delineated in Table 6.2. It is important to differentiate between transient, intermittent, orthostatic, and persistent proteinuria. Transient proteinuria is occasionally seen with high fever, dehydration, strenuous exercise, exposure to cold or emotional stress. Urine protein returns to normal after recovery from the precipitating event.

Intermittent proteinuria refers to proteinuria which is detected in some but not in all urine samples, without an identifiable cause. It is the most common form of proteinuria and is usually not associated with organic renal disease. False positive results should always be excluded.

Orthostatic (postural) proteinuria[12] is defined by the presence of proteinuria only when the child is in the upright position. Characteristically, the proteinuria is absent when the child is at rest. Proteinuria may be found in some (transient) or in all (persistent) urine specimens collected in the upright position. Total protein excretion is extremely variable but rarely exceeds 1 g/m^2/24 hr. It is generally observed in children above six years of age, and occurs more frequently in girls than in boys. The

Table 6.2 Differential diagnosis of isolated proteinuria

Transient
Fever
Dehydration
Exercise
Exposure to cold
Emotional stress

Intermittent

Orthostatic (postural)

Persistent

Primary
    Benign persistent proteinuria
    Tubular proteinuria, familial or non-familial

Secondary
    Idiopathic nephrotic syndrome
    Membranous glomerulonephritis
    Hereditary nephritis
    Tubulointerstitial disease
    Dent's disease and other tubular disorders

patients with minimal change idiopathic nephrotic syndrome. Persistent proteinuria for more than one year, with or without other renal symptoms or signs, is an important sign of renal parenchymal disease, and its presence should dictate a detailed diagnostic evaluation, which may include a renal biopsy. Lesions of focal segmental glomerulosclerosis, focal global glomerulosclerosis, or membranous nephropathy may be found.[13]

The term benign persistent proteinuria refers to a group of patients with glomerular proteinuria, without nephrotic syndrome, in whom glomeruli are completely normal or show segmental thickening of basement membranes or segmental effacement of foot processes.[14] In other circumstances, the proteinuria presents a tubular pattern and may be sporadic or familial. Study of urinary calcium excretion is mandatory in these cases to rule out the diagnosis of Dent's disease. Obviously, isolated persistent proteinuria of unrecognized origin does not represent a homogenous entity, although globally it may have a benign prognosis.

WORKUP OF PROTEINURIA

A diagnostic approach to a child with proteinuria is presented in Figure 6.4.[15] Following the initial discovery of proteinuria, at least two additional first-morning voided urine specimens should be examined. As stated previously, it is important that the child empties the bladder before going to bed. If the morning sample is negative (UPr/UCr <0.2), the child probably has transient or orthostatic proteinuria.

The confirmation of clinical proteinuria (UPr/UCr >0.2) in the morning sample excludes orthostatic proteinuria and makes it necessary to complete the workup searching for symptoms and signs of parenchymal renal disease. The assistance of laboratory and imaging studies may help to establish a definitive diagnosis. The presence of an abnormal sediment (hematuria, etc.) excludes the diagnosis of isolated proteinuria and obliges the physician to follow the workup recommended for a child with hematuria. If the proteinuria remains isolated and the Upr/Ucr ratio is >2.0, the proteinuria

exact pathophysiology of this condition remains unknown but it may depend on altered renal hemodynamics. In a few patients the 'nutcracker phenomenon' may be present. It is generally believed that this type of proteinuria has a benign clinical course. However, a long-term follow-up is necessary because occasional lesions of glomerulosclerosis have been demonstrated in adults who were diagnosed during childhood with orthostatic proteinuria. It should be noted that in patients with glomerular disease, the proteinuria has also a postural component. Therefore, the diagnosis of orthostatic proteinuria should be reserved for patients who have completely normal excretion of protein when supine.

Persistent or fixed proteinuria refers to proteinuria which is found in every urine specimen. Although the actual amount of protein may vary from specimen to specimen in a given patient, the proteinuria persists indefinitely or for a recognizable length of time. It may also resolve after therapy of the underlying renal disorder, as occurs in

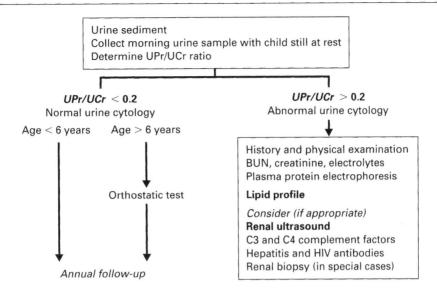

Figure 6.4 Diagnostic workup of a child presenting with proteinuria

probably indicates idiopathic nephrotic syndrome. Evaluation should be completed with quantification and electrophoresis of blood proteins and immunoglobulins, lipid profile, and determination of C3 and C4 fractions of the complement. Renal biopsy should, in general, be reserved for children presenting with persistent proteinuria, especially when a low plasma C3 value is present.

REFERENCES

1. Foreman JW, Chan JC. 10-year survey of referrals to a pediatric nephrology program. Child Nephrol Urol 1990; 10:8–13.
2. Fairley KF, Birch DF. Hematuria: a simple method of identifying glomerular bleeding. Kidney Int 1982; 21:105–108.
3. Lettgen B, Hestermann C, Rascher W. Differentiation of glomerular and non-glomerular hematuria in children by measurement of mean corpuscular volume of urinary red cells using a semi-automated cell counter. Acta Paediatr 1994; 83:946–949.
4. Wendel RG, Crawford ED, Hehman KN. The Nutcracker phenomenon: an unusual cause for renal varicosities with hematuria. J Urol 1980; 123:761–763.
5. West DC. Asymptomatic hematuria and proteinuria in pediatric patients. Diagnostic approach. Urology 1978; 11:205–214.
6. Vehaskari VM, Rapola J, Koskimies O, Savilahti E, Vilska J, Hallman N. Microscopic hematuria in school children: epidemiology and clinico-pathological evaluation. J Pediatr 1979; 95:676–684.
7. Benbassat J, Gergawi M, Offringa M, Drukker A. Symptomless microhematuria in schoolchildren: causes for variable management strategies. Q J Med 1996; 89:845–854.
8. Murakami M, Yamamoto H, Ueda Y, Murakami K, Yamauchi K. Urinary screening of elementary and junior high-school children over a 13-year period in Tokyo. Pediatr Nephrol 1991; 5:50–53.
9. Houser M. Assessment of proteinuria using random urine samples. J Pediatr 1984; 104:845–848.
10. Parsons M, Newman DJ, Pugia M, Newall RG, Price CP. Performance of a reagent strip device for quantification of the urine albumin: creatinine ratio on a point of care setting. Clin Nephrol 1999; 51:220–227.
11. Vehaskari VM, Rapola J. Isolated proteinuria: analysis of a school-age population. Pediatr 1982; 101:661–668.
12. Vehaskari VM. Orthostatic proteinuria. Arch Dis Child 1982; 57:729–730.
13. Trachtman H, Bergwerk A, Gauthier B. Isolated proteinuria in children. Natural history and indications for renal biopsy. Clin Pediatr 1994; 33:468–472.
14. McLaine PN, Drummond NK. Benign persistent asymptomatic proteinuria in childhood. Pediatrics 1970; 46:548–552.
15. Hogg RJ, Portman RJ, Milliner D, Lemley V, Eddy A, Ingelfinger J. Evaluation and management of proteinuria and nephrotic syndrome in children: Recommendations from a Pediatric Nephrology Panel established at the National Kidney Foundation Conference on proteinuria, albuminuria, risk, assessment, detection and elimination (PARADE). Pediatrics 2000; 105:1242–1249.

7. The nephrotic syndrome

Raymond AMG Donckerwolcke and Johan Vande Walle

The nephrotic syndrome (NS) is a clinical entity that is characterized by massive urinary protein losses, resulting in hypoalbuminemia and usually associated with edema formation. The idiopathic form of NS (INS) is present in the large majority of children who are diagnosed with this condition. The incidence of INS is 2–7 new cases per 100,000 child population per year with a sex ratio of 2:1 (M/F). Age at onset is between two and five years. In 10% of patients, INS persists into adulthood.

CLINICAL FEATURES

The major clinical symptom of the NS is edema formation. Abnormal fluid accumulation starts in regions that are gravity dependent, such as pedal edema, and in areas with the least tissue resistance, such as the periorbital region, labia majora or scrotum, and may become more generalized if fluid retention is in excess of 10% of body weight, with the subsequent development in some patients of ascites and pleural effusions. If edema is generalized, grossly edematous genitalia may cause severe discomfort and cellulitis. Rapidly developing NS may result in functional hypovolemia, characterized by abdominal pain, diarrhea, peripheral vasoconstriction with cold extremities, and oliguria. Paradoxically, hypovolemia may be associated with hypertension. Other common clinical symptoms are lethargy, irritability, and poor appetite.

LABORATORY FINDINGS

In the NS there is heavy proteinuria with protein excretion in excess of 40 mg/m^2/hr. For practical purposes, proteinuria is often estimated from an early morning urine specimen. The urinary protein/creatinine (UP/C) ratio in these specimens shows an excellent correlation with overnight protein excretion rate and exceeds 2.0 mg/mg in patients with abnormally high ("nephrotic-range") rates of protein excretion.[1]

Nephrotic-range protein losses result in plasma albumin levels less than 2.5 g/dl. While the hematocrit is often raised as a result of hemoconcentration that is secondary to volume contraction, in some patients hyponatremia is noticed. This may be a spurious finding, consequent to hyperlipidemia, but sometimes is related to non-osmotic antidiuretic hormone (ADH) release. The serum creatinine is initially raised in 30% of the patients, usually transiently. Hematuria (most often microscopic) is a relatively common finding in patients with the NS.

PATHOGENESIS OF EDEMA FORMATION

The pathogenesis of edema formation in the NS is not entirely understood. Based on our observations in children with the NS, we reformulated the sequence of events leading to renal water and sodium retention in the NS.[2] According to the level of development of the NS, different stages were identified: incipient NS, edema forming stage, stable nephrotic syndrome, and incipient remission, all of which were associated with differences in renal sodium handling.

In children with the NS, renal sodium retention starts at the onset of the disorder when the plasma albumin concentration is only slightly decreased. An abnormality in renal solution handling is considered to be the cause of sodium retention (primary sodium retention). As the NS becomes more severe, continued urinary protein losses will result in a decrease in plasma oncotic pressure. As a result, the normal oncotic pressure balance between plasma water and interstitial fluid is disturbed, and there is increased passage of fluid out of the capillaries into the interstitium. This passage of fluid is limited by redistribution of interstital albumin to the blood thereby reducing the change in transcapillary oncotic gradients. Fluid movement out of the vessels effectively decreases plasma volume. This reduction of plasma volume activates the sympathetic nervous system and the renin angiotensin axis, promotes ADH secretion, and suppresses atrial natriuretic peptide (ANP). Interaction of these systems stimulates renal sodium and water retention, and increases plasma volume. In many patients, primary sodium retention and redistribution of albumin will be sufficient to maintain blood volume.[3] However, some patients, especially children with minimal change NS in early relapse, will experience temporary hypovolemia.

If the progression to the nephrotic stage is very fast, with a steep reduction of plasma albumin, compensatory mechanisms are often insufficient to maintain the normal transcapillary oncotic pressure gradient, resulting in massive edema formation and hypovolemia. At this stage, blood volume can only be maintained by secondary stimulation of vasoactive hormones maximizing renal sodium retention. As a consequence of renal sodium retention associated with mechanisms aimed at limitation of edema formation, the majority of patients eventually achieve a new equilibrium characterized by edema, low plasma albumin levels, and stable blood volume (stable nephrotic syndrome). A persistently unstable circulation is found only if the plasma oncotic pressure decreases below a critical level ($\pm$ 8 mmHg). This is found in patients with persistent massive proteinuria such as those with congenital nephrotic syndrome.[2] Evaluation of a patient's overall volume status has important implications for the treatment of the NS. Patients who are hypovolemic may require iv albumin administration to maintain blood volume, while in patients with appropriate maintenance of blood volume, such treatment may result in hypervolemia that may in turn result in severe hypertension.

Hypovolemia can be detected by the assessment of aldosterone bioactivity and measured by the index $U_{K^+}/U_{K^+} + U_{Na^+}$. In the presence of sodium retention [fractional excretion of sodium less than 0.5%], an index in excess of 0.60 indicates hyperaldosteronism and hence hypovolemia.[4] In the majority of nephrotic patients, a decreased GFR and increased or normal renal plasma flow (RPF) is found. These changes may be determined by modifications in blood volume, and oncotic pressure but mainly by a decrease in glomerular membrane permeability.

DEFINITIONS

Nephrotic syndrome:
urine protein excretion $>$ 40 mg/m^2/hr BSA or UP/C $>$ 2.0 mg/mg and plasma albumin $<$ 2.5 g/dl.

Remission:
urinary remission: urinary protein excretion less than 4 mg/m^2/hr BSA, or UP/C less than 0.2 mg/mg, or negative/trace on a reagent strip (albustix) for three consecutive days.
Complete remission: urinary remission associated with normalization of serum albumin.

Relapse:
urinary protein excretion $>$ 4 mg/m^2/hr BSA, UP/C, ratio $>$ 0.2 on three consecutive days, or urine dipstick $\geq$ 2 + proteinuria.

Frequent relapses:
two or more relapses within six months of initial treatment or four or more relapses within any 12 month period.

Steroid dependent NS (SDNS):
patients in whom two consecutive relapses occurred after prednisone doses given for an earlier relapse has been reduced to an alternate day schedule, or within 14 days after the end of a course of steroid therapy (fast relapses), or in whom two of four relapses in a period of six months are fast relapses.

Steroid resistant NS (SRNS):
• Failure to achieve response in spite of 4–6 weeks of 60 mg/m^2/day prednisone therapy (maximum 80 mg/day).

- Primary SRNS: resistance during the first course of corticosteroid treatment.
- Secondary SRNS: resistance to steroids following initial response to a previous course of steroids.
- Late responder: remission following more than 8–12 weeks of corticosteroid therapy (time depending on initial treatment chosen).
- Pulse responder: failure to remit following initial treatment, but with response following intravenous pulses of methyl prednisolone therapy.
- Incomplete responder: increase of serum albumin concentration, resolution of edema, decreased but still significant proteinuria (UP/C decreased by more than 25%).

CLASSIFICATION OF IDIOPATHIC NEPHROTIC SYNDROME

NS is often subdivided into idiopathic, congenital and/or familial and secondary forms (Tables 7.1 and 7.2). The most common form, idiopathic nephrotic syndrome, includes a heterogenous group of diseases with genetic and immunologic factors playing a role in the pathogenesis. Because the causal agent is most often unknown, and there is a need for a rationalized diagnostic approach, many classifications have been developed, all with their own benefits and shortcomings. The factors on which these classifications are based are clinical symptoms, steroid response, histology, genetic factors, and recurrence following transplantation.

The most commonly used classification of NS is based on steroid responsiveness (see definitions in previous section). Approximately 70% of all children with INS respond to a short course of daily corticosteroids. The majority of children with a good response to steroids have minimal change disease (MCD). Much less consistent responses are found in patients with other renal biopsy findings, such as diffuse mesangial proliferation (DMP) and focal segmental glomerulosclerosis (FSGS). Unfortunately, the relapse rate in patients who are steroid responsive is high. 60% of the patients have a relapse within one year of onset of the disease, and 80% relapse by two years. 40% of the patients with

relapses will become frequent relapsers or steroid dependent (see definitions above). Children who relapse only once during the first six months after the initial course of the NS have a 10% risk of becoming frequent relapsers. Predictive factors for SDNS are prevalence of relapses associated with upper respiratory tract infections, and duration of initial treatment needed to induce remission following therapy; all patients still proteinuric following 21 days of treatment become steroid dependent.[5]

Early relapses following initial NS and short remission period before relapse are risk factors for subsequent relapses. The initial steroid response also helps to determine the response to alternative immunosuppressive therapy in the event that this needs to be employed. Steroid responders have a better response to other drugs. If the patient is a primary steroid responder, he/she will likely have a good prognosis for renal function, while many of the primary non-responders will progress to end stage renal disease (ESRD).[6]

Histologic examination shows three different morphologic patterns on light microscopy. The most common form of MCD is characterized by the presence of relatively normal glomeruli on light microcopy. Immunofluorescence shows no accumulation of immunoglobins or complement. Electron microscopy shows loss of foot processes, flattening of epithelial cell surface and microvilli transformation. Pathology of FSGS shows segmental glomerular scars involving some but not all glomeruli. The involved glomerular capillaries are obliterated by a collagenized scar and collapsed, wrinkled basal membranes. Sometimes a fibrous scar involving both a glomerular segment and Bowman's capsule is found. Electron microscopy shows foot process effacement of both involved and uninvolved glomeruli.

Mesangial cell proliferation (hypercellularity): focal (involving less than 50% of glomeruli), or diffuse mesangial cell proliferation, and increase in the synthesis of mesangial matrix. There are either no immune deposits or focal or diffuse IgM-containing deposits in the mesangial areas.

At first biopsy, 95% of patients with INS show MCD, 3% have FSGS, and 2% DMP. Repeat renal

Table 7.1 Diseases associated with idiopathic and genetic forms of NS

A. IDIOPATHIC NS

Clinical syndrome	Pathologic lesion(s)
MCD variants	Minimal change disease (MCD)
	Diffuse mesangial proliferation (DMP)
	IgM/C1q – nephropathies
	Focal segmental glomerulosclerosis (FGS)

B. CONGENITAL OR INFANTILE NS

Clinical syndrome	Pathologic lesion(s)
Congenital or infantile NS without other abnormalities	Diffuse mesangial sclerosis
Denys–Drash syndrome = male pseudohermaphroditism; Wilms tumor	Diffuse mesangial sclerosis
Frazier syndrome = XY gonadal dysgenesis, gonadal tumors	Focal glomerulosclerosis
Finnish type congenital NS = nephrosis starts in utero; mutations nephrin gene	Dilated proximal tubules, foot process effacement
Nephrotic syndrome associated with eye abnormalities = congenital glaucoma, strabismus, nystagmus, cataract, meiosis, buphthalmus	Diffuse mesangial sclerosis
Nephrotic syndrome associated with hypothyroidism and/or hypoadrenocorticism	Diffuse mesangial sclerosis
Nail patella syndrome = dysplastic nails; hypoplastic patellae; variable evolution of renal disease	Disease of basement membrane and podocytes
Charcot-Marie Tooth disease = familial peripheral neuropathy	Focal glomerulosclerosis
Schimke's syndrome: autosomal recessive spondyloepiphysical dysplasia, immunodeficiency	Focul glomerulosclerosis

C. FAMILIAL NS

Clinical syndrome	Pathologic lesion(s)
Steroid resistant NS = autosomal recessive; mutations podocin (see genetics), rapid ESRD	Focal glomerulosclerosis
Steroid sensitive NS = autosomal recessive	MCD and focal glomerulosclerosis
Adult-onset steroid resistant NS = autosomal dominant, mutation α-actin 4, variable disease progression	Focal glomerulosclerosis

biopsies have shown transition between the different histologic patterns. 90% of patients with MCD will respond to steroids, while fewer than 47% of patients with FSGS will respond to (combined forms) of treatment. If proteinuria persists, patients usually progress to ESRD.[7]

Some clinical features and biochemical parameters provide a warning that renal disease with histology other than MCD may be present. These are macroscopic hematuria, persistently reduced GFR, reduced complement levels, persistent hypertension, age below one or more than 12 years at diag-

---

Table 7.2 Diseases associated with the nephrotic syndrome (secondary NS)

Renal diseases associated with the nephrotic syndrome

- Acute proliferative glomerulonephritis
- IgA nephropathy
- Henoch-Schönlein purpura nephritis
- Membranoproliferative glomerulopathy
- Membranous glomerulonephropathy

Nephrotic syndrome associated with generalized diseases

- Congenital rubella
- Neonatal cytomegalovirus infection
- Congenital syphilis
- Congenital toxoplasmosis
- HIV associated NS
- Mercury intoxication
- Lithium intoxication
- Mediterranean fever associated with amyloidosis
- Systemic lupus erythematosus

---

nosis, and a familial nephrotic syndrome. Presence of two or more of these findings are arguments to consider a renal biopsy before starting treatment. However 34% of patients who fulfill the criteria for biopsy still have MCD at pathologic examination.[8] Associated clinical abnormalities often suggest that the NS may be part of a polymalformative syndrome, some of which are listed in Table 7.1.

It is known that genetic factors play a major role in some patients with steroid resistant nephrotic syndrome.[9,10] Several genes and proteins are involved: nephrin, podocin, and actinin. Mutations in the nephrin gene (NPHS1) mapped to chromosome 19q13.1 are present in the Finnish type congenital nephrotic syndrome.[11]

Mutations in the podocin gene (NPHS2) mapped to chromosome 1q25–32 are responsible for a sizable fraction of early onset, familial, and non-familial cases of steroid resistant nephrotic syndrome with FSGS and rapid progression to ESRD.[12] The Denys-Drash syndrome is associated with the WT1 gene located on chromosome 11p. In autosomal dominant, adult onset, steroid resistant NS associated with FSGS, two loci were identified: the alpha actinin 4 gene, located on chromosome

19q13 and a locus located on chromosome 11q. In familial NS associated with FSGS, genetic studies should be performed before onset of treatment, because of known resistance to any form of treatment.

In 44% of patients with FSGS the disease recurs in the transplanted kidney. Except for patients with genetic factors involved in whom no recurrence occurs, there are no symptoms to predict recurrence. In some of these patients a circulating factor affecting glomerular permeability has been identified.[13,14]

INITIAL TREATMENT OF INS

Treatment aims to induce remission, prevent relapses, and avoid side effects. The treatment should induce remission as soon as possible to avoid complications, maintain longstanding remission, and should be as non-toxic as possible to avoid side effects.

Corticosteroid treatment is the first choice of drug for most patients with INS. Several derivatives of glucocorticoids, with varying dosages and duration of therapy, have been proposed. They include a number of liquid preparations, some of which are well tolerated by small children. While disappearance of significant proteinuria almost always occurs within two weeks of continuous prednisone treatment, complete remission is obtained following 4–6 weeks of treatment. The Arbeitsgemeinschaft für Pädiatrische Nephrologie has shown when initial treatment is continued only until achievement of complete remission, it is associated with an 81% relapse rate, while prolonged treatment (12 weeks of treatment: six weeks of daily prednisone treatment followed by six weeks of alternate day treatment) results in only a 36% relapse rate within 12 months.[15] While the need for prolonged continuous steroid treatment has been questioned, most investigators recommend an initial corticosteroid treatment of 60 mg prednisone/m^2/day in three divided doses for four to six weeks (maximum dose 80 mg/day), followed by alternate day treatment with 40 mg/m^2 for another four to six weeks.

If there is no response after the initial six weeks of daily prednisone therapy, some centers recommend that patients should be given three pulses of 1 g methylprednisolone/1.73 m^2 (max 1 g) on alternate days. If there is still no response, the patient is considered to be steroid resistant and treatment with alternative therapy should be considered, as discussed below.

TREATMENT OF RELAPSE

While the relapses of NS are usually as steroid responsive as the initial attack of the NS, the duration/intensity of prednisone treatment for the relapse has no further influence on the subsequent risk of relapses. Therefore standard relapse treatment consisting of 60 mg/m^2 prednisone in one to three divided doses until the urine is protein free for three days, followed by four weeks of alternate day prednisone (40 mg/m^2 as a single dose) is recommended. In infrequent relapsers this standard treatment should be repeated for each relapse.

TREATMENT OF STEROID DEPENDENT OR FREQUENTLY RELAPSING NS

Children with frequent relapses usually remain steroid responsive. In some of these patients, frequent relapses of NS may be treated with low doses of alternate day prednisone therapy. The lowest dose that is enough to prevent relapses should be given. This treatment should be reconsidered if the required dose to prevent relapses is in excess of 0.5 mg/kg on alternate days, duration of treatment exceeds 18 months, or the patients show side effects of steroid treatment such as growth failure, osteoporosis, cataract, and psychologic disturbances.

ALTERNATIVE FORMS OF THERAPY FOR INS

In many studies the use of alkylating agents such as cyclophosphamide and chlorambucil to treat patients with SDNS and FRNS has been favored.[16] Cyclophosphamide is the drug of choice because of the lesser life-threatening side effects that occur with this treatment compared with chlorambucil. Treatment with cytotoxic agents often results in sustained remission with a remission rate of 72% at two years and 36% at five years in FRNS, but with lesser results in SDNS with sustained remission in 40% at two years and of 24% at five years.[17] A daily dose of 2–2.5 mg/kg given for 8–12 weeks is recommended. This may be given on two occasions if a patient responds well to the first course, but then reverts back to SDNS or FRNS.

The most common side effect with the cytotoxic drugs is leucopenia (32%). However, combining cyclophosphamide with low dose alternate day therapy prednisone seems to reduce significantly this complication (15%). A reduction of the daily dose is required if the leukocyte count falls below 4000/mm^3 or if the absolute neutrophil count falls below 1500/mm^3 and treatment should be temporarily interrupted if leukocytes are lower than 2500/mm^3. Alternate day steroid therapy should be continued until the end of cyclophosphamide treatment. Any severe infection, bacterial or viral, should lead to discontinuation of treatment.

Other important side effects are gonadal toxicity, liver toxicity, loss of hair, and hemorrhagic cystitis.[17] Gonadal toxicity is more common in males and is dependent on cumulative dose and duration of treatment. A cumulative dose up to 170–250 mg/kg is considered to be safe, but occasionally azoospermia has been reported at lower doses. Hemorrhagic cystitis most often can be avoided if treatment is delayed until remission has occurred and a stable fluid balance is achieved. A major concern is the development of malignancies following treatment with cytotoxic therapy. Because of the lack of longterm follow-up in nephrotic patients treated with cyclophosphamide, the true incidence of malignancies is not yet known. As stated above, second courses of cytotoxic therapy may be given to patients who relapsed after the first treatment, to increase the rate of long-lasting remissions. However, the risk of long-term morbidity, such as gonadal toxicity and malignancies, is an argument to avoid repeated treatment courses.

Patients who relapse again on a frequent basis after cytotoxic treatment, may be treated by cyclosporine A or mycophenolate mofetil. Cyclosporine has been shown to maintain remission in patients with frequent relapsing, or steroid dependent nephrotic syndrome, and allowing withdrawal of steroids.[18] 80% of steroid sensitive patients will respond to this treatment, but almost all patients will relapse following discontinuation of treatment. Therefore, cyclosporine must be administered for prolonged periods of time. When a patient relapses following withdrawal of cyclosporine, subsequent treatment courses with the same drug will be less effective, and may require additional steroid treatment to maintain remission. The recommended daily dosage is 5–6 mg/kg divided in two oral doses. The oral dose should be adjusted to maintain whole blood trough levels between 80 and 150 mg/ml. The major long-term side effect of cyclosporine treatment is nephrotoxicity. Unfortunately, neither monitoring of cyclosporine blood levels nor serum-creatinine concentrations is sensitive enough to indicate the presence of renal damage. Therefore, during long-standing treatment, repeated renal biopsies are often required to evaluate if continuation of treatment is acceptable. Other common side effects are gum hypertrophy, hirsutism, and hypertension. Currently we only advise cyclosporine after failure of treatment with alkylating agents.

More recently, mycophenolate mofetil (MMF) has been used to treat steroid-dependent and frequent relapsing nephrotic syndrome.[19] Most studies include only small numbers of patients, but have shown that MMF is effective in preventing relapses in these patients. The appropriate dose required to prevent relapses is not well known, and therefore, a similar dose as given to renal transplant patients is administered: 1200 mg/m²/24 hrs in two doses. Side effects include bone marrow suppression and gastrointestinal disturbances. Awaiting the results of larger studies we recommend MMF only in patients relapsing following treatment with alkalizing drugs and if prepubertal.

Note: It is important to stress that use of the various agents described above should only be conducted in consultation with a pediatric nephrologist. This caveat is even more important when considering the treatment of children with SRNS, as we will now describe.

TREATMENT OF STEROID RESISTANT NEPHROTIC SYNDROME

1) Methyl prednisolone iv pulse therapy

If no remission is obtained after 4–6 weeks of daily oral prednisone therapy (60 mg/m²/day), a series of iv methyl prednisolone pulses may be considered. Most commonly, three doses of 1 g MP/1.73m² are given on alternate days. Mendoza et al. have extended the protocol by giving 30 mg/kg iv (maximum dose 1 gram), three days a week for two weeks, followed by one dose/week for eight weeks, then monthly for nine months and finally once every two months for another six months. MP was given with low dose alternate day oral prednisone and/or alkyl-ating agents.[21] The authors reported remission rates of more than 60% in steroid resistant children with FSGS. The same degree of success has not been experienced by others.[21]

2) Alternative treatment options are the same as in steroid responsive NS patients. However, the response to these treatments has been disappointing. Cytotoxic therapy induced complete remission in only 17% of the patients, while a 21% success rate was observed in patients receiving CsA.[6] Prolonged continuation of CsA treatment is required to maintain remission. CsA should be given with steroids and doses should aim at high trough blood levels.[22] The therapy should start early after establishing steroid resistance. If a response to CsA is not observed by six months, it is unlikely to occur subsequently.

MMF has been used in adults with steroid resistant FSGS, and was associated with improvement in proteinuria and stabilization of renal function.[23] Confirmation of these results is required before a firm evaluation can be made.

3) Plasmapheresis

In those patients in whom a circulating plasma factor increasing the permeability of the glomeruli to albumin is found, plasmapheresis may be considered. While plasmapheresis has been successful in patients with recurrence of FSGS following transplantation, its role as rescue treatment for steroid resistant nephrotic syndrome in native kidneys has yet to be shown.[24]

SYMPTOMATIC TREATMENT OF THE NEPHROTIC SYNDROME

In most children with INS, the management of the symptoms that characterize this condition need only be employed on a temporary basis, because most children will go into remission in response to treatment with prednisone after a few weeks. However, there is a small subset of patients who do not respond to specific therapy. The following approaches are particularly useful for such patients. In patients who have incomplete remission following specific therapy, an attempt should be undertaken to reduce proteinuria because proteinuria by itself is an important risk factor for the development of renal failure. Angiostensin converting enzyme (ACE) inhibitors will not only decrease systemic blood pressure but especially intraglomerular pressure by their effect on efferent arteriolar resistance. In children, enalapril has been used to decrease proteinuric. The antiproteinuric effect of ACE-inhibitors is dose dependent, and is also effected by sodium intake. A high sodium intake nullifies the antiproteinuric effect of ACE-inhibitors. Enalapril should be started at a low dose (0.2 mg/kg in two doses) and increased as tolerated. ACE-inhibitors are considered renoprotective by decreasing glomerular fibrosis and hence prevent glomerulosclerosis. While ACE-inhibitors are well tolerated in nephrotic children, the possibility of a decline in GFR requires regular assessment of kidney function.[25]

When edema formation is severe, symptomatic treatment is often required. In patients with normovolemia a low sodium intake and the use of diuretics is recommended. Furosemide is the drug of choice; this may be administered in intermittent doses or by a continuous intravenous infusion, and the recommended dose is 2 mg/kg. For chronic edema, spironolactone (5 mg/kg/day) or amiloride (0.5 mg/kg/day) have been recommended.

In patients with hypovolemia, intravenous albumin administration is required. In these patients, a salt-free albumin infusion (0.5 to 1.0 g/kg of a 20–25% solution over four hours) can safely be administered. While intravenous albumin has little effect in inducing diuresis in patients with the nephrotic syndrome, simultaneous intravenous furosemide administration may induce diuresis. This combination should be used with care in patients with normovolemia to avoid circulatory overload and hypertension.

COMPLICATIONS OF THE NEPHROTIC SYNDROME

Abnormalities in lipid metabolism

Hyperlipidemia occurs in the majority of children with the nephrotic syndrome, hence its name 'lipoid nephrosis' and is characterized by increased levels of cholesterol, both free and cholesterol esters. Increased levels of fasting triglyceride concentrations are also found. The profile of lipoproteins, mixtures of apolipoprotein, and lipids is characterized by increased VLDL, IDL, and of LDL, while HDL concentrations are usually normal. Lipoprotein (a) concentrations are also increased. The abnormalities disappear with remission of the NS.

Hyperlipidemia is the result both of increased synthesis and decreased catabolism. Major abnormalities are related to impaired conversion of VLDL, increased hepatic LDL secretion, increased Lp(a) production by the liver, and impaired HDL maturation. Longstanding nephrotic hyperlipidemia may induce vascular damage, and aortic atheroma has been reported in nephrotic children. Elevated plasma triglyceride levels may be associated with a faster deterioration of renal function in patients with glomerular disease. Influx of lipoproteins into the mesangium through a damaged endothelial barrier will lead to proliferation and sclerosis.

Bacterial infections

Although no longer a major problem in nephrotic children, primary peritonitis still remains a threat.

The predominance of pneumococcal infections is striking. The clinical infection rate is higher in children treated with cytotoxic drugs than in those treated with prednisone alone, being highest in those treated with chlorambucil (6.5%) compared with cyclophosphamide (1.5%). The onset may be insidious, but should be suspected in a nephrotic child who develops abdominal pain. A gram stain performed on ascitic fluid removed by a needle may be required to confirm the diagnosis. Treatment of a bacterial infection should begin quickly. Parenteral antibiotics should always be used. A broad-spectrum antibiotic should be used as initial treatment.

Viral infections

Relapses of MCNS often follow viral upper respiratory infections, but a major threat is either varicella or measles, especially to children receiving steroids or cytotoxic agents. Active varicella zoster infection should be treated with iv acyclovir. Cytoxic therapy should be discontinued and additional steroid be given in patients with severe infections.

Thromboembolic complications

Evident thrombosis in the arterial or venous circulation occurs in 3% of nephrotic children. Common sites include the femoral artery and deep veins of the leg. However, subclinical thrombotic complications, especially pulmonary emboli, have been reported in 28% of the children. No simple etiology can be given. The complex balance of coagulant, fibrinolytic, and regulatory proteins is disturbed in nephrotics. Also alterations in platelet and endothelial cell function seem to be involved. Administered drugs (steroids and diuretics) may play a role. Evident thrombosis should be treated with anticoagulation. The benefit of prophylactic anticoagulation with warfarin remains unclear, but has been recommended in unstable steroid resistant nephrotic syndrome.

Loss of vitamins and hormones in the urine

The losses of vitamin D binding proteins in the urine seldom result in clinical problems, and vitamin D and/or calcium supplementation is not necessary. Despite losses of thyroid binding globulin in the urine, plasma concentration of T3, T4 and TSH are usually normal in MCNS. However, hypothyroidism is a regular feature of the Finnish type congenital nephrotic syndrome.

Acute renal failure

Acute renal failure is very rare (0.8%) and usually follows sepsis, especially peritonitis.[27] While acute tubular necrosis has been found in nephrotic children with ARF, important changes in the permeability of the glomerular membrane may have an important role. Recovery has been usual but urgent hemofiltration may be required to remove fluid overload.

SUMMARY

It is apparent that the evaluation and management of a child with NS requires close attention from multiple caregivers. It is especially important that primary care physicians and pediatric nephrologists work together in developing treatment plans for children with NS and for managing any complications as they occur.

REFERENCES

1. Elises JS, Griffiths PD, Hocking MD, Taylor CM, White RHR. Simplified quantification of urinary protein excretion in children. Clinical Nephrol 1988; 20:255–229.
2. Vande Walle JGJ, Donckerwolcke RA. Pathogenesis of edema formation in the nephrotic syndrome. Pediatr Nephrol 2001; 16:283–293.
3. Humphreys MH. Mechanisms and management of nephrotic edema. Kidney Int 1994; 45:266–281.
4. Koomans HA, Kortlandt W, Geers AB, Dorhout-Mees EJ. Lowered protein content of tissue fluid in patients with the nephrotic syndrome. Nephron 1985; 40:391–395.
5. Yap HK, Han EJS, Heng CK, Gong WK. Risk factors for steroid dependency in children with the idiopathic nephrotic syndrome. Pediatr Nephrol 2001; 16:1049–1052.
6. Niaudet P. Treatment of childhood steroid-resistant idiopathic nephrosis with a combination of cyclosporine and prednisone. French Society of Pediatric Nephrology. J Pediatr 1994; 125:981–986.
7. Korbet S. Treatment of primary focal segmental glomerulosclerosis. Kidney Int 2002; 62:2301–2310.
8. Gulati S, Sharma AP, Sharma RK, Gupta A, Gupta RK. Do current recommendations for kidney biopsy in nephrotic syndrome need modifications. Pediatr Nephrol 2002; 17:404–408.
9. Pollak MR. Inherited podocytopathies: FSGS and nephrotic syndrome from a genetic viewpoint. J Am Soc Nephrol 2002; 13:3016–3023.

10. Antignac C. Genetic models: clues for understanding the pathogenesis of idiopathic nephrotic syndrome. J Clin Invest 2002; 109:447–449.

11. Ruotsalainen, Ljunberg P, Wartiovaara J, Lenkkeri U, Jalanko H, Holmberg C, Tryggvasson K. Nephrin is specially located at the slit diaphragm of glomerular podocytes. Cell Biology 1996; 14:7962–7967.

12. Karle SM, Uetz B, Ronner V, Glaeser L, Hildebrandt F, Fuchshuber A. Novel mutations in NPHS2 detected in both familial and sporadic steroid resistant nephrotic syndrome. J Am Soc Nephrol 2002; 13:388–393.

13. Savin VJ, Sharma R, Sharma M. Circulating factor associated with increased glomerular permeability to albumin in recurrent focal segmental glomerulosclerosis. N Eng J Med 1996; 334:878–883.

14. Hoyer J, Vernier R, Najarian S, Simmons R, Michael A. Recurrence of idiopathic nephrotic syndrome after transplantation. J Am Soc Nephrol 2002; 22:69–72.

15. Ehrich JHH, Brodehl J. Arbeitsgemeinschaft für Pädiatrische Nephrologie. Long versus standard prednisone therapy for initial treatment of idiopathic nephrotic syndrome in children. Eur J Pediatr 1993; 152:357–361.

16. Durkan AM, Hodson EM, Willis NS, Craig JC. Immunosuppressive agents in childhood nephrotic syndrome: A meta-analysis of randomised controlled trials. Kidney Int 2001; 59:1919–1927.

17. Latta K, von Schnakenburg C, Ehrich JHH. A meta-analysis of cytotoxic treatment for frequently relapsing nephrotic syndrome in children. Pediatr Nephrol 2001; 16:271–282.

18. Niaudet P and the French Society of Pediatric Nephrology. Comparison of cyclosporine and chlorambucil in the treatment of steroid dependent idiopathic nephrotic syndrome: A multicenter randomised controlled trial. Pediatr Nephrol 1992; 6:1–3.

19. Choi MJ, Eustace JA, Gimenez LF, Atta MG, Schul PJ, Sothinathar R, Briggs WA. Mycophenolate mofetil treatment of primary glomerular disease. Kidney Int 2002; 61:1098–1114.

20. Tune BM, Lieberman E, Mendoza SA. Steroid resistant nephrotic focal segmental glomerulosclerosis: A treatable disease. Pediatr Nephrol 1996; 10:772–778.

21. Yorgin PD, Krasher J, Al Uzri AY. Pulse methylprednisolone treatment of idiopathic steroid resistant nephrotic syndrome. Pediatr Nephrol 2001; 16:245–250.

22. Niaudet P, Fuchsuber A, Gagnadoux MF, Habib R, Broyer M. Cyclosporine in the therapy of steroid resistant idiopathic nephrotic syndrome. Kidney Int Suppl 1997; 58:S85–90.

23. Day JD, Cockwell P, Lipkin G, Savage C, Howie A, Adu D. Mycophenolate mofetil in the treatment of resistant idiopathic nephrotic syndrome. Nephrol Dial Transplant 2002; 17:2011–2013.

24. Feld SM, Figueroa P, Savin V, Nast CC, Sharma R, Sharma H, Hirschberg R, Adler SG. Plasmapheresis in the treatment of steroid resistant focal glomerulosclerosis in native kidneys. Am J Kidney Dis 1998; 32:230–237.

25. Milliner DS, Morgenstern BZ. Angiotensin converting enzyme inhibitors for reduction of proteinuria in children with steroid-resistant nephrotic syndrome. Pediatr Nephrol 1991; 5:587–590.

26. Abrass CK. Clinical spectrum and complications of the nephrotic syndrome. J Invest Med 1997; 45:143–153.

27. Cavagnaro F, Lagomarisino E. Peritonitis as a risk factor of acute renal failure in nephrotic children. Pediatr Nephrol 2000; 15:248–251.

8. Acute nephritis

Rosanna Coppo and Alessandro Amore

DEFINITION

Acute nephritis may be defined as inflammation of the nephrons of the kidney, which develops over a short period of time, i.e. a few days. The primary site of this inflammation is generally the glomerulus, in which case the condition is referred to as acute glomerulonephritis (AGN). However, acute tubulo-interstitial nephritis (ATIN) may also occur, although this is much less common in children. Hence, when a patient is described as having 'acute nephritis', it may be assumed that the disorder is AGN unless specified otherwise.

The most common clinical manifestations of AGN are: reduced urine volume (oliguria); hematuria (with the urine usually being very dark – often referred to as 'coke colored'); edema, and hypertension. However, incomplete presentations are common, and the distinction between an acute inflammatory process that is destined to resolve, and an acute onset or exacerbation of a chronic nephritis that will persist, is often ill defined. The most frequent cause of AGN is acute post-infectious glomerulonephritis (APIGN),[1] which usually follows streptococcal infection (post-streptococcal glomerulonephritis), but a similar initial clinical picture may occur with some forms of chronic glomerulonephritis (CGN), such as primary IgA nephropathy,[2] or those related to systemic diseases such as Henoch-Schönlein purpura nephritis, or Alport syndromes (Table 8.1).

PATHOLOGY AND PATHOPHYSIOLOGY OF AGN

Although renal biopsies are rarely indicated in children with the clinical picture of AGN, it is occa-

Table 8.1 Most common types/causes of acute glomerulonephritis in childhood

Primary GN	Secondary GN
Acute post-infectious GN	Henoch-Schönlein purpura GN
IgA nephropathy	Lupus GN
Membranoproliferative GN	Systemic vasculitides
	GN associated to
	• Polyarteritis nodosa
	• Wegener's granulomatosis
	• Churg-Strauss syndrome
Pauci-immune crescentic GN	Anti-glomerular basement
	membrane GN
	(Goodpasture syndrome)
	Alport syndrome GN

sionally necessary to define the renal lesion in order to distinguish AGN from CGN. The dominant histologic feature in APIGN is diffuse proliferation of endothelial, mesangial, and often epithelial cells associated with lympho-mononuclear cell infiltration. In the most severe cases, there may be intracapillary thrombi, segmental tuft necrosis, and crescent formation. The precise histologic diagnosis requires immunofluorescence (IF) analysis of the renal tissue, showing the predominant pattern of capillary and mesangial staining of C3 (complement), corresponding to humps detected on electron microscopy (EM).[3] Characteristic IF patterns also provide for the definite identification of many forms of chronic GN that may present with an acute onset (Table 8.2).

The dominant clinical features in children with APIGN result from decrease in the glomerular filtration rate (GFR). The GFR is reduced due to swelling of the glomerulus and thickening of the filtration barrier. These events are triggered by deposition of immune complexes within the glomerular

Table 8.2 Immunoglobulins and complement fractions detected by immunofluorescence in renal biopsy tissue

Primary and secondary (GN) glomerulonephritis	IgG	IgA	IgM	C3	C4	C1q	Fibrinogen
Acute post-infectious GN	Subepithelial +++ (humps)	−	−	Subepithelial +++ (humps)	−	−	−
IgA nephropathy	Mesangial ++	Predominant Mesangial +++	±	Mesangial +++	−	−	±
Membranoproliferative GN	Sub-endothelial +++	++	±	Subendothelial +++	±	±	
Paucimmune crescentic GN	−	−	−	−	−	−	Crescentic/ necrotic areas ++
Henoch-Schönlein purpura GN	Mesangial ++	Mesangial +++	±	Mesangial +++	±	±	Necrotic areas ++
Lupus GN	Sub-endothelial, subepithelial, mesangial +++	Sub-endothelial, subepithelial, mesangial ++	++	++	++++	++++	
Anti-glomerular basement membrane (GBM) GN	Linear along GBM +++	−	−	Linear along GBM ++	−	−	Crescents ++
Microscopic polyarteritis GN	−	−	−	−	−	−	Necrotic areas ++
Alport syndrome	−	−	−	−	−	−	−

structures (subendothelial space, epithelial filtration barrier, mesangial area) in APIGN. This may result in a sudden decrease in GFR that is associated with sodium retention, edema, and hypertension. In addition, most patients usually have moderate degrees of proteinuria and hematuria. The hematuria is most often gross, but may be microscopic in some patients. In cases of ATIN, the process starts with an immune reaction in the tubules and interstitium due to the sudden influx of lymphocytes and monocytes which may be sensitized to a specific drug.

EPIDEMIOLOGY AND TRIGGERING FACTORS

The epidemiology of APIGN varies around the world according to the social conditions in different areas. In well-developed countries, the disease is usually sporadic, although it is likely that genetic factors may play a role in determining the susceptibility to the condition. The incidence of APIGN in the Western World is about 1/500 children, mostly aged 2–12 years, with a 2/1 male predominance. Whereas the incidence of APIGN in the USA and Europe is reported to have decreased significantly over the last 50 years, it appears to be higher in undeveloped countries.[7,8] However, it is difficult to be precise on this matter since it is known that incomplete or sub-clinical forms may occur, especially during epidemics of the condition.

APIGN can follow bacterial, viral, or parasitic infections (Table 8.3) although it is clear that streptococcal infections have the highest frequency of association with this condition. So-called "nephritogenic" strains include M-types 12, 1, 24, which are often responsible for a rather non-specific form of acute upper-respiratory tract acute infection. If the streptococcus produces erythrogenic toxin, the child develops scarlet fever. Streptococcal M-types 47, 49, 57, 55 have been isolated in impetiginous skin lesions, that are usually vesicular and often pustular. However, it is not simply a matter of a child being infected by a nephritogenic strain; the process needs particular host immune response characteristics to trigger the development of APIGN.[5]

The role of infections or other etiologic events appears to be less important in other forms of GN that may present with an acute nephritis. Therefore, it is tempting to speculate that although environmental factors may trigger the nephritogenic process, subsequent development and progression of renal damage are regulated by unknown factors, among which genetics might be of relevance. However, it is worth noting that persistence of a focus of infection (e.g. an unresolved skin infection or a peritonsillar abscess) may represent the source for the development of CGN in some patients.[1,3–6]

Table 8.3 Infections that may precipitate acute post-infectious glomerulonephritis

- Bacterial
  - β-hemolytic streptococcus
  - *Streptococcus viridans*
  - *Staphylococcus aureus*
  - *Diplococcus pneumonia*
  - Klebsiella pneumonia
  - Leptospira
  - *Salmonella typhosa*
- Viral
  - Hepatitis B
  - Cytomegalovirus
  - Varicella
  - Epstein-Barr
  - Coxsackie
  - Rubella
  - Mumps
- Fungal
  - *Coccidiodes immitis*
- Parasitic
  - Plasmodium malaria and falciparum
  - *Toxoplasma gondii*
  - Filaria
  - *Schistosoma mansonii*

CLINICAL FEATURES AND DIFFERENTIAL DIAGNOSIS

The presentation of APIGN typically occurs 7–14 days after an acute infectious episode. At the time the AGN develops, the signs of the infection may still be present or may have completely healed. During the silent interval, the child is asymptomatic. It is of paramount importance to obtain a comprehensive past history including questions regarding the results of any prior urinalyses in case microscopic hematuria may have been present earlier. Dental granuloma or parodontopathies must be searched for, as well as other less common causes of acute or chronic infections.

Extrarenal systemic signs may be important for a correct diagnosis, particularly if a patient has purpura, arthritis, or abdominal pain. These are the characteristic features of Henoch-Schönlein purpura (HSP). Patients with HSP nephritis have palpable purpura, mostly often affecting ankles, buttocks, and lower limbs. It is also important to evaluate the possibility of a collagen disease: the detection of arthralgia/arthritis affecting medium-sized or small joints should raise the possibility of systemic lupus erythematosus (SLE) or primary systemic vasculitis. The presence of a time lag between the symptoms and signs of an acute infection and the development of AGN is important to distinguish between APIGN and the presentation or exacerbation of a chronic glomerular disease such as primary IgA nephropathy. In APIGN, the infectious episodes generally occur 7–14 days before the clinical onset of nephritis whereas acute presentations or exacerbations of CGN often develop within 12–24 hours of an acute infection, such as an upper respiratory infection.

In patients with APIGN, the urinary sediment usually shows many red blood cells, most of which are dysmorphic, varying numbers of white blood cells of inflammatory origin, and cellular casts. The urine volume is often reduced, and the subsequent salt and water retention leads to facial puffiness, generalized edema, volume-dependent hypertension, and dilutional anemia. The urine is very concentrated (SG usually > 1.025) and often contains mild to moderate amounts of protein (1–3 g/m²/day).[1,4–7]

In APIGN, a β-hemolytic streptococcal strain can often be identified by tonsillar cultures (Table 8.4). Antistreptolysin O (ASO) titers are generally elevated, with the highest levels occurring after 3–5 weeks; however they are unrelated to incidence, severity, and prognosis of renal damage. AntiDNAse B levels are increased in up to 100% of the cases. Serum immunoglobulins are increased, mostly IgG and IgM. This polyclonal immunoglobulin response may lead to detectable rheumatoid factor, or immune complexes, and cryoglobulins. Complement factor measurement in the blood is of great value, since C3 and C4 consumption leads to marked reductions in serum C3/C4 levels in 90% and 20% of the cases respectively. There is at first a depression of both factors, since the complement activation follows the classical pathway, but the process is then maintained mostly by the alternative pathway, hence the depression of serum C3 complement levels lasts longer, usually for up to six weeks after the onset of disease.[10]

Serum complement measurements may provide particularly useful information for distinguishing between APIGN and other acute nephritic presentations due to chronic disorders, such as membranoproliferative GN (which usually has persistently low levels of C3), or SLE nephritis (profoundly depressed C4 levels in addition to persistently low levels of C3). The diagnosis is further supported by specific tests such as anti-DNA antibodies (SLE) or ANCA (systemic or renal-limited vasculitides). Even though neither of these tests has a 100% specificity and sensitivity, the combination of the laboratory results and the recent past history usually leads to a specific clinico-laboratory diagnosis.[9,10]

In some cases, however, the patient may not present with completely clear clinical or laboratory features. For example, if the history of a prior infectious episode is not clear, the depression of the C3/C4 complement levels is only moderate, or the serology is not specific, the diagnosis may be uncertain. In such children, it may be appropriate to consider a renal biopsy, which makes the diagnosis certain. The need for a child with AGN to have a precise diagnosis is based on the possibility that it may define more appropriate therapy, especially in patients who have potentially progressive renal lesions.

In APIGN, laboratory parameters should be followed sequentially in order to identify an atypical course, which would define who may need a renal biopsy. Table 8.5 reports the expected evolution of clinical and laboratory data in APIGN. When the evolution of the syndrome does not fit with the usual course, a renal biopsy should be considered (Table 8.6).

NATURAL HISTORY

A precise diagnosis of the specific renal disease in a child with persistent features of AGN is of importance, since it permits the distinction between a self-limited form of glomerular inflammation and

---

Table 8.4 Laboratory abnormalities observed in patients with APIGN

- Positive tonsil culture for Group A (hemolytic streptococcus (40–70%)
- ASO titers elevated (70–80%), except in case of pyoderma
- AntiDNAse B levels elevated in 100% of children
- Reduced levels of serum C3 (90%) and C4 (20%) complement
- Elevated serum IgG and IgM (90%)
- Positive for rheumatoid factor (40%), circulating immune complexes (60–80%), ANCA (5%)
- Coagulation cascade activation in some patients, increased d-dimer and factor XIII levels

---

Table 8.5 Expected rate of normalization of laboratory and clinical features in patients with APIGN

- Serum C3 levels in 2–4 weeks (70% of the cases), in eight weeks (94%)
- Gross hematuria usually resolves in 2–3 days
- Microscopic hematuria in 6–12 months
- Proteinuria in 2–7 days
- Full acute nephritic syndrome in 2–7 days
- Hypertension in 14–30 days

Table 8.6 Indications for renal biopsy in children with acute nephritis

- Age < 2 years and > 12 years
- Positive family history of chronic nephritis
- Past history of urinary abnormalities in the patient
- No infections in the 1–4 weeks preceding the onset of acute nephritis
- Coincidence of upper respiratory tract infection and nephritis
- Systemic symptoms (fever, arthralgia, abdominal pain, pleuritis, pericarditis)
- Nephritic syndrome with acute renal failure lasting > 2 weeks
- Gross hematuria for > 3 weeks
- Hypertension for > 3 weeks
- Persistent C3 hypocomplementemia for > 6 weeks
- Persistent proteinuria and/or hematuria for > 6 weeks

diseases which may progress to end stage renal failure (ESRD).[11] APIGN has a favorable prognosis in the majority of patients. The early mortality is less than 0.5%. Hypertensive encephalopathy and left ventricular failure are the major complications occurring during the peak of the acute nephritic syndrome, if fluid overload is not recognized and treated promptly. Children who have severe diuretic-resistant fluid retention should be followed in intensive care units, to treat hypertensive crises and fluid overload. This may even require the institution of acute dialysis in a small number of patients. Another 1% of cases with APIGN present with a rapidly progressive course with extensive crescent formation, which can progress in rare instances to glomerular sclerosis and ESRD. There are controversial reports as far as the long-term evolution is concerned, but some reports indicate that in 1–5% of the cases, reduced renal function and/or urinary abnormalities can be detected after 10–20 years.[11,12]

The natural history of other forms of GN that may have an acute nephritic onset varies according to the specific diagnosis. For instance, HSP nephritis accounts for 5% of children with chronic renal failure in Europe, and progression after an acute nephritic onset can be observed in up to 25% of these children, even in patients who have complete normalization of their urine. In such patients, persistent proteinuria is the most predictable risk factor for progression. Similarly, children who present with features of AGN, but are subsequently diagnosed with primary IgA nephropathy, may have a progressive course.[2] The most sensitive risk factors in this disease are presence of glomerulosclerotic changes, high percentage of epithelial crescents, Afro-American race, hypertension, proteinuria, and male gender. These factors play a similar role in the progression of these forms of chronic GN that present with an acute onset, and then show signs of persistent activity. For instance, Alport syndrome often has a relentless progression to ESRD that occurs about five years after the development of significant proteinuria. However, the natural history of ANCA associated vasculitides, SLE nephritis, and Goodpasture syndrome is much more unpredictable.

MANAGEMENT OPTIONS

The initial treatment of patients with APIGN should involve measures to control fluid overload, edema, and hypertension. Loop diuretics such as furosemide may be used for this purpose, particularly when there is reduced urinary output together with hypertension. Doses of 1–4 mg/kg usually given intravenously may be useful in such patients. If hypertension is severe, calcium channel blockers, such as nifedipine or amlodipine, or angiotensin converting enzyme inhibitors (ACE-I), such as lisinopril, can be used.[12]

In patients with APIGN it may also be relevant to eliminate the antigen when the infection source is apparent, but frequently the infection has resolved when the child presents to the physician. Indeed, in experimental models of acute serum sickness, induced by injecting exogenous bovine serum albumin into rabbits, the animal develops acute nephritis with gross hematuria and histologic features mimicking APIGN about 10 days after the antigen injection, at the time when antigen clearance has reached maximal effectiveness due to immune complex removal by phagocytic cells. Similarly, when patients present with features of APIGN, the infection which stimulated the immune complex disease is likely to be over. For these reasons there is no strict need for antibiotic treatment. On the contrary, antibiotics are indicated in cases of persistent infection (such as pyoderma[4,10,12]).

Since APIGN is generally a benign disease, there is usually no need to use immunosuppressive drugs or other potent medications that have potential side effects. However, it should be noted that a small percentage of patients with APIGN may present with rapidly declining renal function that is due to extensive crescent formation in their glomeruli, which may lead to glomerular obliteration and obsolescence. In these cases, identified by renal biopsy, the treatment may be more aggressive, using methylprednisolone pulses (e.g. 10–30 mg/kg/day per 3–5 days) followed by prednisone 1 mg/kg/day, and/or immunosuppressive drugs such as cyclophosphamide (2 mg/kg/day)[12] sometimes in association with plasma exchange.

Some children with AGN and impaired renal function that is associated with HSP nephritis and extensive crescents in the glomeruli, may also need an aggressive therapeutic regimen (e.g. methylprednisolone 20–30 mg/kg/iv pulses for three days followed by six months of prednisone, dipyridamole, and cyclophosphamide for 2–3 months). This has been associated with a favorable outcome in 60% of severe cases with up to 90% glomeruli with crescents. Plasma exchange, in association with corticosteroids and cytotoxic drugs, can be used in the most severe cases; however, the expected effects are time-limited with subsequent renal relapses leading to ESRD, even though with some years of delay. Similarly, in children with HSP nephritis presenting with crescentic nephritis in 50–75% of glomeruli, prednisone for four months in association with cyclophosphamide and heparin or warfarin can be effective.[12] The management of these patients must be with the direct involvement and guidance of a pediatric nephrologist.

In primary IgA nephropathy, the onset is generally characterized by gross hematuria, sometimes associated with a decrease in renal function. Some of these patients recover their renal function rapidly without the need for specific therapy, whereas others need the treatment approach described for patients with severe crescentic HSP nephritis, which shares the same histologic pattern of mesangial proliferation with IgA deposits.[8] Once again, the decisions regarding this aggressive form of therapy must be made by, or with a pediatric nephrologist.

LONG-TERM COURSE AND OUTCOME OF APIGN

APIGN has a benign course in most, if not all children, although some follow-up studies in adults have suggested a higher frequency of subclinical renal scars following APIGN in childhood than was previously recorded. However, such long-term data are difficult to interpret since it is not easy properly to relate non-specific sclerotic glomerular changes to an episode of APIGN suffered decades before. Indeed, data obtained on prospective cohorts, gathered from the follow-up of epidemics of APIGN, do not suggest that chronic damage is a feature of APIGN. It is thought that only 1–5% of the patients who present with APIGN will show persistent and significant urinary abnormalities or reduced renal function in adulthood.[11,12]

The long-term course and outcome of chronic GN presenting with acute nephritis is completely different from that of APIGN, hence it is important to make a precise diagnosis of these clinico-pathologic entities to present correctly to the child's parents the probable natural history of the disease, and the possible influence of therapy on the disease course. A careful follow-up of children is the most effective means to detect progressive deterioration of renal status that may need further attention. In such cases, a repeat renal biopsy may be needed to detect lesions that are more severe than expected from the clinical features. Since proteinuria is one of the most sensitive risk factors and hence treatment is usually attempted in cases with persistent significant proteinuria (≥ 1 g/m^2/day) after the acute phase.[12]

From the above considerations, it is evident that acute nephritis is not always a benign disease, since the same clinical onset can hide a chronic renal disease, which has the potential of progressing to ESRD. Hence the follow-up of a child with acute nephritis must be extremely careful, especially in the atypical cases. The long-term prognosis of children with chronic GN of various types can vary from persistent urinary abnormalities to a more progressive course leading, in some cases, to end stage renal failure. This is discussed further in Chapters 7 and 9.

SUMMARY AND THOUGHTS FOR THE FUTURE

Top list of take home messages:

1. Never forget a careful family history.
2. Consider the possibility of a previous infection or allergic reaction.
3. Chronic nephritis may present with the clinical features of APIGN, which usually has a benign course. It is important to remember that atypical short-term course is not uncommon, and the risk of severe hypertension, fluid overload, and pulmonary edema may result.
4. APIGN and HSP acute nephritis may apparently recover completely, but scars can develop, accounting for some functional detriment of renal function even decades later.
5. The persistence of proteinuria and trace hematuria may be a sign that the initial process was not a true APIGN, but the beginning of a chronic glomerular disease, needing careful follow-up.
6. There is a need to distinguish patients with progressive chronic GN from the benign ones, even with similar clinical and histologic data: hopefully genetic markers will define the genetic trait of the potentially progressor children who need intensive treatment.

CYBER SOURCES FOR INFORMATION:

http://www.principalhealthnews.com/topic/apsgneph
http://www.emedicine.com/med/byname/glomerul onephritis-poststreptococcal.htm
http://www.gpnotebook.co.uk/simplepage.cfm?ID=-1026555892
http://www.nt.gov.au/health/cdc/treatment_proto col/apsgn.pdf

http://www.hhs.state.ne.us/epi/epiimpet.htm
http://www.kernanhospital.com/ency/article/0005 03sym.htm
http://www.continuingeducation.com/nursing/strepto/strepto.pdf
http://medicine.ucsd.edu/peds/Pediatric%20Links/Links/Infectious%20Disease/Toxic%20Shock%20Syndromes%20Infect%20Dis%20Clin%20of%20NA%20Dec%201996.htm
http://www.findarticles.com/cf_0/m3225/7_61/61432932/p9/article.jhtml?term=
http://www.coloradohealthsite.org/chnqna.html?Kidney%20Disease?Types?all
http://www.kumc.edu/instruction/medicine/pathology/ed/CAI_text_Documents/kidney95.doc
http://www.ucsfhealth.org/childrens/adam/data/003522.html
http://www.hc-sc.gc.ca/fnihb/ons/nursing/resources/pediatric_guidelines/chapter_13.htm
http://student.ttuhsc.edu/PeerTutoring/msii/path/block%20v/blk5_96.rtf
http://www.ucihs.uci.edu/adolescent/Quiz.htm
http://www.keepkidshealthy.com/welcome/conditions/hematuria.html
http://www.sunmb.com/family/problems_pediatrics.htm

REFERENCES

1. Dodge WF, Spagro BH, Travis LB. Poststreptococcal glomerulonephritis: a prospective study in children. N Engl J Med 1972; 2836:273–278.
2. Hogg RJ. Prognostic indicators and treatment of childhood IgA nephropathy. Contrib Nephrol, Benè MC, Faure GC, Kessler M (eds). IgA Nephropath: the 25 years. Basel, Karger. 1995; 104:1–5.
3. Richards J. Acute post-streptococcal glomerulonephritis. WV Med J 1991; 87:61–65.
4. Simckes AM, Spitzer A. Poststreptococcal acute glomerulonephritis. Pediatr Rev 1995; 16(7):278–9.
5. Nordstrand A, Norgren M, Holm SE. Pathogenic mechanism of acute post-streptococcal glomerulonephritis. Scand J Infect Dis 1999; 31(6):523–37.
6. Garcia R, Rubio L, Rodriguez-Iturbe B. Long-term prognosis of epidemic poststreptococcal glomerulonephritis in Maracaibo: follow-up studies 11–12 years after the acute episode. Clin Nephrol 1981; 15(6):291–8.
7. Rodriguez-Iturbe B. Epidemic poststreptococcal glomerulonephritis. Kidney Int 1984; 25(1):129–36.
8. Coppo R, Amore A. The nephritis of Henoch-Schoenlein papura. In: Oxford Textbook of Clinical Nephrology (3rd ed) ed by AM Davison. Oxford University Press. Oxford. 2005.

9. Rodriguez-Iturbe B, Carr RI, Garcia R, Rabideau D, Rubio L, McIntosh RM. Circulating immune complexes and serum immunoglobulins in acute poststreptococcal glomerulonephritis. Clin Nephrol 1980; 13(1):1–4.

10. Parra G, Romero M, Henriquez-La Roche C, Pineda R, Rodriguez-Iturbe B. Expression of adhesion molecules in post-streptococcal glomerulonephritis. Nephrol Dial Transplant 1994; 9(10):1412–1417.

11. Baldwin DS. Poststreptococcal glomerulonephritis. A progressive disease? Am J Med 1977; 62(1):1–11.

12. Rodriguez-Iturbe B. Postinfectious glomerulonephritis. Am J Kidney Dis 2000; 35(1):XLVI-XLVIII.

9. Chronic nephritis in children – with emphasis on IgA nephropathy

Norishige Yoshikawa and Koichi Nakanishi

INTRODUCTION

The term chronic nephritis may be defined as a slow but persistent form of renal disease that is often accompanied by proteinuria, hematuria, and/or hypertension.[1-4] In most cases the primary disease affects the glomeruli, although in others the tubules or interstitium may be the initial 'target'. The time period over which chronic nephritis evolves is usually measured in years or decades. Ultimately, the process may lead to irreversible end-stage renal disease (ESRD) and necessitate renal replacement therapy, i.e. dialysis and/or a renal transplant. The glomerular lesions that underlie chronic nephritis vary widely[1] (Table 9.1). The most common form of chronic nephritis that results in ESRD in both children and adult patients around the world is IgA nephropathy, which will be the primary focus of this chapter.[2-4] Some other glomerular lesions that may cause chronic nephritis, such as focal segmental glomerulosclerosis, which usually presents as the nephrotic syndrome, are discussed elsewhere. In addition some general features of children with various types of chronic nephritis will be discussed in this chapter.

Table 9.1 Common histopathologic patterns in children with chronic nephritis

Mesangial proliferative glomerulonephritis including IgA nephropathy
Membrano-proliferative glomerulonephritis
Membranous glomerulonephritis
Focal segmental glomerulosclerosis
Lupus nephritis
Diabetic glomerulosclerosis
Alport syndrome
Diffuse mesangial sclerosis

IGA NEPHROPATHY

IgA nephropathy was first described in adults in 1968 by Berger and Hinglais.[2] It was initially considered to be a benign condition, but extended follow-up of patients indicated that 20–50% of adults will progress to ESRD if left untreated. Likewise, the favorable prognosis initially attributed to children with IgA nephropathy must be questioned in the light of more recent studies.[5-9]

EPIDEMIOLOGY

Although IgA nephropathy has been diagnosed all over the world, its prevalence varies widely from one country to another. The explanation for this apparent variability is uncertain, but it may be due to genetic/racial differences in the basic underlying pathology of IgA nephropathy, or to differences in patterns of referral and biopsy selection practices.[10] It has also been proposed that the high incidence of IgA nephropathy in certain countries may reflect the practice of routine urinalysis. In Japan, for example, all children between the ages of six and 18 years are screened annually, and those found to have urinary abnormalities are referred for further investigation. Thus, IgA nephropathy is the most common primary glomerulopathy diagnosed in children seen in Kobe University and Wakayama Medical University Hospitals, where it is detected in about 30% of biopsy specimens. In the Pacific Rim (Japan, Singapore, Australia, and New Zealand), IgA nephropathy accounts for as many as one half of the cases of primary glomerular disease. In Europe, it accounts for between 20 and 30% of all primary glomerular diseases, whereas in North America it is responsible for only 2–10% of patients who undergo renal biopsies and are found to have renal disease.

Genetic factors and environmental influences could contribute to these geographic differences in prevalence. A lower prevalence in African-Americans compared to Caucasians has been reported in the USA. However, in American children, similar incidences of IgA nephropathy have been reported in Caucasian and African-American children from Shelby County, Tennessee.[11] In Australia, where the population is heterogeneous and includes many immigrants from Third World countries, all racial groups seem to be affected equally.[12]

PATHOLOGY

The histopathologic lesions that are found in renal biopsies of patients with various forms of chronic nephritis provide the means by which a patient is given one of the specific diagnoses. In some cases, the light microscopy findings are most relevant. However, the diagnostic feature in the kidney biopsy of children with IgA nephropathy is the presence of immunoglobulin A in the glomerular mesangium as the dominant or co-dominant immunoglobulin,[1,2,4,5] (Fig. 9.1). There may also be less prominent deposits of C3 complement, IgG, and/or IgM.

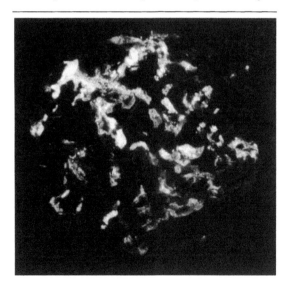

Figure 9.1 Immunofluorescence micrograph showing mesangial IgA deposits in a patients with IgA nephropathy. (See color plate section)

However, the early classical complement components, C4 or C1q, are usually absent.

ETIOLOGY

Because IgA is the main immunoglobulin directed against antigens (viral and bacterial) in the exocrine system, and because of the frequent association between upper respiratory tract or gastrointestinal infection, clinical exacerbations of IgA nephropathy, it has been suggested that certain viral or bacterial infections may lead to IgA nephropathy, and that IgA may act as the antibody to viral or bacterial antigens. The observation of numerous antigenic substances in the glomeruli indicates that the antigenic materials in IgA nephropathy may be heterogeneous. These are listed in Table 9.1.

PATHOGENESIS

Although the pathogenesis of IgA nephropathy remains uncertain, there is substantial evidence that it is an immune complex disease.[2] Granular electron-dense deposits are observed in the glomerular mesangial areas by electron microscopy, and confirmed as containing IgA and C3 by immunofluorescence microscopy. Circulating IgA immune complexes have been detected by several different specific assays, often associated with IgG immune complexes. Many immunologic abnormalities that may lead to the formation of IgA immune complex have been reported in patients with IgA nephropathy. Recurrences of IgA nephropathy occur frequently in allografted kidney,[20] and the rapid disappearance of glomerular IgA deposits is observed when kidneys with mesangial IgA deposits are transplanted into patients without IgA nephropathy.[21] Although much of this work was performed in adults there is no reason to suggest that the findings cannot be extrapolated to children.

PREDISPOSING GENETIC FACTORS

Predisposing genetic factors have recently been suggested as important determinants in the development of IgA nephropathy.[13–19] Moreover, it has been suggested that genetic factors, such as ACE genotyping and defective o-glycosylation of the IgA1 molecule (Fig. 9.2), may not only determine susceptibility to this and other forms of glomerulonephritis, but also influence the pathologic severity and natural course of IgA nephropathy.[14–19]

MECHANISM OF PROGRESSION OF DISEASE IN THE KIDNEYS

IgA alone appears to be sufficient to provoke injury among susceptible individuals,[22] and deposition of polymeric IgA, but not of monomeric IgA, can initiate glomerulonephritis.[23] There is little to suggest that the mechanisms of mesangial proliferative glomerulonephritis, progression, and scarring are distinct in IgA nephropathy compared with other types of chronic glomerulonephritis. Extensive studies in vitro and in animal models of mesangial proliferative glomerulonephritis have shown the key role of cytokines and growth factors, particularly platelet-derived growth factor (PDGF) and transforming growth factor β (TGFβ), in the induc-tion and progression of mesangial injury, and there is some evidence that these are also involved in IgA nephropathy (Fig. 9.3).[24–26] Studies on children with IgA nephropathy suggest that mesangial proliferation might be partially the result of local production of cytokines; IL-1, IL-6, tumor necrosis factor, platelet-derived growth factor, transforming growth factor-β, and vascular permeability factor/endothelial growth factor.[27–29] Although much has been learned about the fundamental abnormalities of the IgA molecule in IgA nephropathy, there is still no imminent prospect of these insights providing approaches to treatment that can prevent glomerular IgA deposition or the subsequent inflammation and injury.

LIGHT MICROSCOPY FINDINGS

Various glomerular changes are observed. The most characteristic abnormality is mesangial enlargement, caused by various combinations of hypercellularity and increase in matrix (Fig. 9.4). Individual biopsies can be graded according to the amount of

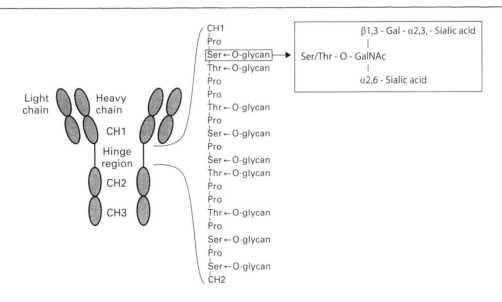

Figure 9.2 IgA1 molecule with hinge region O-glycosylation sites

IgA1 molecule with two heavy chains, each having three constant region domains CH1 to CH3, and a hinge region between CH1 and CH2. Each serine (Ser) and threonine (Thr) residue is a potential site for an O-glycan side chain. O-glycosylation sites consist of N-acetylgalactosamine (GalNAc) O-linked to the serine or threonine residues of hinge region

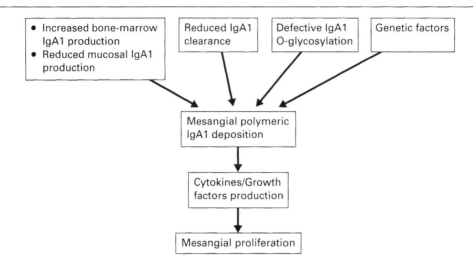

Figure 9.3 Proposed pathogenesis of IgA nephropathy

mesangial cell proliferation on the basis of the World Health Organization criteria.[1]

1. Minimal glomerular lesions. The majority of glomeruli appear optically normal, although a few may show a slight increase of mesangial matrix, with or without accompanying hypercellularity. The number of mesangial cells per peripheral mesangial area does not exceed three. There are also small foci of tubular atrophy and interstitial lymphocyte infiltration in some patients.

2. Focal mesangial proliferation. Up to 80% of glomeruli show moderate or severe mesangial cell proliferation, that is, more than three cells per peripheral mesangial area. The degree of mesangial cell proliferation varies considerably among glomeruli as well as segmentally within individual glomeruli. The proliferation is usually associated with increased matrix. Small cellular or fibrocellular crescents are frequently found, but rarely affect more than 20% of the glomeruli. Capsular adhesions are frequently seen, overlying lobules showing mesangial proliferation. Segmental capillary collapse is often observed in association with crescents. A small number of glomeruli showing global sclerosis are often present. Tubular atrophy, interstitial fibrosis and interstitial lymphocyte infiltration are frequently present but are not extensive.

3. Diffuse mesangial proliferation. More than 80% of glomeruli show moderate or severe mesangial cell proliferation, which varies in intensity in different regions of the mesangium in a given glomerulus, as well as from one glomerulus to another. Mesangial cell proliferation is always accompanied by increased mesangial matrix. Cellular and fibrocellular crescents (Fig. 9.5) are often found, usually affecting less than 50% of the glomeruli, although in about 10% of patients more than 50% are involved. Capsular adhesions are frequently seen in the absence of crescents. A small number of globally sclerosed glomeruli are often present. Tubular atrophy, interstitial fibrosis, and interstitial lymphocyte infiltration are frequently present, and are extensive in 10% of patients.

Progression of IgA nephropathy is associated with a gradual reduction of mesangial hypercellularity and an increase of matrix, associated with the gradual development of sclerosis. The severity of tubulointerstitial changes usually reflects the severity of glomerular damage. Vascular lesions such as

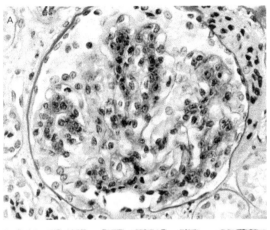

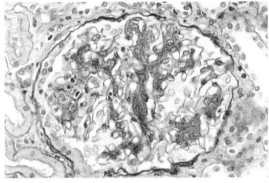

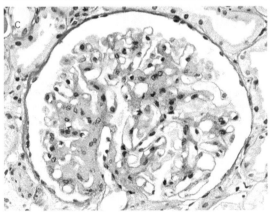

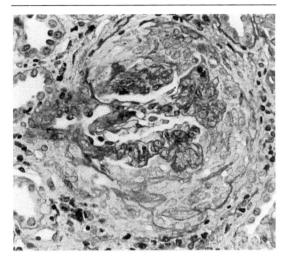

Figure 9.5 Fibrocellular crescent (PAS). (See color plate section)

Figure 9.4 Light micrograph showing mesangial proliferation in patients with IgA nephropathy

Three types of mesangial change are identified: (A) mesangial hypercellularity is more prominent than the increase in matrix (PAS stain); (B) the degrees of mesangial hypercellularity and matrix increase are similar (PAS stain), and (C) the increase in matrix is more prominent than the mesangial cellularity (PAS stain). (See color plate section)

arterial or arteriolar sclerosis are common in adults, but are very unusual in children with IgA nephropathy. This difference may be related to the age at biopsy and the duration of disease before biopsy.

ELECTRON MICROSCOPY

Electron microscopic abnormalities are mainly observed in the mesangium, which is variably enlarged by a combination of increased cytoplasm and matrix. Electron-dense deposits in the mesangium are the most constant and prominent feature and are seen in almost all patients (Fig. 9.6). They are granular masses situated immediately beneath the lamina densa in the perimesangial region and expanded mesangium. The size and extent of mesangial deposits varies from patient to patient.

CLINICAL FEATURES OF IGA
NEPHROPATHY

FINDINGS AT PRESENTATION

IgA nephropathy occurs at all ages but is most common during the second and third decades of life; it

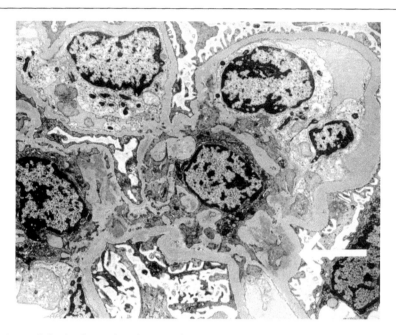

Figure 9.6 Electron micrograph showing electron-dense deposits in the mesangium in a patient with IgA nephropathy (white arrow)

affects males more often than females, the reported male:female ratio varying from under 2:1 to 6:1. In a study of Japanese children,[30] the age at initial presentation was 9.3 years in boys and 10.3 years in girls, and the male:female ratio was 3:2. As in patients with other forms of chronic nephritis, the clinical presentation of IgA nephropathy varies, ranging from asymptomatic urinary abnormalities to acute renal failure. However, there are five clinical presentations that generally can be identified in patients with chronic nephritis/IgA nephropathy:

1. Macroscopic hematuria – usually intermittant.
2. Asymptomatic microscopic hematuria and/or proteinuria.
3. Acute nephritic syndrome, defined as hematuria associated with hypertension and/or renal insufficiency.
4. Nephrotic syndrome.
5. Mixed nephritic-nephrotic syndrome.

Sixty-two percent of our 258 Japanese children were found to have microscopic hematuria and/or asymptomatic proteinuria.[30] Twenty-six percent presented with macroscopic hematuria and 12% with an acute nephritic syndrome and/or nephrotic syndrome. Several studies of IgA nephropathy in children from Europe and the United States have shown that more than 80% of all patients have macroscopic hematuria, and recurrent macroscopic hematuria is traditionally regarded as the hallmark of childhood IgA nephropathy.[31–34] However, it was presumably the initial feature in only 26% of our series, because of the school-screening program which detected a high prevalence of asymptomatic urinary abnormalities, rather than regional variation in the expression of IgA nephropathy. During the observation period, 60% of patients had one or more episodes of macroscopic hematuria, but the other 40% remained asymptomatic without macroscopic hematuria. The incidence of macroscopic hematuria is lower in adults than children with IgA nephropathy.

Episodes of macroscopic hematuria often occur in association with upper respiratory tract infections in children with IgA nephropathy. These episodes are sometimes associated with unilateral or bilateral loin pain which can be severe. The interval between the precipitating infection and the appearance of hematuria occurs within one to two days. Although children and adolescents with IgA nephropathy often have recurrent episodes of macroscopic hematuria, adults with IgA nephropathy do not usually have such episodes and are often asymptomatic.

In asymptomatic patients of all ages, microscopic hematuria is almost always present and persistent. Proteinuria is found in approximately 50% of patients and is an important prognostic feature in IgA nephropathy – as well as in other forms of chronic nephritis (Fig. 9.7). The blood pressure and renal function at onset are normal in most patients, but when abnormal the prognosis is more guarded.

Patients who present with the most severe clinical abnormalities usually have the most severe glomerular damage. Nephrotic range proteinuria and edema are reported in about 10% of patients. Acute renal failure is a rare event that may be associated with episodes of macroscopic hematuria; this is usually reversible. However, a number of investigators have documented a subset of patients with IgA nephropathy that is characterized by extensive crescents and a rapidly progressive course.[35,36] The other forms of chronic nephritis that are listed in Table 9.1 may also be associated with the spectrum of clinical abnormalities described above. The capacity for each of these features to occur in more than one glomerular disease is the reason why a renal biopsy is often needed to clarify the specific diagnosis. A review of published cases of crescentic IgA nephropathy revealed that 41% of patients with this rapidly progressive form of disease were 16 years of age or younger.[36]

LABORATORY INVESTIGATION

There are no laboratory studies that are specific for IgA nephropathy, but this is not always the case with some other forms of chronic nephritis. For example, serum complement component concentrations are usually normal in IgAN, but the serum C3 complement level should be measured routinely in patients who have clinical features of chronic nephritis, or even after the first attack of hematuria, to eliminate a diagnosis of membranoproliferative glomerulonephritis and poststreptococcal nephritis. Likewise, antistreptococcal antibody titers should be determined following the initial episode of hematuria. The serum creatinine should be measured routinely to estimate the GFR, as discussed in Chapter 1. The plasma proteins, including the serum albumin, should be measured routinely, especially in the presence of heavy proteinuria.

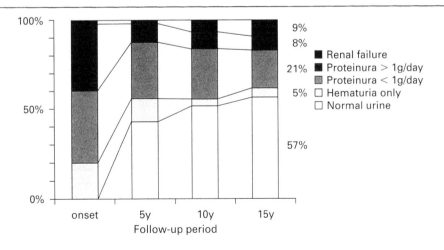

Figure 9.7 Long-term prognosis of the 169 Japanese children with IgA nephropathy followed more than 10 years

DIFFERENTIAL DIAGNOSIS

As in the case of all forms of chronic nephritis, the diagnosis of IgA nephropathy must be based on specific findings on renal biopsy. In patients with IgA nephropathy, the presence of IgA as the dominant or co-dominant immunoglobulin in the glomerular mesangium is the diagnostic feature. However, since diffuse mesangial IgA deposits are observed in a variety of other disorders (Table 9.2), the diagnosis of IgA nephropathy can be made only by interpreting the biopsy features in conjunction with the clinical and laboratory results. These associated disorders include Henoch-Schönlein purpura and systemic lupus erythematosus, both of which have characteristic clinical and laboratory features.

Table 9.2 Diseases associated with diffuse mesangial IgA deposits

Primary
IgA nephropathy
Secondary
Multisystem disease
  Henoch-Schönlein purpura
  Systemic lupus erythematosus
  Cystic fibrosis
  Celiac disease
  Crohn's disease
  Dermatitis herpetiformis
  Ankylosing spondylitis
Neoplasms
  Carcinomas of the lung and colon
  Monoclonal IgA gammopathy
  Mucosis fungoides
  Non-Hodgkin's lymphoma
Infectious diseases
  Mycoplasma infections
  Leprosy
  Toxoplasmosis
Others
  Chronic liver disease
  Thrombocytopenia
  Pulmonary hemosiderosis
  Mixed cryoglobulinemia
  Polycythemia
  Scleritis

HENOCH-SCHÖNLEIN PURPURA NEPHRITIS

The relationship between IgA nephropathy and Henoch-Schönlein purpura nephritis is complex.[37] The morphologic and immunopathologic features are similar in the two conditions,[38,39] and the two disorders have been reported to coexist in different members of the same family,[40,41] including a pair of monozygotic twins who developed them simultaneously following a well-documented adenovirus infection. Moreover, the evolution of IgA nephropathy into Henoch-Schönlein purpura nephritis in the same patient is described in both adults[42] and children.[43] It has been suggested that the two conditions are variants of the same process. However, Henoch-Schönlein purpura nephritis occurs mostly in young children, and is rare in adulthood, whereas IgA nephropathy affects mainly older children and young adults. It is therefore reasonable that IgA nephropathy and Henoch-Schönlein purpura nephritis are treated as different clinicopathologic entities until the pathogenesis of the two conditions is better understood.[44]

NATURAL HISTORY AND PROGNOSIS OF IGA NEPHROPATHY

Most forms of chronic nephritis follow an insidious course with some patients showing a progressive fall in kidney function over years or decades, whereas other patients remain stable for even longer. In long-term follow-up of adult patients with IgA nephropathy, 30–35% were found to develop progressive renal insufficiency 20 years after the initial discovery of disease.[45] Similarly, the long-term prognosis of 169 Japanese children with IgA nephropathy followed more than 10 years, showed that 9% of the patients had developed chronic renal failure after 15 years (Fig. 9.6).

Because of this variable rate of progression to chronic renal failure in patients with IgA nephropathy and other forms of chronic nephritis, there have been attempts to identify features present at the time of diagnosis that would predict the ultimate outcome. The following clinical findings are regarded as poor prognostic indicators in adult patients with IgA nephropathy: persistent hypertension, persistent heavy proteinuria, and reduced glomerular filtration rate at presentation.[45–48] In children, several studies have shown that the degree of proteinuria correlates with the severity of morphologic glomerular lesion, and heavy proteinuria at the time of biopsy predicts a poor outcome (Fig. 9.7).[49–51] Hypertension and acute renal failure at onset are usually reversible in children. Male sex has also been considered an unfavorable prognostic feature by some investigators, but we and others could not confirm it in a large cohort of adult and pediatric patients. Recently, Schena et al. reported an increased risk of end-stage renal disease in familial IgA nephropathy.[52]

Among the pathologic features analyzed in patients with IgA nephropathy, as well as other forms of chronic nephritis, a high proportion of glomeruli showing sclerosis, crescents, or capsular adhesions, and the presence of moderate or severe tubulointerstitial changes are indicative of a poor prognosis (Fig. 9.8). Patients with diffuse mesangial proliferation have been reported to have a signifi-

cantly worse prognosis than those with focal proliferation, or with minimal lesions by light microscopy in adults.[53] In many adult studies, glomerular sclerosis and crescents have also been associated with poor renal outcome. Since the severity of the tubulointerstitial changes usually corresponds with the severity of the glomerular changes, tubulointerstitial changes in IgA nephropathy are thought to be secondary to the glomerular injury. Vascular lesions such as arterial or arteriolar sclerosis have been reported to play an important role in the progression of IgA nephropathy in adults. However, vascular changes are very unusual in children. This difference may be related to the age at biopsy and the duration of disease before biopsy.

TREATMENT OF IgA NEPHROPATHY

IgA nephropathy is a leading cause of chronic renal disease and end-stage renal disease in adult patients, and recent long-term studies assessing the prognosis in children have challenged earlier views that the condition represents a benign disorder.

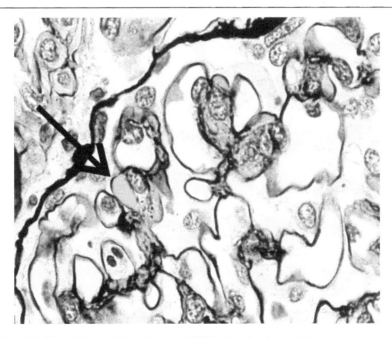

Figure 9.8 Eosinophilic nodular 'fibrinoid' mesangial deposits (arrow) (PASM). (See color plate section)

Thus IgA nephropathy presents a therapeutic challenge in both adults and children. Because of the variable rate of progression to renal failure, and because of the probable multifactorial pathogenesis of the disease, the effectiveness of any treatment can only be properly evaluated by means of a randomized controlled trial.[54] When considering treatment protocols, an issue of great importance is the selection of appropriate patients in whom the treatment is to be evaluated. Patients with heavy proteinuria at biopsy, and most severe glomerular lesions on renal biopsy, appear to be at greatest risk of progressive renal deterioration and, therefore, the most appropriate candidates for specific therapeutic interventions. However, patients with longstanding disease and extensive, irreversible glomerular damage are unsuitable for such treatments.

A controlled double-blind trial in adult patients with IgA nephropathy[55,56] showed that treatment with fish oil for two years retarded the rate at which renal function was lost, but a meta-analysis showed that there was only a 75% probability that fish oil was beneficial.[57] Recent studies have indicated that angiotensin-converting enzyme inhibitors and angiotensin-II receptor antagonists reduce urinary protein excretion and preserve renal function in adult patients with IgA nephropathy.[58] High-dose oral and intravenous methylprednisolone was shown to delay development of renal failure in a randomized controlled trial in adult patients.[59] However, there is mixed evidence in the reports that have been published to date with respect to the use of fish oil, angiotensin-converting enzyme inhibitors and/or prednisone, and other immuno-suppressive agents for the treatment of children with IgA nephropathy, and at present there is no consensus on the most appropriate therapy for IgA nephropathy or most of the other forms of chronic nephritis listed in Table 9.1.[60]

It should be understood, however, that there are some very encouraging reports on approaches using these medications. For example, in a recent controlled trial by the Japanese Pediatric IgA Nephropathy Treatment Study Group, 78 children with severe IgA nephropathy were randomly assigned to receive either the combined therapy of prednisolone, azathioprine, heparin-warfarin, and dipyridamole for two years (group 1) or the combination of heparin-warfarin and dipyridamole for two years (group 2). The results showed more significant benefits from treatment with the combination of prednisolone, azathioprine, heparin-warfarin and dipyridamole; this was accompanied by relatively few serious side effects specifically attributable to the drugs.[61] Mesangial IgA deposits had completely disappeared by the end of treatment in 7 of the 33 group 1 patients examined, but persisted in all 25 group 2 patients examined (Fig. 9.7). These 7 patients showed clinical remission defined as complete disappearance of proteinuria and hematuria with normal renal function and serum IgA levels, and marked improvement of the glomerular changes with minimal mesangial proliferation, minimal glomerular sclerosis, and no crescents at the end of treatment (Fig. 9.9). Previous studies demonstrating therapeutic benefit have not described loss of mesangial IgA deposits. However, it is likely that administration of prednisolone, aza-thioprine, heparin-warfarin, and dipyridamole for two years does achieve remission in these patients. A controlled trial is currently in progress to compare the effects of prednisolone, azathioprine, heparin-warfarin, and dipyridamole with those of prednisolone alone in children with severe IgA nephropathy.

Progression of IgA nephropathy leads to a gradual resolution of mesangial hypercellularity and an increase of matrix, associated with the development of sclerosis. The majority of patients with IgA nephropathy in our series were diagnosed early in the course of the disease, and the asymptomatic period before the discovery of urinary abnormalities was short. Patients with long-standing disease and extensive glomerulosclerosis are unsuitable for treatment. In our controlled trial, average interval between onset or discovery of disease and start of treatment was 11 months, and no patient showed predominant matrix increase or extensive glomerulosclerosis. Early diagnosis and early treatment are very important in IgA nephropathy.

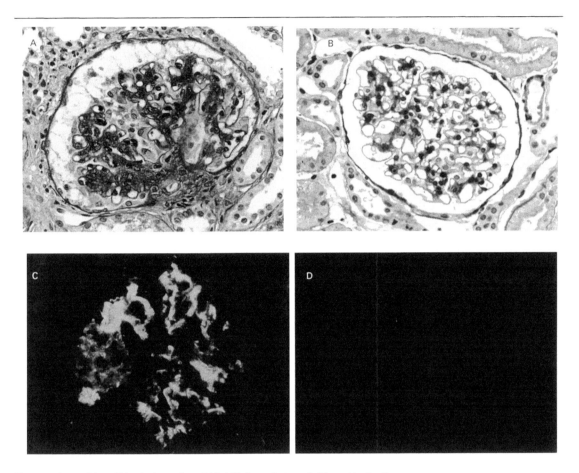

Figure 9.9 Sequential renal biopsies in a patient with IgA Nephropathy treated with combination therapy

(A) First renal biopsy from patient treated with prednisolone, azathioprine, heparin-warfarin, and dipyridamole, glomerulus showing moderate mesangial proliferation (PAS). (B) Second renal biopsy from the same patient. The extent of mesangial proliferation decreased (PAS). (C) First renal biopsy from the same patient with intense mesangial IgA deposits. (D) Second renal biopsy from the same patient showing that the mesangial IgA deposits completely disappeared. (See color plate section)

Recurrence of mesangial IgA deposits is often observed in transplant recipients whose original disease was IgA nephropathy. Such recurrences are mild or even asymptomatic and despite this risk of recurrent glomerulonephritis, graft survival in patients with IgA nephropathy is considered good.

At the present time, there are multiple factors that must be considered when deciding whether to treat a child with IgAN or some other form of chronic nephritis. Hence it is not appropriate for a primary care physician to embark on such therapy without seeking pediatric nephrology consultation. As such, the various therapeutic permutations and combinations that are possible for patients with these chronic conditions will not be discussed in this text. Such information is available in texts designed for pediatric nephrologists.

REFERENCES

1. Churg J, Bernstein J, Glassock RJ. Renal Disease: Classification and Atlas of Glomerular Diseases, 2nd edn. Igaku-shoin Medical Publishers: Tokyo, 1995.
2. Berger J, Hinglais N. Les depots intercapillaire d'IgA-IgG. J Urol Nephrol 1968; 74:694–695.
3. D'Amico G. The commonest glomerulonephritis in the world: IgA nephropathy. Q J Med 1987; 64: 709–727.
4. Donadio J, Grande J. IgA nephropathy. N Eng J Med 2002; 347:738–748.
5. Yoshikawa N, Ito H, Yoshiara S et al. Clinical course of IgA nephropathy in children. J Pediatr 1987; 110:555–560.
6. Yoshikawa N, Iijima K, Maehara K et al. Mesangial changes in IgA nephropathy in children. Kidney Int 1987; 32:585–589.
7. Yoshikawa N, Iijima K, Matsuyama S et al. Repeat renal biopsy in children with IgA nephropathy. Clinical Nephrol 1990; 33:160–167.
8. Wyatt RJ, Kritchevsky SB, Woodford SY et al. IgA nephropathy: long-term prognosis for pediatric patients. J Pediatr 1995; 127:913–919.
9. Hogg RJ, Silva FG, Wyatt RJ et al. Prognostic indicators in children with IgA nephropathy – report of the Southwest Pediatric Nephrology Study Group. Pediatr Nephrol 1994; 8:15–20.
10. Rodicio JL. Idiopathic IgA nephropathy. Kidney Int 1984; 25:717–729.
11. Sehic AM, Gaber LW, Roy S 3rd et al. Increased recognition of IgA nephropathy in African-American children. Pediatr Nephrol 1997; 11:435–437.
12. Clarkson AR, Woodroffe AJ, Aarons I. IgA nephropathy and Henoch-Schönlein purpura. In: Schrier RW, Gottschalk CW, eds. Diseases of the Kidney. Little, Brown, Boston: 1996, 1645–1670.
13. Hsu SI, Ramirez SB, Winn MP et al. Evidence for genetic factors in the development and progression of IgA nephropathy. Kidney Int 2000; 57:1818–1835.
14. Rambausek MH, Waldherr R, Ritz E. Immunogenetic findings in glomerulonephritis. Kidney Int 1993; 43: S3–8.
15. Schmidt S, Ritz E. Genetic factors in IgA nephropathy. Ann Med Interne 1999; 150: 86–90.
16. Julian BA, Quiggins PA, Thompson JS et al. Familial IgA nephropathy. Evidence for an inherited mechanism of disease. N Engl J Med 1985; 312:202–208.
17. Wyatt RJ, Rivas ML, Julian BA et al. Regionalization in hereditary IgA nephropathy. Am J Hum Genet 1987; 41:36–50.
18. Scolari F, Amoroso A, Savoldi S et al. Familial clustering of IgA nephropathy: Further evidence in an Italian population. Am J Kidney Dis 1999; 33:857–865.
19. Hsu SI, Ramirez SB, Winn MP et al. Evidence for genetic factors in the development and progression of IgA nephropathy. Kidny Int 2000; 57: 1818–1835.
20. Andresdottir MB, Hoitsma AJ, Assmann KJ, et al, Favorable outcome of renal transplantation in patients with IgA nephropathy, Clin Nephrol 2001;56:279–288.
21. Koselj M, Rott T, Kandus A, et al, Donor-transmitted IgA nephropathy: long-term follow-up of kidney donors and recipients, Transplant Proc 1997;29:3406–3407.
22. Allen AC, Barratt J, Feehally J. Immunoglobulin A nephropathy. In: Neilson EG, Couser WG, eds, Immunologic renal diseases, 2nd edn. Lippincott Williams & Wilkins: Philadelphia, 2001; 931–947.
23. Stad RK, Bruijn JA, van Gijlswijk-Janssen DJ et al. An acute model for IgA-mediated glomerular inflammation in rats induced by mono-clonal polymeric rat IgA antibodies. Clin Exp Immunol 1993; 92:514–521.
24. Niemir ZI, Stein H, Noronha IL et al. PDGF and TGF-beta contribute to the natural course of human IgA glomerulonephritis. Kidney Int 1995; 48:1530–1541.
25. Stein-Oakley AN, Maguire JA, Dowling J et al. Altered expression of fibrogenic growth factors in IgA nephropathy and focal and segmental glomerulosclerosis. Kidney Int 1997; 51:195–204.
26. Taniguchi Y, Yorioka N, Masaki T et al. Localization of transforming growth factors beta1 and beta2 and epidermal growth factor in IgA nephropathy. Scand J Urol Nephrol 1999; 33:243–247.
27. Yoshioka K, Takemura T, Murakami K et al. Transforming growth factor-β protein and mRNA in glomeruli in normal and diseased human kidneys. Lav Invest 1993; 68:154–163.
28. Yoshioka K, Takemura T, Murakami K et al. In situ expression of cytokines in IgA nephritis. Kidney Int 1993; 44:825–833.
29. Iijima K, Yoshikawa N, Connolly DT et al. Human mesangial cells and peripheral blood mononuclear cells produce vascular permeability factor. Kidney Int 1993; 44:959–966.
30. Yoshikawa N, Ito H, Nakamura H. IgA nephropathy in children from Japan. Child Nephrol Urol 1989; 9:191–199.
31. Michalk D, Waldherr R, Seelig HP et al. Idiopathic mesangial IgA-glomerulonephritis in childhood. Eur J Pediatr 1980; 134:13–22.
32. Linné T, Aperia A, Broberger O et al. Course of renal function in IgA glomerulonephritis in children and adolescents. Acta Paediatr Scand 1982; 71:735–743.
33. Lévy M, Gonzalez-Buschard G, Broyer M et al. Berger's disease in children. Medicine 1985; 64:157–180.
34. Southwest Pediatric Nephrology Study Group. A multicenter study of IgA nephropathy in children: Report of the Southwest Pediatric Nephrology Study Group. Kidney Int 1982; 22:643–652.
35. Silva FG, Hogg RJ. IgA nephropathy. In: Tisher CC, Brenner BM, eds. Renal Pathology: with Clinical and Functional Correlations. Lippincott: Philadelphia, 1989:434–493.
36. Abuelo JG, Esparza AR, Matarese RA et al. Crescentic IgA nephropathy. Medicine (Baltimore) 1984; 63:396–406.
37. Davin JC, Ten Berge IJ, Weening JJ. What is the difference between IgA nephropathy and Henoch-Schönlein purpura nephritis? Kidney Int 2001; 59:823–834.
38. Habib R, Niaudet P, Levy M. Henoch-Schönlein purpura nephritis and IgA nephropathy. In: Tisher C, Brenner B, eds. Renal Pathology: with Clinical and Functional Correlations, 2nd edn. JB Lippincott: Philadelphia,1994:472–523.
39. Yoshikawa N, Nakanishi K, Iijima K. Henoch-Schönlein nephritis. In: Neilson EG, Couser WG, eds. Immunologic Renal Diseases, 2nd edn. Lippincott Williams & Wilkins: Philadelphia, 2001:1127–1140.
40. Montoliu J, Lens XM, Torras A et al. Henoch-Schönlein purpura and IgA nephropathy in father and son. Nephron 1990;54:77–79.
41. Meadow SR, Scott DG. Berger disease: Henoch-Schönlein syndrome without the rash. J Pediatr 1985; 106:27–32.
42. Araque A, Sanchez R, Alamo C et al. Evolution of immunoglobulin A nephropathy into Henoch-Schönlein purpura. Am J Kidney Dis 1995; 25:340–342.
43. Silverstein DM, Greifer I, Folkert V et al. Sequential occurrence of IgA nephropathy and Henoch-Schönlein purpura: support for common pathogenesis. Pediatr Nephrol 1994; 8:752.
44. Yoshikawa N, Ito H, Yoshiya K et al. Henoch-Schönlein nephritis and IgA nephropathy: A comparison of clinical course. Clin Nephrol 1987; 27:233–237.
45. D'Amico G. Natural history of idiopathic IgA nephropathy: Role of clinical and histological prognostic factors. Am J Kidney Dis 2000; 36:227–237.

46. Glassock RJ, Adler SG, Ward HJ et al. Primary glomerular diseases. In: Brenner BM, Rector FCJr, eds. The Kidney. Saunders: Philadelphia, 1991:1182–1279.

47. Neelakantappa K, Gallo GR, Baldwin DS. Proteinuria in IgA nephropathy. Kidney Int 1988; 33:716–721.

48. Bartosik LP, Lajoie G, Sugar L et al. Predicting progression in IgA nephropathy. Am J Kidney Dis (2001)38:728–735.

49. Hattori S, Karashima S, Furuse A et al. Clinicopathological correlation of IgA nephropathy in children. Am J Nephrol 1985; 5:182–189.

50. Andreoli SP, Yum MN, Bergstein JM. IgA nephropathy in children: Significance of glomerular basement membrane deposition of IgA. Am J Nephrol 1986; 6:28–33.

51. Hogg RJ. Prognostic indicators and treatment of childhood IgA nephropathy. Contrib Nephrol (1995); 111:194–200.

52. Schena FP, Cerullo G, Rossini M et al. Increased risk of end-stage renal disease in familial IgA nephropathy. J Am Soc Nephrol 2002; 13:453–460.

53. Haas M. Histologic subclassification of IgA nephropathy: A clinico-pathologic study of 244 cases. Am J Kidney Dis 1997; 29:829–842.

54. Wyatt RJ, Hogg RJ. Evidence-based assessment of treatment options for children with IgA nephropathies. Pediatr Nephrol 2001; 16:156–167.

55. Donadio JJ, Bergstralh EJ, Offord KP et al. A controlled trial of fish oil in IgA nephropathy. Mayo Nephrology Collaborative Group. N Engl J Med 1994; 331:1194–1199.

56. Donadio JV Jr, Grande JP, Bergstralh EJ et al. The long-term outcome of patients with IgA nephropathy treated with fish oil in a controlled trial. Mayo Nephrology Collaborative Group. J Am Soc Nephrol 1999; 10:1772–1777.

57. Dillon JJ. Fish oil therapy for IgA nephropathy: Efficacy and inter-study variability. J Am Soc Nephrol 1997; 8:1739–1744.

58. Perico N, Remmuzzi A, Sangalli F et al. The antiproteinuric effect of angiotensin antagonism in human IgA nephropathy is potentiated by indomethacin. J Am Soc Nephrol 1998; 9:2308–2317.

59. Pozzi C, Bolasco PG, Foggazzi GB et al. Corticosteroids in IgA nephropathy: a randomised controlled trial. Lancet 1999; 353:883–887.

60. Schlöndorff D, Dendorfer U, Brumberger V et al. Limitations of therapeutic approaches to glomerular diseases. Kidney Int 1995; 48(Supp):19–25.

61. Yoshikawa N, Ito H, Sakai T et al. A controlled trial of combined therapy for newly diagnosed severe childhood IgA nephropathy. J Am Soc Nephrol 1999; 10:101–109.

10. Hypertension: evaluation, monitoring, and therapy

Vera Hermina Koch and Ronald Portman

INTRODUCTION

International epidemiologic studies on blood pressure among children and adolescents have revealed that blood pressure levels in childhood are the strongest predictor of adult blood pressure levels.[1] In the adult population, hypertension causes a two to threefold increase in an individual's risk of cardiovascular morbidity.[2] The relationship between hypertension and cardiovascular disease seems to be continuous; cardiovascular risk depends on blood pressure itself, coexistent risk factors, and whether there is hypertensive end-organ damage.

BLOOD PRESSURE EVALUATION IN CHILDREN

METHODOLOGIC ISSUES

CASUAL BLOOD PRESSURE

As accuracy in determining blood pressure is essential, a standardized protocol should be utilized for blood pressure measurement. Observers should be trained and certified to minimize measurement bias. Ideally, standardized approaches should be taken regarding equipment factors such as an appropriate cuff bladder size, or the alternative use of mercury manometers or oscillometric devices. Technical factors such as the recording of fourth, fifth or both Korotkoff sounds for diastolic blood pressure need to be taken into consideration. Also, the number of measurements needed for estimating a child's blood pressure and the influence on its level of environmental factors such as the time of the day and ambient temperature must be considered.[3]

In order to obtain an accurate blood pressure measurement, a cuff bladder width of approximately 40% of the upper arm circumference should be chosen because it most closely approximates intra-arterial readings. The bladder length should be at least 90% of arm circumference to avoid overestimation of blood pressure.[4] Another less-known effect of the cuff size change occurs when, in accordance with the above-mentioned instructions for cuff selection, the cuff size is changed to a larger one. In this case, the cuff change may lead to a fall in the value of measured blood pressure that is not arm-dependent, but cuff-dependent.[5]

Another important issue to consider is the number of measurements that should be repeated within a visit and between visits in order to determine a child's blood pressure. For example, using a Dinamap model in 106 children aged 9 to 13 years, systolic blood pressure values obtained after three weekly visits with four measurements per visit demonstrated that the first of several measurements during one particular visit was generally higher than the following ones. The values obtained started to level off after 4–5 measurements within a visit, with the 'first measurement effect' being reproducible even after three consecutive visits.

There has been an ongoing controversy over whether the muffling (Korotkoff 4 – K4) or disappearance of sounds (K5) should be used preferentially for the determination of diastolic blood pressure in children.[6] Neither value correctly defines intra-arterial diastolic blood pressure. Although K5 is approximately 9 mmHg higher than direct diastolic blood pressure, it is much easier for the human ear to discern than K4.[7] Current recommendations therefore favor the use of K5.

NORMATIVE BLOOD PRESSURE DATA FOR CHILDREN

The first age-related norms for blood pressures in children and adolescents were developed in 1977 by the Task Force on Blood Pressure Control in Children,[8] a group sponsored by the National Institutes of Health. These standards were revised in 1987 by a second task force, which evaluated data from more than 70,000 children.[9] Rosner et al. in 1993 emphasized the lack of homogeneous methodology that was used to collect the data on which the Second Task Force of Blood Pressure Measurement in Children based its recommendations.[10]

In a more recent revision of the guidelines that was published in 1996, height was added as a category, along with age and gender.[11] Data from the National Health and Nutrition Examination Survey, 1988–91 NHANES III study[12], was also incorporated, enabling the recognition of obesity as an important independent risk factor for hypertension in children. The update redefined diastolic blood pressure as the fifth rather than the fourth Korotkoff sound for children in all age groups. All measurements that were used in constructing the tables were first measurements that were made with a standard mercury sphygmomanometer on the child's right arm. The cuff size covered 80% to 100% of the circumference of the arm, and the data were obtained in over 60,000 children aged 1 to 17 years of age. A fourth set of guidelines was published recently.[13]

Standards for infants younger than 1 year of age are available in the 1987 Task Force report[9] and in two more recent studies.[14,15] In children younger than 1 year of age, systolic blood pressure has been used to define arterial hypertension.

The blood pressure measurement methodology recommended by the 1996 update states that blood pressure in children is most conveniently measured with a standard clinical sphygmomanometer, using the stethoscope placed over the brachial artery pulse, proximal and medial to the cubital fossa, with the bottom edge of the cuff placed approximately 2 cm above the cubital fossa.[11]

The equipment necessary to measure BP in children aged 3 years through adolescence includes three pediatric cuffs of different sizes as well as a standard adult cuff, an oversized cuff, and a thigh cuff for leg BP measurement. The latter two cuffs may be needed for use in obese adolescents. BP should be measured in a controlled environment

and after three to five minutes of rest in the seated position with the cubital fossa supported at heart level. The cuff should be inflated at a pressure approximately 20 mm greater than that at which the radial pulse disappears, and then allowed to deflate at a rate of 2–3 mmHg/second.

BP should be recorded at least twice on each occasion, and the average of the systolic and diastolic BP measurements should be used to estimate the blood pressure level. Systolic BP is determined by the onset of the 'tapping' Korotkoff sounds (K1), and diastolic BP by the disappearance of the Korotkoff sounds (K5). In some children, Korotkoff sounds can be heard to 0 mmHg. When this occurs, it excludes diastolic hypertension. Doppler and oscillometric techniques can be used in children in whom auscultatory blood pressure measurements are difficult to obtain; infants should have their blood pressure evaluated in the supine position.

Systolic blood pressure in the lower extremities must be measured whenever elevation of the systolic blood pressure in the upper extremities is noted. Blood pressure evaluation in the lower extremities should be made with the patient in the supine position; the cuff should be placed on the calf, and it should be wide enough to cover at least two thirds of the distance from knee to ankle. A common artifact of distal pulse amplification may cause the value of systolic blood pressure at the brachial artery to be less than that at the posterior tibial or dorsalis pedis artery. This difference may be only a few millimeters in the infant but can rise to 10–20 mmHg in the older child or adult, but the systolic pressure in the arm should *never* exceed that in the foot. If systolic pressure in the arm consistently exceeds that in the foot, the presence of an aortic coarctation should be suspected.

Tables 10.1 and 10.2 show the blood pressure levels by height percentiles, corresponding to the 90th and 95th percentiles of blood pressure for boys and girls respectively, age 1 to 17 years of age.[13] Further details, including the 50th and 99th BP percentiles are available in Ref 13. Height percentiles should be obtained from a standard growth chart. Figures 10.1 and 10.2 show standards for infants younger than one year of age.[9]

Table 10.1 Blood pressure levels for the 90th and 95th percentiles of blood pressure for boys aged 1 to 17-years by percentiles of height* Data extracted from Table 3 in Ref 13

Age (Year) ↓	BP† Percentile	Systolic BP (mm Hg) ← Percentile of Height →							Diastolic BP (mm Hg) ← Percentile of Height →						
		5th	10th	25th	50th	75th	90th	95th	5th	10th	25th	50th	75th	90th	95th
1	90th	94	95	97	99	100	102	103	49	50	51	52	53	53	54
	95th	98	99	101	103	104	106	106	54	54	55	56	57	58	58
2	90th	97	99	100	102	104	105	106	54	55	56	57	58	58	59
	95th	101	102	104	106	108	109	110	59	59	60	61	62	63	63
3	90th	100	101	103	105	107	108	109	59	59	60	61	62	63	63
	95th	104	105	107	109	110	112	113	63	63	64	65	66	67	67
4	90th	102	103	105	107	109	110	111	62	62	64	65	66	66	67
	95th	106	107	109	111	112	114	115	66	67	68	69	70	71	71
5	90th	104	105	106	108	110	111	112	65	66	67	68	69	69	70
	95th	108	109	110	112	114	115	116	69	70	71	72	73	74	74
6	90th	105	106	108	110	111	113	113	68	68	69	70	71	72	72
	95th	109	110	112	114	115	117	117	72	72	73	74	75	76	76
7	90th	106	107	109	111	113	114	115	70	70	71	72	73	74	74
	95th	110	111	113	115	117	118	119	74	74	75	76	77	78	78
8	90th	107	109	110	112	114	115	116	71	72	72	73	74	75	76
	95th	111	112	114	116	118	119	120	75	76	77	78	79	79	80
9	90th	109	110	112	114	115	117	118	72	73	74	75	75	76	77
	95th	113	114	116	118	119	121	121	76	77	78	79	80	81	81
10	90th	111	112	114	115	117	119	119	73	73	74	75	76	77	78
	95th	115	116	117	119	121	122	123	77	78	79	80	81	81	82
11	90th	113	114	115	117	119	120	121	74	74	75	76	77	78	78
	95th	117	118	119	121	123	124	125	78	79	79	80	81	82	82
12	90th	115	116	118	120	121	123	123	74	75	75	76	77	78	79
	95th	119	120	122	123	125	127	127	78	79	80	81	82	83	83
13	90th	117	118	120	122	124	125	126	75	75	76	77	78	79	79
	95th	121	122	124	126	128	129	130	79	79	80	81	82	83	83
14	90th	120	121	123	125	126	128	128	75	76	77	78	79	79	80
	95th	124	125	127	128	130	132	132	80	80	81	82	83	84	84
15	90th	122	124	125	127	129	130	131	76	77	78	79	80	80	81
	95th	126	127	129	131	133	134	135	81	84	82	83	84	85	85
16	90th	125	126	128	130	131	133	134	78	78	79	80	81	82	82
	95th	129	130	132	134	135	137	137	82	83	83	84	85	86	87
17	90th	127	128	130	132	134	135	136	80	80	81	82	83	84	84
	95th	131	132	134	136	138	139	140	84	85	86	87	87	88	89

*Height percentile determined by standard growth curves
†BP, Blood pressure percentile determined by a single measurement
90th percentiles is 1.28 SD above the mean; 95th percentiles is 1.645 SD above the mean

AMBULATORY BLOOD PRESSURE MONITORING

Ambulatory blood pressure monitoring (ABPM) is a technique that is based on the principle that repeated measurements of blood pressure through-out a 24-hour period provide a better approximation of true blood pressure level than is afforded by a single measurement. The procedure has been used extensively to document and monitor hypertension in adults, but there is less experience with this form

Table 10.2 Blood pressure levels for the 90th and 95th percentiles of blood pressure for girls aged 1 to 17-years by percentiles of height* Data extracted from Table 4 in Ref 13

Age (Year)	BP† Percentile	Systolic BP (mm Hg) ← Percentile of Height →							Diastolic BP (mm Hg) ← Percentile of Height →						
		5th	10th	25th	50th	75th	90th	95th	5th	10th	25th	50th	75th	90th	95th
1	90th	97	97	98	100	101	102	103	52	53	53	54	55	55	56
	95th	101	101	102	104	105	106	107	56	57	57	58	59	59	60
2	90th	98	99	100	101	103	104	105	57	58	58	59	60	61	61
	95th	102	103	104	105	107	108	109	61	62	62	63	64	65	65
3	90th	100	100	102	103	104	106	106	61	62	62	63	64	64	65
	95th	104	104	105	107	108	109	110	65	66	66	67	68	68	69
4	90th	101	102	103	104	106	107	108	64	64	65	66	67	67	68
	95th	105	106	107	108	110	111	112	68	68	69	70	71	71	72
5	90th	103	103	105	106	107	109	109	66	67	67	68	69	69	70
	95th	107	107	108	110	111	112	113	70	71	71	72	73	73	74
6	90th	104	105	106	108	109	110	111	68	68	69	70	70	71	72
	95th	108	109	110	111	113	114	115	72	72	73	74	74	75	76
7	90th	106	107	108	109	110	112	113	69	70	70	71	72	72	73
	95th	110	110	112	113	115	116	117	73	74	74	75	76	76	77
8	90th	108	109	110	111	113	114	114	71	71	71	72	73	74	74
	95th	112	112	114	115	116	118	118	75	75	75	76	77	78	78
9	90th	110	110	112	113	114	116	116	72	72	72	73	74	75	75
	95th	114	114	115	117	118	119	120	76	76	76	77	78	79	79
10	90th	112	112	114	115	116	118	118	73	73	73	74	75	76	76
	95th	116	116	117	119	120	121	122	77	77	77	78	79	80	80
11	90th	114	114	116	117	118	119	120	74	74	74	75	76	77	77
	95th	118	118	119	121	122	123	124	78	78	78	79	80	81	81
12	90th	116	116	117	119	120	121	122	75	75	75	76	77	78	78
	95th	119	120	121	123	124	125	126	79	79	79	80	81	82	82
13	90th	117	118	119	121	122	123	124	76	76	76	77	78	79	79
	95th	121	122	123	124	126	127	128	80	80	80	81	82	83	83
14	90th	119	120	121	122	124	125	125	77	77	77	78	79	80	80
	95th	123	123	125	126	127	129	129	81	81	81	82	83	84	84
15	90th	120	121	122	123	125	126	127	78	78	78	79	80	81	81
	95th	124	125	126	127	129	130	131	82	82	82	83	84	85	85
16	90th	121	122	123	124	126	127	128	78	78	79	80	81	81	82
	95th	125	126	127	128	130	131	132	82	82	83	84	85	85	86
17	90th	122	122	123	125	126	127	128	78	79	79	80	81	81	82
	95th	125	126	127	129	130	131	132	82	83	83	84	85	85	86

*Height percentile determined by standard growth curves
†BP, Blood pressure percentile determined by a single measurement
90th percentiles is 1.28 SD above the mean; 95th percentiles is 1.645 SD above the mean

of BP monitoring in children. The overall success rate for ABPM in pediatric patients is about 70% to 80%; older pediatric patients seem to be more receptive to ABPM than are younger patients.[16] A recent study compared casual blood pressure and ambulatory blood pressure monitoring parameters among normotensive and hypertensive adolescents.[17] Contrary to findings in adult populations, the mean casual systolic/diastolic blood pressure measured in the clinic was lower than the mean

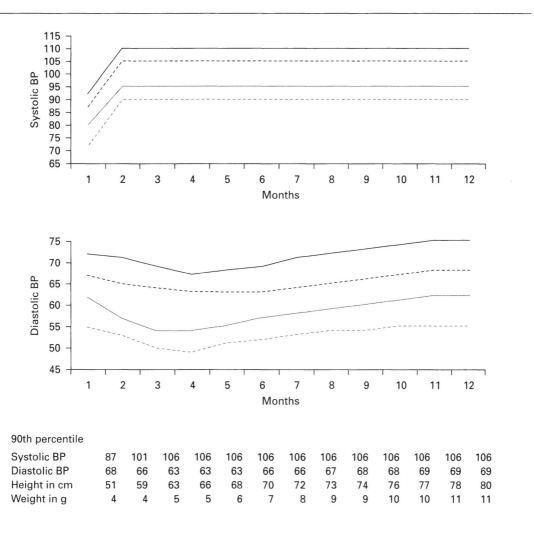

90th percentile													
Systolic BP	87	101	106	106	106	106	106	106	106	106	106	106	106
Diastolic BP	68	66	63	63	63	66	66	67	68	68	69	69	69
Height in cm	51	59	63	66	68	70	72	73	74	76	77	78	80
Weight in g	4	4	5	5	6	7	8	9	9	10	10	11	11

Figure 10.1 Blood pressure levels in boys from birth until 1 year of age[9]

ambulatory blood pressure monitoring parameters while awake, for normotensive and hypertensive adolescents.

The current general indications for ambulatory blood pressure monitoring are: identification of white coat hypertension, borderline hypertension, identification of nocturnal hypertension, drug resistant hypertension, indication of antihypertensive medication, hypertension of pregnancy, and identification of hypotension.[18] Among the current issues for ambulatory blood pressure monitoring use in pediatrics, the main problem is the lack of robust normative data. The methodology is promising, since recordings show good accuracy and reproducibility in children.[16] The white coat effect on BP that is well known with adults has also been confirmed in the pediatric population.[19–21] Recent studies have shown that left ventricular mass index

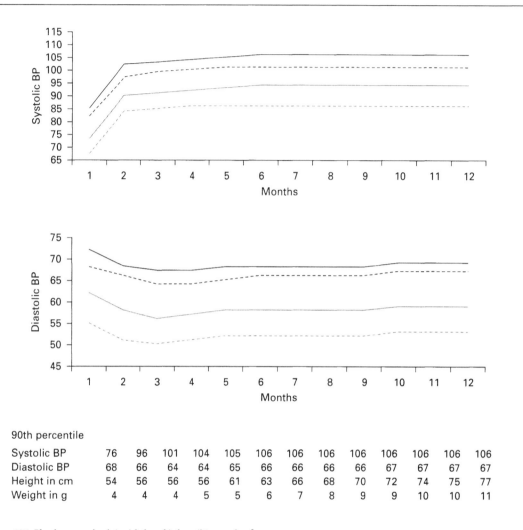

90th percentile												
Systolic BP	76	96	101	104	105	106	106	106	106	106	106	106	106
Diastolic BP	68	66	64	64	65	66	66	66	66	67	67	67	67
Height in cm	54	56	56	56	61	63	66	68	70	72	74	75	77
Weight in g	4	4	4	5	5	6	7	8	9	9	10	10	11

Figure 10.2 Blood pressure levels in girls from birth until 1 year of age[9]

and left ventricular hypertrophy are better correlated with ABPM confirmed hypertension than with casual systolic blood pressure in children[22] – as in adults. According to Kapuku et al., left ventricular hypertrophy can even be predicted by initial ambulatory systolic parameters.[23]

One of the major limitations to the use of ABPM in children has been the lack of reliable reference values. The Task Force data are derived exclusively from daytime casual measurements, and are of uncertain applicability to 24-hour blood pressure interpretation. One of the first studies to provide specific pediatric ABPM reference data was by Soergel et al. who performed ABPM on 1141 normal mid-European children.[24] From these data, percentile values for 24-hour awake and asleep periods were derived based on gender and height. Lurbe et al. recently presented data on 750 healthy children aged 4 to 18 years to further establish reference ambulatory blood pressure values stratified by gender and height.[25] Although these large normative ABPM data sets are useful, they still remain relatively small when one considers tthat pediatric databases must be stratified by age and height to account for the normal age-related rise in blood pressure in children.[26] Table 10.3 shows oscillometric mean ABPM values in healthy children according to Soergel et al.[24]

CLINICAL DIAGNOSIS AND MONITORING OF HYPERTENSIVE PEDIATRIC PATIENTS

Any child who is found to have a blood pressure that exceeds the 90th percentile for height, age and gender requires repeated evaluations; several measurements of blood pressure should be made at weekly intervals to determine whether the elevation is sustained. If the average measurement is between the 90th and 95th percentiles, the child's blood pressure should be monitored at six-month inter-

vals and consideration should be given to lifestyle changes that may be relevant. If the average systolic or diastolic blood pressure is consistently above the 95th percentile, the child should be regarded as being hypertensive and should be further evaluated and considered for therapy.

Clinical evaluation of a child with hypertension starts with a well-taken history and careful physical examination. The history should include information on the items listed in Table 10.4. Presenting symptoms and signs in neonates and infants may be mild or severe, although usually they are not specific. They range from failure to thrive, irritability and feeding problems to more specific signs of cardiovascular compromise such as cardiac failure, seizures, and respiratory distress. In older children, hypertension is frequently silent unless the blood pressure elevation is rapid and severe. The younger the child and the higher the blood pressure, the greater the chance that the hypertension is secondary to a potentially identifiable cause. An underlying cause can be found in most children with hypertension who are 1 to 10 years old. In the majority of cases the cause will be related to renal disease, although there are a number of other, less common causes.[27] Table 10.5 presents the main causes of hypertension in neonates, children, and adolescents.

Physical examination should try to identify signs indicative of secondary hypertension, including the

Table 10.3 Oscillometric mean ABPM values in healthy children: summary for clinical use[24]

Height in cm (n)	Percentile for 24 hr period		Daytime*
	50th	95th	50th
Boys			
120 (33)	105/65	113/72	112/73
130 (62)	105/65	117/75	113/73
140 (102)	107/65	121/77	114/73
150 (108)	109/66	124/78	115/73
160 (115)	112/66	126/78	118/73
170 (83)	115/67	128/77	121/73
180 (69)	120/67	130/77	124/73
Girls			
120 (40)	103/65	113/73	111/72
130 (58)	105/66	117/75	112/72
140 (70)	108/66	120/76	114/72
150 (111)	110/66	122/76	115/73
160 (156)	111/66	124/76	116/73
170 (109)	112/66	124/76	118/74
180 (25)	113/66	124/76	120/74

*Daytime: 8 am to 8 pm

Table 10.4 Important aspects of the history in a patient with hypertension

- Prematurity
- Low birth weight
- Bronchopulmonary dysplasia
- History of umbilical artery catheterization
- Failure to thrive
- Episodes of febrile urinary tract infections
- Unexplained bouts of fever
- History of head or abdominal trauma
- Use of drugs potentially affecting blood pressure such as amphetamines, nasal decongestants, steroids, tricyclic antidepressants
- Substance abuse
- Family history of heritable diseases

Table 10.5 Some causes of hypertension in pediatric patients – according to age

Infants
- Renal artery thrombosis
- Coarctation of the aorta
- Congenital renal disease
- Bronchopulmonary dysplasia
- Patent ductus arteriosus
- Intraventricular hemorrhage

Children and adolescents

Renal disorders
- Renal artery stenosis
- Neurofibromatosis
- Glomerulonephritis of various types
- Post-urologic surgery

Endocrine disorders
- Neurogenic tumors
- Pheochromocytoma
- Mineralocorticoid excess
- Liddle syndrome
- Hyperthyroidism

Cardiovascular disorders
- Coarctation of the disorder

Miscellaneous causes
- Hypercalcemia

Table 10.6 Physical abnormalities and specific disorders leading to hypertension in children

Physical sign	Diagnostic possibilities
• *Café au lait* spots	neurofibromatosis/pheochromocytoma
• Abdominal mass	Wilms tumor, neuroblastoma
• Abdominal bruit	coarctation of the aorta, renal vascular abnormalities
• Blood pressure lower legs	coarctation of the aorta
• Thyroid enlargement	hyperthyroidism
• Virilization	adrenal disorders

BUN, serum creatinine, uric acid, fasting cholesterol and its fractions, triglycerides, serum electrolytes, urinalysis and urine culture, renal sonography, and target organ damage evaluation, which would include a careful fundoscopic examination. Target organ damage evaluation is important even in patients with mild to moderate degrees of hypertension. Hence, consideration should be given to obtaining an echocardiogram, determination of microalbuminuria, and evaluation of carotid artery intimal-medial thickness. Mild-to-moderate blood pressure elevation in children may be accompanied by increased left ventricular mass,[29,30] glomerular hyperfiltration[30] and retinovascular abnormalities[30] in a significant number of patients. Recently, Sorof et al., in a study of 32 untreated pediatric hypertensive patients, found that carotid artery intimal-medial thickness and left ventricular mass index (LVMI) were positively associated after accounting for age, gender, and body mass index.[31] These findings raise the possibility that carotid duplex ultrasound, by indicating the presence of early arterial wall changes, may be useful for predicting other cardiovascular sequelae in hypertensive children.

Yiu et al.[32] recently emphasized the importance of a low peripheral plasma renin activity (< 1 ng/ml/hour) as a critical marker in pediatric hypertension, as it is a feature shared by a number of inherited disorders, such as glucocorticoid remediable aldosteronism, Liddle syndrome, and apparent mineralocorticoid excess, whose diagnosis is presently possible by molecular biology assays.

abnormalities listed in Table 10.6. Systolic hypertension is more common in children, whether examining an unselected sampling of patients by routine screening or a selected sampling of referred hypertensive patients.[28,29] The presence of fundoscopic changes, cardiomegaly, heart failure, or neurologic deficits usually points to the chronicity and severity of hypertension.

An extensive family history is a valuable part of the evaluation of pediatric hypertension. Emphasis should be given to age of occurrence of cardiovascular events, peripheral vascular disease, and diabetes in first- and second-degree relatives. Parents' and siblings' blood pressure should be measured. In this way, primary or secondary familial hypertension can be identified from an index case.

For individuals with mild hypertension and an innocent history and physical examination, a basic diagnostic work up should consist of: a complete blood cell count with differential and platelet count,

Controversy persists about the need for extensive investigations to exclude identifiable causes in all pediatric patients with hypertension. In the evaluation of the hypertensive child, it is important to recognize that the likelihood of identifying a secondary cause of hypertension is directly related to the level of blood pressure, and inversely related to the age of the child. Severe elevations of blood pressure, regardless of age, warrant aggressive evaluation. In contrast, the approach to children with mild elevations of blood pressure (i.e. those slightly above the 95th percentile), which are usually not associated with secondary disease, should be more restrained and focused mainly on non-invasive studies that are conducted in an attempt to identify renal disease.[27]

Other diagnostic studies are available for selected patients, especially those who have moderate to severe elevations of blood pressure. In patients with a previous history of urinary tract infection, a 99m Tc dimercaptosuccinic acid (DMSA) scan is advisable to exclude renal cortical scarring. In suspected urinary malformations, additional tests may include a voiding cystourethrogram (VCUG). The presence of arterial hypertension in association with hematuria and/or proteinuria may indicate the need for a renal biopsy to determine if the patient has renal parenchymal disease.

If a pheochromocytoma is suspected, diagnosis depends on biochemical evidence of catecholamine production by the tumor. However, confirmation of this diagnosis may be complicated as pheochromocytomas may secrete catecholamines intermittently or in low amounts, and the best test to establish the diagnosis has not been determined. Measurements of urinary metanephrines were initially performed by spectrophotometric methods. These methods have recently been replaced by techniques involving liquid chromatography that allow separation of nor-metanephrine and metanephrine into fractionated components that can be measured individually as 'urinary fractionated metanephrines'. Measurements of the fractionated metabolites are superior to measurements of total metenephrines.[33,34] More recent developments include liquid chromatographic measurements of plasma-free metanephrines, the single largest source of which are adrenal chromaffin cells.[35]

The prevalence of renovascular disease is estimated to be 3–5% in pediatric patients with hypertension. The main described causes are neurofibromatosis[36] and fibromuscular dysplasia.[37] The utility of non-invasive imaging tests has not been evaluated in children, and renal arteriography remains the diagnostic test of choice. Shahdadpuri et al.[38] reviewed the yield of renal arteriography in pediatric patients if the test was performed based on the following two criteria: 1) severe hypertension exceeding the 99th percentile for age and sex, 2) failure to control high blood pressure with one antihypertensive drug. The authors concluded that the prevalence of renovascular disease in a population of hypertensive children subjected to renal arteriography is approximately 40%, and the criteria that are quoted above were useful guides for the application of renal arteriography in children with hypertension.

THERAPY

Most pediatricians agree that anti-hypertensive therapy should be instituted in children who have persistent elevation of blood pressure above the 99th percentile. However, as there are currently no long-term studies to evaluate the effect of treatment on end-organ damage in children, it is difficult to provide evidence that treating children for this disorder results in a reduction in their risk for cardiovascular disease.[39] Even less clear is the appropriate approach to the therapeutic management of children and adolescents with blood pressure between the 95th and 99th percentiles, although attempts to improve the exercise level and dietary habits of such children should be adopted. Indeed, the initial treatment for all children with hypertension should involve weight reduction, exercise, and dietary intervention. Body size which is the major determinant for blood pressure among children and blood pressure is directly related to the degree of physical fitness. Weight reduction, although difficult to achieve, has been shown to be an effective therapy for obese children with hypertension.[40] Exercise is helpful in reducing weight and blood pressure levels as well, with better effects on systolic than on diastolic blood pressure levels.[41,42]

The effect of sodium restriction on blood pressure reduction in children with borderline hypertension was evaluated by the Minneapolis Children's Blood Pressure Study.[43] Study participants were randomized either to a family intervention involving a low-sodium diet or to no therapy. Despite achieving a reduction in the sodium intake in the study group, as shown by measured urinary sodium excretion, no significant reduction in blood pressure was observed in patients in the treatment arm compared with the control group. Other possible dietary interventions, including potassium and calcium supplements, have been suggested but lack evidence of efficacy.[44]

PHARMACOLOGIC TREATMENT

Pharmacologic therapy should be administered to children who have severe hypertension, have evidence of end-organ damage, or do not respond to non-pharmacologic measures. However, it is not clear when drug therapy should be started in asymptomatic patients with mild or moderate elevation of BP. When pharmacologic therapy is instituted, the goal is to reduce blood pressure to levels below the 95th percentile. Table 10.7 shows the dosages of most of the commonly prescribed agents used to manage chronic pediatric hypertension. Antihypertensive drug treatment should be individualized, depending on the level of blood pressure, degree of response, occurrence of side effects, and patient's medical history. Children with secondary hypertension, which may or may not be cured, should have therapy directed at the underlying cause of the hypertension if this is feasible.

CALCIUM CHANNEL BLOCKERS

Calcium channel blockers reduce blood pressure by dilating peripheral arterioles in a dose-dependent fashion. Nifedipine, amlodipine, nicardipine, and felodipine are the most commonly prescribed cal-

Table 10.7 Common oral antihypertensive drugs and dosage regimens[a] for treatment of pediatric hypertension

Drug	Initial dose (mg/kg/dose)	Maximum dose (mg/kg/day)	Dosing interval
Amlodipine	0.1	0.34	q24h
Nifedipine XL	0.25	3 mg (up to 120 mg/day)	q12–24h
Captopril	0.3	2	q8–q12h
Enalapril	0.08 (max 5 mg)	0.6 (up to 40 mg/day)	q12–24h
Lisinopril	0.07	0.6 (up to 40 mg/day)	q24h
Benazepril	0.2	0.6 (up to 40 mg/day)	q25h
Losartan	0.7	1.4 (up to 100 mg/day)	q24h
Propranolol	1	4 (up to 640 mg/day)	q6–q12h
Atenolol	0.5–1	2 (up to 100 mg/day)	q12–24h
Labetalol	1	10–12 (up to 1200 mg/day)	q12h
Hydrochloro-thiazide	1	3	q12h
Metalozone	0.1	3	q12h
Spironolactone	1	3	q12–24h
Hydralazine	0.75	7.5 (up to 200 mg/day)	q6–12h
Minoxidil	0.2	Maximum 50 mg/day	q8–q24h
Chlorothiazide	10–20 p.o.	20–40 p.o.	q12h
Infants <6 mo	1–4 i.v.	2–8 i.v.	q12h
Infants 6–12 mo	10 p.o.	20	q12h
and children	4	4	q24h

[a]Dosage regimens are based on limited published data and thus are not definitive[55]

cium channel blockers in children. Unfortunately there are only a few controlled studies available to define optimal dosages and long-term safety and efficacy profiles for these drugs.[45–47]

ANGIOTENSIN-CONVERTING ENZYME INHIBITORS

Angiotensin-converting enzyme (ACE) inhibitors decrease blood pressure by inhibiting formation of angiotensin II and by inactivating the kinases that degrade bradykinin, a potent vasodilator. Captopril is the most widely studied ACE inhibitor in children.[48] It reduces both systemic vascular resistance and left ventricular pressure, and causes negative inotropic and chronotropic effects. As inhibition increases, a precipitous drop in blood pressure may occur.[49] Neonates and infants respond to ACE inhibitors to a greater extent and for a longer duration than older children.[49] This increased sensitivity may be explained by the higher renin levels in the first few months of life, or by renal and hepatic immaturity leading to decreased drug clearance. In premature infants and those up to six months of age, 0.1–0.2 mg/kg/dose is recommended by the International Collaborative Study Group.[48] Enalapril and lisinopril are two newer ACE inhibitors with longer elimination half-lives that allow dosing once/day. Enalapril has similar efficacy to captopril in controlling blood pressure. ACE inhibitors seem to be better tolerated by children, with fewer side effects that adults.[48,49] ACE inhibitors should be avoided in the presence of bilateral renal artery stenosis or in cases where renal artery stenosis of a transplanted kidney is suspected, because these agents may significantly reduce renal function.

β-BLOCKERS

β-adrenergic blockers decrease cardiac output, inhibit renin secretion, reduce plasma volume, reduce peripheral vascular resistance, and reset baroreceptor levels. These agents are not as widely used for treatment of pediatric hypertension as calcium channel blockers or ACE inhibitors predominantly because of their potential side effects in patients with asthma and chronic obstructive lung disease. There is extensive pediatric experience with the use of propranolol[50,51] and other β-blockers.[52,53] Cardioselective agents such as atenolol and metoprolol may be given in patients with diabetes mellitus or congestive heart failure as well as in patients experiencing night terrors with propranolol[52] with the advantage of once daily dosing and cardioselectivity at low doses. Metoprolol blunts the response of systolic blood pressure and heart rate to aerobic exercise and mental stress in children, with significant reductions of systolic blood pressure, diastolic blood pressure, and heart rate. It was not associated with limitation in endurance capacity and heart rates increased to maximum levels; it is suggested that this agent could be useful for an athletic adolescent patient.[52]

DIURETICS

Diuretics reduce intra-vascular volume, decrease peripheral vascular resistance, and reduce systemic blood pressure. Thiazide diuretics are frequently prescribed in children for treatment of hypertension if multiple-drug treatment is required. Their adverse effects are mostly related to electrolyte disorders, such as hypokalemia, hyponatremia, hypomagnesemia, and hyperuricemia. Although it is commonly assumed that thiazide diuretics are ineffective in patients with advanced renal failure (GFR < 30 ml/min/1.73 m^2), the co-administration of a thiazide diuretic and a loop diuretic was found to be synergistic in advanced chronic renal failure.[54] Furosemide is a loop diuretic frequently prescribed in children. Spironolactone is a potassium-sparing diuretic commonly given to children. Its principal indication is for hypertension due to mineralocorticoid excess. Pediatric experience with other potassium sparing diuretics, such as eplerenone and amiloride, is still very limited.

SPECIAL CONSIDERATIONS

In some clinical situations, the decision to adopt pharmacologic intervention should be considered at lower levels of blood pressure; this seems to be the case for chronic renal failure and for children with diabetes mellitus. In these groups of patients, an effort should be made to keep blood pressure levels below the 95th percentile. Patients who have severe hypertension, often associated with symptoms, should be referred to a pediatric cardiologist or nephrologist for immediate attention. Surgical treatment of renovascular hypertension in carefully selected young patients is an important possibility that should be considered when evaluating a patient with severe hypertension.

REFERENCES

1. Lauer RM, Clarke WR. Childhood risk factors for high adult blood pressure: The Muscatine Study. Pediatrics 1989; 84:633–641.
2. Klag MJ, Whelton PK, Randall BL. Blood pressure and end-stage renal disease in men. N Engl J Med 1996; 334:13–18.

3. Gillman MW, Cook NR. Blood pressure measurement in childhood epidemiological studies. Circulation 1995; 92:1049–57.

4. Vyse TJ. Sphygmomanometer bladder length and measurements of blood pressure in children. Lancet 1987; 1:561–562.

5. Whincup PH, Cook DG, Shaper AG. Blood pressure measurement in children: the importance of cuff bladder size. J Hypertens 1989; 7:845–850.

6. Prineas RJ, Jacobs D. Quality of Korotkoff sounds: bell vs diaphragm, cubital fossa vs brachial artery. Prev Med 1983; 12:715–719.

7. Stolt M, Sjönell G, Aström H et al. Factors affecting the validity of the standard blood pressure cuff. Clin Physiol 1993; 13:611–620.

8. National Heart, Lung and Blood Institute. Report of the Task Force on Blood Pressure Control in Children. Pediatrics 1977; 59:797–820.

9. Report of the Second Task Force on Blood Pressure Control in Children – 1987. Task Force on Blood Pressure Control in Children. National Heart, Lung and Blood Institute, Bethesda, Maryland. Pediatrics 1987; 79:1–25.

10. Rosner B, Prineas RJ, Loggie JM et al. Blood pressure nomograms for children and adolescents, by height, sex and age, in the United States. J Pediatr 1993; 123:871–886.

11. Update on the 1987 Task Force Report on High Blood Pressure in Children and Adolescents: a working group report from the National High Blood Pressure Education Program. National High Blood Pressure Education Program Working Group on Hypertension Control in Chldren and Adolescents. Pediatrics 1996; 98:649–658.

12. Centers for Disease Control and Prevention, National Center for Health Statistics. National Health and Nutrition Examination Survey NHANHES III; 1988–1991, data computed for the National Heart, Lung and Blood Institute, Atlanta, GA: Centers for Disease Control and Prevention.

13. The Fourth Report on the Diagnosis, Evaluation, and Treatment of High Blood Pressure in Children and Adolescents. National High Blood Pressure Education Program Working Group on High Blood Pressure in Children and Adolescents. Pediatrics 2004; 114:555–576

14. Hulman S, Edwards R, Chen YQ et al. Blood pressure patterns in the first three days of life. J Perinatol 1991; 11:231–234.

15. Zubrow A, Hulman S, Kushner H et al. Determinants of blood pressure in infants admitted to neonatal intensive care units: a prospective multicenter study. J Perinatol 1995; 15:470–479.

16. Lurbe E, Cremades B, Rodriguez C et al. Factors related to quality of ambulatory blood pressure monitoring in a pediatric population. Am J Hypertens 1999; 12:929–933.

17. Koch VH, Colli A, Saito MI et al. Comparison between casual blood pressure and ambulatory blood pressure monitoring parameters in healthy and hypertensive adolescents. Blood Press Monit 2000; 5:281–289.

18. O'Brien E, Beevers G, Lip GY. ABC of hypertension. Blood pressure measurement. Part III – automated sphygmomanometry: ambulatory blood pressure measurement. BMJ 2001; 322:1110–1114.

19. Sorof JM, Portman RJ. White coat hypertension in children with elevated casual blood pressure. J Pediatr 2000; 137:493–497.

20. Vaindirlis I, Peppa-Patrikiou M, Dracopoulou M et al. 'White coat hypertension' in adolescents: Increased values of urinary cortisol and endothelin. J Pediatr 2000; 136:359–364.

21. Koch VH, Furusawa EA, Ignes E et al. Ambulatory blood pressure monitoring of chronically dialyzed pediatric patients. Blood Press Monit 1999; 4:213–216.

22. Belsha CW, Wells TG, McNiece KL et al. Influence of diurnal blood pressure variations on target organ abnormalities in adolescents with mild essential hypertension. Am J Hypertens 1998; 11:410–417.

23. Kapuku GK, Treiber FA, Davis HC et al. Hemodynamic function at rest, during acute stress, and in the field: predictors of cardiac structure and function two years later in youth. Hypertension 1999; 34:1026–1031.

24. Soergel M, Kirschstein M, Busch C et al. Oscillometric twenty-four-hour ambulatory blood pressure values in healthy children and adolescents: a multicenter trial including 1141 subjects. J Pediatr 1997; 130:178–184.

25. Lurbe E, Cremades B, Torro MI et al. Reference values of ambulatory blood pressure in children and adolescents [abstract]. Am J Hypertens 2000; 13:265.

26. Sorof JM, Portman RJ. Ambulatory blood pressure measurements. Curr Opinion Pediatr 2001; 13:133–137.

27. Sinaiko AR. Current concepts: hypertension in children. N Engl J Med 1996; 335:1968–1973.

28. Sorof JM. Systolic hypertension in children: benign or beware? Pediatr Nephrol 2001; 16(6):517–525.

29. Sorof JM. Prevalence and consequence of systolic hypertension in children. Am J Hypertens 2002; 15:57S–60S.

30. Daniels SR, Meyer RA, Strife CF et al. Distribution of target-organ abnormalities by race and sex in children with essential hypertension. J Hum Hypertens 1990; 4:103–104.

31. Sorof JM, Alexandrov AV, Cardwell G et al. Carotid artery intimal-medial thickness and left ventricular hypertrophy in children with elevated blood pressure. Pediatrics 2003; 111:61–66.

32. Yiu VWY, Dluhy RP, Lifton RP et al. Low peripheral plasma renin activity as a critical marker in pediatric hypertension. Pediatr Nephrol 1997; 11:343–346.

33. Rosano TG, Swift TA, Hayes LW. Advances in catecholamine and metabolite measurements for diagnosis of pheochromocytoma. Clin Chem 1991; 37:1854–1867.

34. Gardet V, Gatta B, Simonnet G et al. Lessons from an unpleasant surprise: a biochemical strategy for the diagnosis of pheochromocytoma. J Hypertens 2001; 19:1029–1035

35. Eisenhofer G, Huynh TT, Hiroi M et al. Understanding catecholamine metabolism as a guide to the biochemical diagnosis of pheochromocytoma. Rev Endocrinol Metab Disord 2001; 2:297–311

36. McTaggart SJ, Gulati S, Walker RG et al. Evaluation and long-term outcome of pediatric renovascular hypertension. Pediatr Nephrol 2000; 14:1022–1029.

37. Deal JE, Snell MF, Barratt TM et al. Renovascular disease in childhood. J Pediatr 1992; 121:378–384.

38. Shahdadpuri J, Frank R, Gauthier BG et al. Yield of renal arteriography in the evaluation of pediatric hypertension. Pediatr Nephrol 2000; 14:816–819.

39. Kay J, Sinaiko AR, Daniels SR. Pediatric hypertension. Am J Heart J 2001; 142:422–432.

40. Rocchini AP, Katch V, Anderson J et al. Blood pressure in adolescents: effect of weight loss. Pediatrics 1988; 82:16–23.

41. Hagberg JM, Goldring D, Holloszy JO. Effect of exercise training on the blood pressure and hemodynamic features of hypertensive adolescents. Am J Cardiol 1983; 52:763–768.

42. Hansen HS, Hyldebrandt N, Froberg K et al. Blood pressure and physical fitness in a population of children – the Odense Schoolchild Study. J Hum Hypertens 1990; 4:615–620.

43. Gillum RF, Elmer PJ, Prineas RJ. Changing sodium intake in children: The Minneapolis Children's Blood Pressure Study. Hypertension 1981; 3:698–703.

44. Miller JZ, Wienberger MH, Christian JC. Blood pressure response to potassium supplement in normotensive adults and children. Hypertension 1987; 10:437–442.

45. Sinaiko AR. Clinical pharmacology of converting enzyme inhibitors, calcium channel blockers and diuretics. J Hum Hypertens 1994; 8:389–394.
46. Resnick L. Calcium metabolism, renin activity, and the antihypertensive effects of calcium channel blockade. Am J Med 1986; 81:6–14.
47. Tallian KB, Nahata MC, Turman MA et al. Efficacy of amlodipine in pediatric patients with hypertension. Pediatr Nephrol 1999; 13:304–310.
48. Mirkin BL, Newman TJ. Efficacy and safety of captopril in the treatment of severe childhood hypertension: report of the international collaborative group. Pediatrics 1985; 75:1091–2002.
49. Sinaiko A, Kashtan CE, Mirkin BL. Antihypertensive drug therapy with captopril in children and adolescents. Clin Exp Theory Pract 1986; 8:829–839.
50. Griswold WR, McNeal R, Mendoza SA. Propranolol as an antihypertensive agent in children. Arch Dis Child 1978; 53:594–598.
51. Boertl RC. Effect of propranolol in the treatment of hypertension in children. Pediatr Res 1976; 10:328–332.
52. Falkner B, Lowenthal DT, Affrime MB. The pharmacodynamic effectiveness of metoprolol in adolescent hypertension. Pediatr Pharmacol 1982; 2:49–55.
53. Ishisaka DY, Yonan CD, Housel BF. Labetolol treatment of hypertension in a child. Clin Pharm 1991; 10:500–501.
54. Fliser D, Schroter M, Neubeck M et al. Coadministration of thiazides increases the efficacy of loop diuretics even in patients with advanced renal failure. Kidney Int 1994; 46:482–488.
55. Temple ME, Nahata MC. Treatment of pediatric hypertension. Pharmacotherapy 2000; 20(2):140–50.

11. Cardiovascular disease in patients with kidney disorders in childhood and adolescence

Rulan Parekh, Mark Mitsnefes and Stephen Daniels

INTRODUCTION

Atherosclerosis, previously thought to occur only in adults, has been described in adolescents and young adults from autopsy studies with evidence of a fatty streak or initial plaque formation in the coronary arteries and the aorta. Antecedents of cardiovascular disease in the general pediatric population, including elevated body mass index (BMI), hypertension, and dyslipidemia, have also been shown to track into adulthood, and are associated with the development of atherosclerosis.[1–4] In addition, left ventricular hypertrophy (LVH), an independent predictor of cardiovascular morbidity and mortality in adults, is frequently found in children with essential hypertension.[5,6]

It is well known that adults with chronic kidney disease (CKD) are at high-risk for cardiovascular disease and often die from cardiovascular causes. Children with CKD are also at risk for accelerated rates of cardiovascular disease due to the high burden of cardiovascular risk factors in CKD.

EPIDEMIOLOGY

Cardiovascular disease has been identified as the leading cause of mortality in adult ESRD patients accounting for over 40% of deaths.[7] In children with CKD, the burden of cardiovascular disease is less clear, as the overt clinical manifestations of cardiovascular disease are not common in children, and the early more subtle cardiovascular abnormalities are more difficult to measure. Data from the United States Renal Data System (USRDS), a national registry of End Stage Renal Disease (ESRD) patients, show that approximately 25% of all deaths in this patient population are due to cardiovascular causes with Black and dialysis patients having the highest risk of a cardiac death (Fig. 11.1).[8] Cardiac arrest is one of the leading causes of death in pediatric ESRD patients. Cardiovascular death rates in the pediatric population on dialysis are significantly greater than the nationally reported death rates in the general pediatric population.[8]

Children undergoing chronic dialysis have a prevalence of cardiovascular disease of 31% with cardiac arrhythmia being the most common cardiovascular abnormality.[9] The prevalence of cardiomyopathy has doubled from 1991 to 1996 in the population with ESRD.[9] Echocardiographic studies have shown that children with CKD have a high prevalence and persistence of left ventricular hypertrophy (LVH).[10–14] This is already present in children with mild-to-moderate renal insufficiency (31%) and has been reported in up to 75% of children on dialysis (Fig. 11.2).[15] Unfortunately, cardiac hypertrophy persists even after successful renal transplantation with prevalence rates between 56% and 82%.[14–16] Increased left ventricular mass may initially have the beneficial effect of reducing left ventricular wall stress, but longstanding cardiac hypertrophy might lead ultimately to maladaptive LVH with decreased capillary density, coronary reserve, and subendocardial perfusion, and the subsequent development of myocardial fibrosis.

Studies of cardiac function in children with CKD have demonstrated that children with pre-dialysis stages of renal failure, and those on chronic dialysis, have a hyperdynamic circulation as evidenced by increased contractility of the left ventricle at rest.[15] However, dialysis patients had significantly diminished contractile reserve during exercise tests, which might reflect the early development of a maladaptive stage of LVH with risk of ultimate worsening of

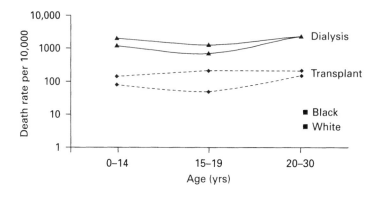

Figure 11.1 Cardiovascular mortality in pediatric ESRD patients: relationship with mode of therapy, age and race (1990–96)
Adapted from Parekh RS, Carrol C, Wolfe RA, Port FK[8], with permission from Elsevier. (See color plate section)

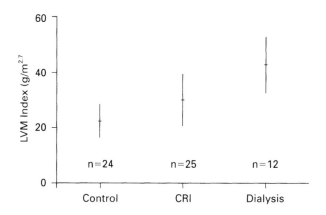

Figure 11.2 Left ventricular mass index (LVMI) in children with CKD and ESRD[15]

cardiac function over time.[15] This emphasizes the importance of routine monitoring of cardiac structure and function in pediatric patients with CKD, especially in children on chronic dialysis. We recommend annual echocardiographic evaluation to assess these children for the presence of LVH and systolic or diastolic dysfunction of the LV.

Due to the difficulty in imaging and screening children for atherosclerosis, there are few data currently available in large cohorts defining and classifying cardiovascular disease. In a small autopsy series of patients with CKD and nephrotic syndrome, there are data revealing that 80% of the patients had moderate to severe atherosclerosis in the coronary arteries.[17] In a study of 12 transplant patients, intimal thickening or atheromatous plaques in the iliac artery was revealed in 33% of subjects with glomerulonephritis, and 100% of subjects with obstructive uropathy. The higher frequency in the latter group was probably due to a longer duration of ESRD in those patients.[18]

Newer imaging techniques suggest an increased prevalence of subclinical atherosclerosis in young adults with onset of ESRD during childhood, as detected by elevated coronary artery calcium scores or intimal medial thickness.[19,20] Up to 90% of these patients have evidence of coronary artery calcifications which may reflect atherosclerosis or medial wall calcification.[20] In addition, there is evidence of abnormal arterial wall compliance in pediatric onset ESRD compared to controls, which may also reflect the development of early atherosclerosis.[21,22]

Another measure of early vascular disease is endothelial dysfunction which has been shown to occur in pediatric patients with CKD, and has been found to be independent of lipid profile abnormalities or hypertension.[21,23,24] It is not currently known how to treat abnormalities of endothelial function. However, this might be improved by lowering homocysteine via dietary folate treatment.[24]

CARDIOVASCULAR RISK FACTORS IN CHILDHOOD CKD

Traditional cardiovascular risk factors such as hypertension and dyslipidemia are highly prevalent in pediatric patients with CKD.[25,26] The progression of kidney failure complicates the pathogenesis of atherosclerosis as the metabolism of novel risk factors such as Lp(a), homocysteine, calcium and phosphorus metabolism requires normal renal function. Despite the young age of the pediatric CKD patients, this subgroup is at particularly high-risk due to the clustering of traditional and non-traditional risk factors (Figs 11.3 and 11.4) in the unique uremic environment, with volume and pressure overload, which may accelerate the process of cardiovascular abnormalities with ultimately the development of symptomatic disease.

TRADITIONAL RISK FACTORS

Dyslipidemias are commonly described in children with CKD.[25] An elevated low density lipoprotein-cholesterol (LDL) is associated with atherosclerotic disease in the general population. In the pediatric population, from cross sectional studies, the prevalence of dyslipidemias is very high in ESRD. Data from studies published after 1980 with a sample

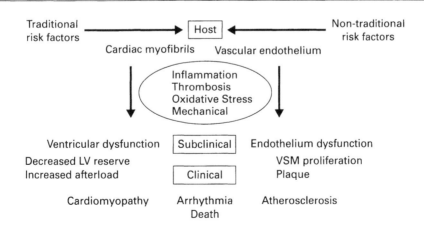

Figure 11.3 Schematic of cardiovascular disease in chronic kidney disease

Rulan S Parekh, Samuel S Gidding.[45] With kind permission of Springer Science and Business Media

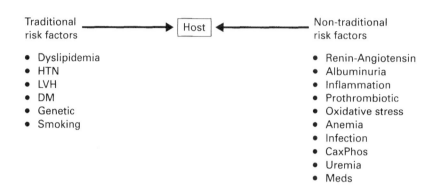

Figure 11.4 Schematic of cardiovascular disease risk factors in chronic kidney disease
RS Parekh, Samuel S Gidding.[45] With kind permission of Springer Science and Business Media

size greater than 15 patients, reported the prevalence of dyslipidemia in patients on dialysis to range from 29% to 87%.[25] An elevated LDL [>100 mg/dl (>2.29 mmol/l)] was reported in 72% to 84% of pediatric kidney transplant recipients.[25] There are no longitudinal studies, however, which have defined the long-term risk of dyslipidemias in children with CKD, particularly as they survive into young adulthood. In addition, nephrotic syndrome is associated with hypercholesterolemia. It is unclear at present if this is associated with the progression of CKD in children. Limited data are available on other lipoproteins, except Lp(a), which is composed of LDL and apolipoprotein(a), and is homologous to plasminogen.[27–29] Lp(a) interacts with macrophages and interferes with the fibrinolytic system. Lp(a) levels are largely genetically determined, but increase with worsening renal function.[27,28] Elevated Lp(a) has been shown to be an independent risk factor for atherosclerotic cardiovascular disease in adults on hemodialysis.[27,28] In the pediatric ESRD population, it has been shown that Lp(a) levels increase in patients receiving growth hormone.[29,30] This may be important since therapy with growth hormone is common in the pediatric CKD. At this time, routine screening

for Lp(a) is not recommended, and no specific treatment options are available for elevated Lp(a) levels.

Hypertension has been a known complication in children with CKD.[31–33] The prevalence of hypertension has not changed and remained high for the last two decades. The 2003 Annual Report from the North American Pediatric Renal Transplant Cooperative Study (NAPRTCS) demonstrated that 38% of children with pre-ESRD, 60% children on chronic dialysis, and 70% of children after transplantation used antihypertensive medications. Recent studies have demonstrated that elevated blood pressure in children and young adults with CKD is associated with cardiac hypertrophy.[10,11,16] Improvement of blood pressure over time with treatment may lead to regression of LVH in these children.[10,34] Hypertension also adversely affects vascular structure and function in children with CKD. Recent studies have shown an association of elevated blood pressure with endothelial dysfunction of the brachial artery[21] and abnormal carotid artery wall compliance[22] in children and young adults on chronic dialysis and after transplantation. These data emphasize the importance of strict blood pressure control to prevent progression or development of hypertension-related cardiovascular injury.

NON-TRADITIONAL RISK FACTORS

Knowledge regarding non-traditional risk factors in children with CKD is limited. Further long-term observational studies are needed to determine the association of these novel risk factors and cardiovascular disease in childhood. These novel risk factors may include homocysteine, inflammation, malnutrition, oxidative stress, proteinuria, anemia, infection, activation of the renin-angiotensin system, and treatment with certain medications.[35] Hyperphosphatemia and hypercalcemia in ESRD patients on hemodialysis has been associated with increased cardiovascular mortality in adults.[36,37] In children, vascular and soft tissue calcification has been reported in many post-mortem studies.[18–20,38,39] In the pediatric CKD population, it is unclear if calcium and phosphorus metabolism may play a role only when the patients are dialysis dependent.

It has been established that homocysteine is significantly elevated in CKD.[40,41] This may predispose to vessel damage, and aid the thrombogenic process and plaque formation. Levels of homocysteine are increased in children with CKD.[24,42,43] Preliminary studies show an association of increased homocysteine with endothelial dysfunction. Homocysteine has been shown to be elevated in >65% children with CKD. Interestingly, the level appears only to increase after seven years of age and the increase is independent of renal function.[43] The higher the homocysteine levels in children with CKD, the lower the vitamin B_{12} and folate levels.[43] This may indicate nutritional deficiencies in the pediatric ESRD population. Despite the high prevalence of homocysteinemia in the CKD population, there are still only preliminary data showing that lowering of homocysteine will have a protective effect on the heart and blood vessels in the pediatric population with CKD.[24] The currently recommended supplementation of vitamins in the dialysis population should have adequate folate and B complex vitamins.[40] At present, routine testing and treatment has not been recommended for the general popula-

tion or patients with ESRD. Randomized controlled trials are under way to study the question of homocysteine lowering and improved survival in the adult transplant population.[44]

MODIFICATION OF PEDIATRIC CARDIOVASCULAR DISEASE (CVD)

Little is known about the natural history of CVD in ESRD patients due to lack of prospective longitudinal studies with long duration of follow-up. In addition, the prevalence of conventional CVD risk factors such as obesity, insulin resistance, and smoking is not known; however, screening of these traditional risk factors would be important. The screening for family history of early coronary disease is also important in the prevention of cardiovascular disease.

Preventive measures in pediatric patients should include routine screening, monitoring, and treatment of traditional cardiovascular risk factors, such as hypertension and dyslipidemias. The current available guidelines on treatment of dyslipidemia should be used for children with CKD stage 1–4; adolescents with stage V CKD should use the NKF K/DOQI guidelines.[25] The strategies in the management of hypertension in many cases will be determined by the causes of elevated BP in children with CKD (see chapter 10). Regardless of the cause, the goal is to keep blood pressure below child's age, sex and height specific 90th percentile. All major classes of antihypertensive medications have been used in the treatment of hypertension in children with CKD. However, angiotensin converting enzyme inhibitors (ACEI) and angiotensin II blockers are being used increasingly as the antihypertensive drugs of choice. The rationale for use of these medications derives from the large body of evidence demonstrating their beneficial effect beyond blood pressure control including renal and cardiac protection in patients with diabetic and non-diabetic chronic kidney diseases.

Children with CKD are at risk for the accelerated development of CVD. There is a window of opportunity for aggressive CVD preventive therapy to be instituted in pediatric patients. Hopefully, these patients will benefit in terms of long-term prognosis and outcome. Prevention of cardiovascular disease should be a top clinical priority in the management of children with CKD.

REFERENCES

1. Berenson GS, Srinivasan SR, Bao W, Newman WP, Tracy RE, Wattigney WA. Association between multiple cardiovascular risk factors and atherosclerosis in children and young adults. The Bogalusa Heart Study. N Engl J Med 1998; 338:1650–1656.
2. Enos WF, Holmes RH, Beyer J. Coronary disease among United States soldiers killed in action in Korea. JAMA 1953; 152:1090–1093.
3. Enos WF, Holmes RH, Beyer J. Landmark article, July 18, 1953: Coronary disease among United States soldiers killed in action in Korea. Preliminary report. By William F. Enos, Robert H. Holmes and James Beyer. JAMA 1986; 256:2859–2862.
4. Strong JPMG, McMahan CA, Tracy RE, Newman WP, Herderick EE, Cornhill JF. Prevalence and Extent of Atherosclerosis in Adolescents and Young Adults for Prevention from the Pathobiological Determinants of Atherosclerosis in Youth Study. JAMA 1999; 281 (8):727–735.
5. Daniels SR, Loggie JM, Khoury P, Kimball TR. Left ventricular geometry and severe left ventricular hypertrophy in children and adolescents with essential hypertension. Circulation 1998; 97:1907–1911.
6. Daniels SR. Cardiovascular sequelae of childhood hypertension. Am J Hypertens 2002; 15:61S–63S.
7. Levey AS. Controlling the epidemic of cardiovascular disease in chronic renal disease: Where do we start? Am J Kid Dis 1998; 32:S5–13.
8. Parekh RS, Carroll CE, Wolfe RA, Port FK. Cardiovascular mortality in children and young adults with end-stage kidney disease. J Pediatr 2002; 141:191–197.
9. Chavers BM, Li S, Collins AJ, Herzog CA. Cardiovascular disease in pediatric chronic dialysis patients. Kidney Int 2002; 62:648–653.
10. Mitsnefes MM, Daniels SR, Schwartz SM, Khoury P, Strife CF. Changes in left ventricular mass in children and adolescents during chronic dialysis. Pediatr Nephrol 2001; 16:318–323.
11. Mitsnefes MM, Daniels SR, Schwartz SM, Meyer RA, Khoury P, Strife CF. Severe left ventricular hypertrophy in pediatric dialysis: prevalence and predictors. Pediatr Nephrol 2000; 14:898–902.
12. Morris KP, Skinner JR, Wren C, Hunter S, Coulthard MG. Cardiac abnormalities in end stage renal failure and anaemia. Arch Dis Child 1993; 68:637–643.
13. Ulmer H. Cardiovascular impairment and physical working capacity in children with chronic renal failure. Acta Paediatrica Scandinavia 1978; 67:43–48.
14. Johnstone LM, Jones CL, Grigg LE, Wilkinson JL, Walker RG, Powell HR. Left ventricular abnormalities in children, adolescents and young adults with renal disease. Kidney Int 1996; 50:998–1006.
15. Mitsnefes MM, Kimball TR, Witt SA, Glascock BJ, Khoury PR, Daniels SR. Left ventricular mass and systolic performance in pediatric patients with chronic renal failure. Circulation 2003; 107:864–8.
16. Matteucci MC, Giordano U, Calzolari A, Turchetta A, Santilli A, Rizzoni G. Left ventricular hypertrophy, treadmill tests, and 24-hour blood pressure in pediatric transplant patients. Kidney Int 1999; 56:1566–1570.
17. Portman RJ, Hawkins E, Verani R. Premature atherosclerosis in pediatric renal patients: Report of the Southwest Pediatric Nephrology Study Group. Pediatr Res 1991; 29:349A.
18. Nayir A, Bilge I, Kilicaslan I, Ander H, Emre S, Sirin A. Arterial changes in paediatric haemodialysis patients undergoing renal transplantation. Nephrol Dial Transplant 2001; 16:2041–2047.
19. Goodman WG, Goldin J, Kuizon BD et al. Coronary-artery calcification in young adults with end-stage renal disease who are undergoing dialysis. N Engl J Med 2000; 342:1478–1483.
20. Oh J, Wunsch R, Turzer M et al. Advanced coronary and carotid arteriopathy in young adults with childhood-onset chronic renal failure. Circulation 2002; 106:100–105.
21. Lilien MR, Stroes ES, Op't Roodt J, de Jongh S, Schroder CH, Koomans HA. Vascular function in children after renal transplantation. Am J Kidney Dis 2003; 41:684–691.
22. Groothoff JW, Gruppen MP, Offringa M et al. Increased arterial stiffness in young adults with end-stage renal disease since childhood. J Am Soc Nephrol 2002; 13:2953–2961.
23. Kari JA DA, Vallance DT, Bruckdorfer KR, Leone A, Mullen MJ, Bunce T, Dorado B, Deanfield JE, Rees L. Physiology and biochemistry of endothelial function in children with chronic renal failure. Kidney International 1997; 52:468–472.
24. Bennett-Richards K, Kattenhorn M, Donald A et al. Does oral folic acid lower total homocysteine levels and improve endothelial function in children with chronic renal failure? Circulation 2002; 105:1810–1815.
25. National Kidney Foundation: K/DOQI Clinical Practice Guidelines for Managing Dyslipidemias in Chronic Kidney Disease. Am J Kidney Dis 2003; 41:S1–S92.
26. Mitsnefes M, Ho PL, McEnery PT. Hypertension and progression of chronic renal insufficiency in children: a report of the North American Pediatric Renal Transplant Cooperative Study (NAPRTCS). J Am Soc Nephrol 2003; 14:2618–2622.
27. Kronenberg F, Neyer U, Lhotta K et al. The low molecular weight apo(a) phenotype is an independent predictor for coronary artery disease in hemodialysis patients: a prospective follow-up. J Am Soc Nephrol 1999; 10(5):1027–1036.
28. Kronenberg F, Utermann G, Dieplinger H. Lipoprotein(a) in renal disease. Am J Kidney Dis 1996; 27:1–25.
29. Querfeld U, Lang M, Friedrich JB, Kohl B, Fiehn W, Scharer K. Lipoprotein(a) serum levels and apolipoprotein(a) phenotypes in children with chronic renal disease. Pediatr Res 1993; 34:772–776.
30. Querfeld U, Haffner D, Wuhl E et al. Treatment with growth hormone increases lipoprotein(a) serum levels in children with chronic renal insufficiency. Eur J Pediatr 1996; 155:913.
31. Drukker A. Hypertension in children and adolescents with chronic renal failure and end-stage renal disease. Child Nephrol Urol 1991; 11:152–158.
32. Baluarte HJ, Gruskin AB, Ingelfinger JR, Stablein D, Tejani A. Analysis of hypertension in children post renal transplantation – a report of the North American Pediatric Renal Transplant Cooperative Study (NAPRTCS). Pediatr Nephrol 1994; 8:570–573.
33. Fivush BA, Jabs K, Neu AM et al. Chronic renal insufficiency in children and adolescents: the 1996 annual report of NAPRTCS. North American Pediatric Renal Transplant Cooperative Study. Pediatr Nephrol 1998; 12:328–337.
34. Miltenyi G. Monitoring cardiovascular changes during hemodialysis in children. Pediatr Nephrol 2001; 16:19–24.

35. Chavers B, Schnaper HW. Risk factors for cardiovascular disease in children on maintenance dialysis. Adv Ren Replace Ther 2001; 8:180–190.

36. Block GA, Hulbert-Shearon TE, Levin NW, Port FK. Association of serum phosphorus and calcium x phosphate product with mortality risk in chronic hemodialysis patients: a national study. Am J Kidney Dis 1998; 31:607–617.

37. Ganesh SK, Stack AG, Levin NW, Hulbert-Shearon T, Port FK. Association of elevated serum PO_4, Ca x PO_4 product, and parathyroid hormone with cardiac mortality risk in chronic hemodialysis patients. J Am Soc Nephrol 2001; 12:2131–2138.

38. Litwin M, Grenda R, Prokurat S et al. Patient survival and causes of death on hemodialysis and peritoneal dialysis – single-center study. Pediatr Nephrol 2001; 16:996–1001.

39. Milliner DA ZA, Lieberman E, Landing B. Soft tissue calcification in pediatric patients with end-stage renal disease. Kidney International 1990; 38:931–936.

40. Bostom AG. Homocysteine: 'expensive creatinine' or important modifiable risk factor for arteriosclerotic outcomes in renal transplant recipients? J Am Soc Nephrol 2000; 11:149–151.

41. Bostom AG, Kronenberg F, Jacques PF et al. Proteinuria and plasma total homocysteine levels in chronic renal disease patients with a normal range serum creatinine: critical impact of true glomerular filtration rate. Atherosclerosis 2001; 159:219–223.

42. Canepa A, Carrea A, Caridi G et al. Homocysteine, folate, vitamin B_{12} levels, and C677T MTHFR mutation in children with renal failure. Pediatr Nephrol 2003; 18:225–229.

43. Merouani A, Lambert M, Delvin EE, Genest J, Jr., Robitaille P, Rozen R. Plasma homocysteine concentration in children with chronic renal failure. Pediatr Nephrol 2001; 16:805–811.

44. Bostom AG, Kronenberg F, Gohh RY et al. Chronic renal transplantation: a model for the hyperhomocysteinemia of renal insufficiency. Atherosclerosis 2001; 156:227–230.

45. Rulan S Parekh, Samuel S Gidding. Cardiovascular complications in pediatric end-stage renal disease. Pediatr Nephrol. 2005; 20(2):125–131.

12. Urinary tract infections and vesico-ureteral reflux in children

Tommy Linné

INTRODUCTION

Urinary tract infection (UTI) is one of the most common bacterial infections during childhood.[1,2] Half of the UTIs involve the kidneys resulting in acute pyelonephritis, with subsequent risk for permanent renal injury (scarring) and possible deterioration of renal function and hypertension in later life. Renal scarring may be avoided, or reduced in many patients, by early treatment and investigation of predisposing factors, such as obstruction and vesico-ureteral reflux. The correct UTI diagnosis in the febrile infant is essential in these efforts. Table 12.1 gives some definitions that are useful in describing UTIs in infants and children.

PATHOPHYSIOLOGY

The urinary tract is under constant threat from bacterial invasion from the fecal flora, but the local defence mechanisms usually provide appropriate protection. However, several host factors may predispose to UTI, and bacteria may express certain virulence factors that favor UTIs in general, and more importantly, infection of the kidneys, i.e. pyelonephritis. Virulence factors may also be important for the risk of permanent damage (renal scarring). Most UTIs are ascending in origin, with bacterial colonization of the urethral orifice being followed by transfer of bacteria up the urethra to the bladder (i.e. urethritis, cystitis, cystourethritis, and ABU), and then up one or both ureters to the renal pelvis and renal parenchyma (i.e pyelonephritis). Vesico-ureteral reflux increases the risk of pyelonephritis in a significant way. A normal periurethral flora is part of the first defence, to avoid colonization of the urethral orifice by pathogens. Abnormalities in the periurethral flora have been shown to precede UTI. Antibiotic treatment for respiratory infection may alter the peri-urethral flora, and increase the risk of a symptomatic infection. The first bacterial colonization under the prepuce in boys may be followed by symptomatic UTI. Early circumcision may prevent UTI, while later circumcision has little value.

PREDISPOSING FACTORS FOR UTI

Most children with a first-time UTI, and also those with recurrent infections, have no evident predisposing factors that increase the risk for UTI. The investigation and follow-up care should, however, focus on a variety of factors in an effort to avoid permanent renal parenchymal damage. The first factor to consider is the presence of residual urine in the bladder post-voiding. This is common in the child with recurrent symptomatic UTI and usually indicates bladder dysfunction. Incomplete emptying of the bladder may be caused by imbalance

---

Table 12.1 Definitions used to describe types of urinary tract infection

- **Bacteriuria**
  Significant: $>10^5$ bacteria/ml
- **Symptomatic UTI**
  Infections involving the renal parenchyma
     Pyelonephritis (PN)
  Infections involving only the lower urinary tract
     Cystitis
     Urethritis
     Cysto-urethritis
- **Asymptomatic bacteriuria (ABU)**
  Bacteriuria in repeated samples without clinical symptoms
- **Pyelonephritic scarring**
  Reduction of parenchyma
  Calyceal clubbing or blunting

between the sphincter and the detrusor activity. Constipation may also influence bladder function, with resulting residual urine. If a child has encopresis, the number of fecal bacteria in the perineal area is increased, with a higher risk of UTI. Infravesical obstruction, bladder diverticula, and calculi may also predispose to infection. Catheterization or cystoscopy may be followed by UTI, even if the child has received antibacterial treatment in connection with the procedure. Recurrent infections may, in rare cases, be caused by a fistula between the urinary and the gastrointestinal tract.

RISK FACTORS FOR RENAL SCARRING

Infections of the renal parenchyma may result in permanent renal scarring. The risk is increased in case of obstruction and in dilated VUR, if the treatment is significantly delayed and if the patient has recurrent episodes of pyelonephritis. Younger patients also run a much higher risk of scarring. The renal parenchyma seems to be more vulnerable during infancy and early childhood, irrespective of urologic abnormality. Some children with VUR also have areas of dysplastic parenchyma which may be more prone to UTI and renal scarring. It is uncommon to find new scars in older children in spite of new episodes of PN.

One major reason for pyelonephritic scarring in the young child with UTI is probably delayed diagnosis. Without a prompt correct diagnosis, treatment of the febrile infant will not be optimal. Virulence factors of the bacteria may also be of importance for the risk of UTI. Not so virulent bacteria seem to have a higher risk of damage than most virulent ones.

MALFORMATIONS

Infravesical obstruction significantly increases the risk of more severe renal scarring. The renal parenchyma may be underdeveloped and dysplastic, and the parenchyma often seems to be more vulnerable to pyelonephritic infections. Vesico-ureteral reflux (VUR) increases the risk of upper UTI, and if the VUR is dilated (Grade III–V) the

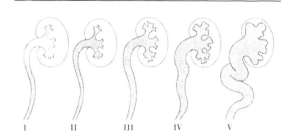

Figure 12.1 Vesico-ureteral reflux: Grading according to the International Reflux Study,[3] modified by Rushton HG[4]

Grade I: Ureter only; *Grade II*: Ureter, pelvis, and calyces, but no dilation, and normal calyceal fornices; *Grade III*: Mild or moderate dilation or tortuosity of the ureter, and mild or moderate dilation of the pelvis, but no or slight blunting of the fornices; *Grade IV*: Moderate dilation or tortuosity of the ureter and mild dilation of renal pelvis and calyces, with complete obliteration of sharp fornice angle, but maintenance of the papillary impressions in most calyces. *Grade V*: Gross dilation and tortuosity of ureter, and gross dilation of renal pelvis and calyces – papillary impressions are not visible in most calyces

risk for pyelonephritic scarring is exaggerated. Figure 12.1 shows the grading system for VUR that was developed by the International Study of VUR.[3,4] Figure 12.2 provides examples of patients with VUR grade III, IV and V, as well as intrarenal reflux.

BACTERIAL VIRULENCE FACTORS

P-fimbriated *E. coli* attach better to the mucus membranes of the urinary tract and are more often found in more serious infection. Thus, 80% of *E. coli* strains isolated from patients with pyelonephritis were P-fimbriated while only 30% of those from patients with cystitis.

GLOBAL SCOPE OF THE PROBLEM

Urinary tract infection is common in children in all parts of the world. However, other infections may get more attention especially in developing countries with a high incidence of gastrointestinal infections. In many countries, the likelihood of obtaining a clear specimen for urinalysis and urine culture is limited. This creates a problem because correct handling of urine samples before culture is

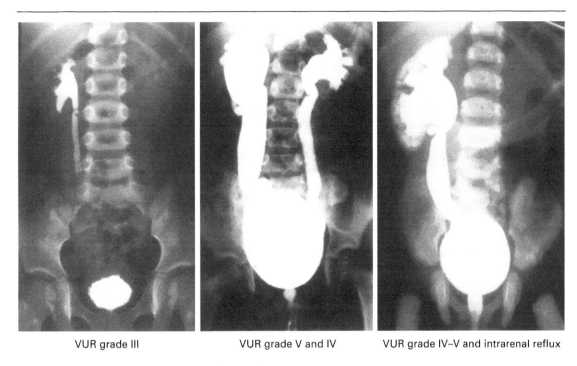

| VUR grade III | VUR grade V and IV | VUR grade IV–V and intrarenal reflux |

Figure 12.2 Vesico-ureteral reflux (VUR). (See color plate section)

crucial for correct diagnosis and management. It is of special importance when evaluating an infant with fever and a possible UTI, since fever is often the only symptom in such a patient, and contamination of urine samples is quite common.

In a Swedish study, 7.8% of the girls and 1.6% of the boys starting school had a history of UTI, and half of the infections had been with fever, i.e. pyelonephritis, with risk of permanent damage, i.e. renal scarring. Similar figures have been in found in the UK.[2]

Different approaches to the use of antibiotics in different countries of the world influence the rates of bacterial resistance. The extensive use of antibiotics in the developing countries, but also elsewhere, has resulted in multi-resistant bacteria. The need for cultures and evaluation of the resistance pattern is therefore of special importance. It is also important to know the local bacterial resistance patterns when acute treatment is started without the benefit of a culture and sensitivities. This is even more important if the result from the culture is delayed for several days, or if the quality of the culture examination is suspect.

The use of trimethoprim-sulfa for respiratory tract infection will select for trimethoprim-resistant, Gram-negative bacteria like *E. coli*. In countries with frequent use of this antimicrobial agent for the treatment of respiratory tract infection, 70–80% resistance may be seen.

CLINICAL FEATURES AND NATURAL HISTORY

SIGNS AND SYMPTOMS IN DIFFERENT AGE GROUPS

In infants who usually have pyelonephritis with risk of pyelonephritic scarring, the symptoms are usually non-specific (Table 12.2A). Most children only have fever in combination with signs that the

Table 12.2 Symptoms of pyelonephritis in infants and older children

A. **Infants**
   Symptoms unspecific
   Fever
   'Not doing well', inactive/irritable
   Gastrointestinal symptoms: vomiting, loose stools
   Weight loss or poor weight gain
   Septic symptoms

B. **Older children**
   Fever
   Abdominal pain
   Flank pain
   Cystitis symptoms
      Urgency
      Frequency
      Voiding pain
      Day-incontinence
      Enuresis

child is not doing well. The child may be pale, have poor appetite, recurrent vomiting, and loose stools. Weight loss of more than 10% of the birthweight during the first week of life may indicate UTI, as well as poor weight gain during the following months. Since these symptoms are nonspecific in the infant with UTI, it is crucial for a correct diagnosis to perform a urinalysis with urine culture in an infant with fever without strong evidence for infection elsewhere. Respiratory infection is very common in children, and a red ear or throat is not enough to avoid investigating the urine!

Septicemia and bacterial meningitis may complicate the picture, and sometimes conjugated hyperbilirubinemia may be seen.

In older children (from 1½–2 years of age) the symptoms more directly indicate a UTI, with voiding pain (dysuria), frequency, urine incontinence during the day and/or night, abdominal pain, which is often localized to the bladder region or the flanks, and tenderness on palpation over the bladder and the kidneys (Table 12.2B).

LEVEL OF INFECTION – LOWER OR UPPER UTI

Infections of the urethra (urethritis) and bladder (cystitis) are also named lower UTI. If the infection spreads to the renal pelvis and renal parenchyma the patient has an upper UTI, i.e. pyelonephritis.

ADDITIONAL DEFINITIONS

Pyelonephritis: Symptoms according to above, no indication of other explaining infection, significant bacteriuria ($>10^5$ bacteria/ml), fever $>38.5°C$ and C-reactive protein (CRP) >20 mg/l. Reduced maximal concentrating ability supports the diagnosis (Table 12.3).

Cystitis: Micturition symptoms, no fever or slightly increased temperature, significant bacteriuria, normal or slightly increased CRP and normal maximal concentrating ability.

ASYMPTOMATIC BACTERIURIA (ABU)

Positive urine cultures without clinical symptoms of UTI are called asymptomatic bacteriuria (ABU). Usually the urine findings are only mild. Asymptomatic bacteriuria is not uncommon in children, with 1–2% of most age groups having positive urine cultures. The ABU strains with time seem to lose virulence factors, but continue to occupy the urinary tract. Studies have shown that the ABU strain does not cause renal parenchymal damage. This seems to be the case also in patients with VUR, with or without renal parenchymal scarring, who have been followed for long periods without evidence of deterioration. The ABU strains of bacteria appear to give protection against more virulent bacteria.

LABORATORY INVESTIGATION (Table 12.3)

URINE INVESTIGATION

Evaluation of the urine by microscopy and dipstick is the first step in the diagnosis of a UTI. Increased number of leukocytes, often in combination with increased number of erythrocytes and slight proteinuria, indicates a UTI. If the urine is nitrite positive, a UTI is likely. However, sometimes the nitrite may come from bacterial colonization under the

Table 12.3 Laboratory investigations in the evaluation of children with an acute UTI

- Urinalysis
  Test strips
  - WBC, RBC, albumin
  - Nitrite
  Urine sediment
  - WBC, RBC, bacteria
- Urine culture
  Dip slide culture
  Quantitative culture
  - Significant bacteriuria ($>10^5$/ml)
- C-reactive protein (CRP)
- Erythrocyte sedimentation rate (ESR)
- Serum creatinine
- Serum urea
- Serum Na
- Maximal urine concentrating capacity

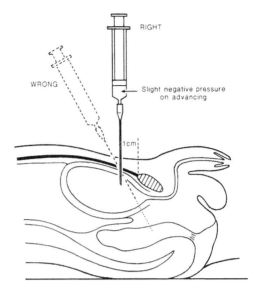

a) Suprapubic aspiration procedure (Reprinted from Taylor, C.M. & Chapman, S.[15] Handbook of Renal Investigations in Children, London: Wright, 1989), with permission from Elsevier

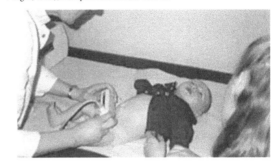

b) Ultrasonography to scan for urine before bladder puncture

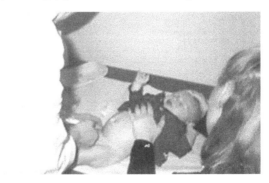

c) Suprapubic aspiration

Figure 12.3 Suprapubic aspiration. (See color plate section for Figs 12.3 b and c)

prepuce only, and only about 50% of the children with pyelonephritis have nitrite positive urine. A negative nitrite test thus does not exclude a UTI.

Urine culture with antibiotic sensitivities is essential for the correct diagnosis and treatment of a UTI. It is important to avoid contamination as much as possible. In the infant, collection of urine by percutaneous bladder puncture is the best way to avoid contamination, and risk of over-diagnosis. Bag-urine (plastic bag stuck to skin) gives a risk for contamination and false positive cultures. Catheterization of the bladder risks introducing bacteria in the child without infection, and a risk of transferring bacteria to the blood in heavy infection. Probably this method should only be used if treatment is immediately started after the catheterization. In older children a mid-stream urine specimen should be collected in order to avoid contamination in the first portion of urine.

The technique of percutaneous bladder puncture is shown in Figure 12.3. The finding of bacteria in a sample obtained with this technique is always considered to be significant. No serious complications have been reported in connection with the use of this technique. It is important that the bladder is relatively full when the procedure is performed.

Since the infant normally has a high urine volume it is usually enough to wait 60 minutes after the child has urinated. If a bladder scan is available, it can be used to determine if enough urine is present in the bladder. An intramuscular needle is used for perforation of the bladder. In the mid-line, 1 cm above the symphysis and at an angle of 90 degrees, the needle is forced slowly toward the bladder. A slight negative pressure in the syringe will help to know when the bladder wall has been passed. The most common reason for no urine is too little urine in the bladder, or that the tip of the needle has not been deep enough (3–4 cm).

A bacterial count of $>10^5$/ml in a clean urine is considered significant. However, sometimes also lower figures may be seen. *Escherichia coli* dominates in both upper and lower UTI (80–90% of the infections). Proteus, enterococci, staphylococci and pseudomonas may also be seen, especially in patients with recurrent infections and urologic malformation (Table 12.4).

STORAGE AND TRANSPORT

If urine is left in room temperature for many hours any bacterial numbers in the original sample will increase significantly. The urine should therefore be immediately refrigerated or be put in ice water and kept cool all the way to the laboratory (Fig. 12.4).

MAXIMAL URINE CONCENTRATING ABILITY

In acute PN the ability to concentrate the urine is reduced, in the order of 100–200 mOsm/kg. Normalization may take 1–2 months. Reduced maximal urine concentrating ability, after overnight thirst or after desmopressin, thus supports the diagnosis of PN.

BLOOD TESTS

Increased blood concentration of C-reactive protein (CRP; >20 mg/l) is indicative of renal involvement (i.e. pyelonephritis). Sometimes the CRP may not be increased until 24 hours after the first sign of disease, and the CRP may also increase the day after the start of bacterial treatment, even if the choice of

Table 12.4 Etiology of urinary tract infections in children

- *Escherichia coli*
  80–90% of first-time infections
- *Proteus mirabilis*
- *Klebsiella*
- *Staphylococcus saprophyticus*

Less virulent bacteria – more common if recurrent infections, malformation and bladder dysfunction
- Enterococci
- Pseudomonas
- *Staphylococcus aureus*
- *Staphylococcus epidermidis*
- Group B streptococci
- *Haemophilus influenzae*

Other infectious agents
- *Mycobacterium tuberculosis*
- *Leptospira icterohaemorrhagiae*
- *Schistosoma haematobium*
- *Echinococcus granulosus*
- *Candida albicans*

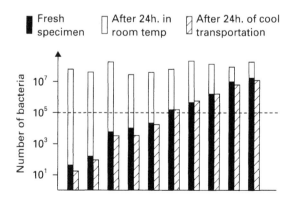

Figure 12.4 Storage influence on outcome of urine culture[16]

drug is correct. The erythrocyte sedimentation rate (ESR) will be increased after a few days of infection. Serum concentrations of creatinine and urea are usually not increased, unless the child has a more severe infection associated with septicemia or dehydration.

RADIOLOGIC INVESTIGATION

Acute pyelonephritic changes may be evaluated with different techniques (Fig. 12.5). Table 12.5 shows advantages and disadvantages with different techniques for evaluating the anatomy of the urinary tract and UTI related damage.[2,5–9] Further details regarding the use of renal sonography and other radiologic techniques that are described in brief in this section are given in Chapter 2.

ULTRASONOGRAPHY

In a child with a first-time pyelonephritis it is important to obtain a renal sonogram to evaluate for obstruction. This is of special importance in infants. An estimation of the renal parenchyma is also provided by this technique. Sometimes the

---

Table 12.5 Methods for morphologic evaluation of the urinary tract – Indications and advantages, and disadvantages and difficulties

	Indications and advantages	Disadvantages and difficulties
Ultrasonography (US)	Evaluation for obstruction and to give a rough estimation of total renal parenchyma and larger local parenchyma loss; acute changes Non-invasive No radiation	Examiner dependent Detailed parenchymal evaluation limited
Intravenous urography (NU)	Evaluation for permanent renal scarring, renal size, renal pelvic changes, obstruction and double collecting system	Radiation Invasive
Computerized tomography (CT)	Difficulties in performing IVU	Heavy radiation dose Invasive
DMSA scintigraphy	Parenchymal evaluation Confirmation of PN in the patient with first time infection Sensitive	Difficult to separate acute and chronic changes The consequences of persistent changes, which are very common, not known
MAG-3 renography	Obstruction evalution Functional distribution between kidneys Local parenchymal damage	Local parenchymal evaluation limited
Magnetic resonance imaging (MRI)	Parenchymal evaluation Non-invasive No radiation	Long registration periods Limited experience
Voiding cysto-urethrography (VCU)	Investigation for VUR and urethral obstruction or abnormality	Radiation Invasive
Indirect isotope cysto-urethrography	Investigation for VUR Follow-up of diagnosed VUR	No evaluation of urethra Invasive

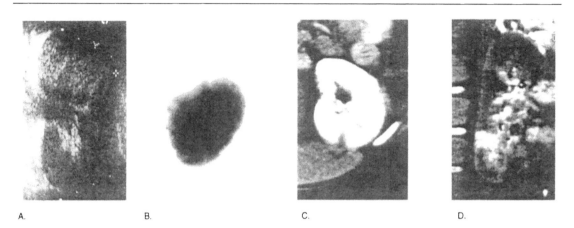

A. B. C. D.

Figure 12.5 Acute pyelonephritic changes visualized by different techniques:

(A) Ultrasonography: Changed echogenicity in the upper pole, not possible to separate cortex and medulla; (B) DMSA scintigraphy: Large uptake defect in the upper pole of the kidney. (C) CT scan with contrast: Note the two areas with reduced circulation. (D) MRI: Multiple areas with changed water content = pylonephritic areas. (See color plate section)

location of the pyelonephritis process will be seen, but usually the kidney is only swollen (this can in most cases only be shown by comparison with a later non-acute examination). Thickening of the renal pelvis is sometimes seen as well as hyperechoic particles in the bladder urine. Small scars are usually not visible by sonography. However, it may be used for screening patients for more severe parenchymal loss and ureteral dilation.

DMSA SCAN

The pyelonephritic process may be localized with DMSA scintigraphy. Areas of decreased isotope uptake reflect disturbed renal circulation and decreased tubular uptake. However, it is often difficult to separate acute from chronic damage. An uneven outline indicates chronic damage (scarring also seen by urography). DMSA scintigraphy is a very sensitive method for detection of renal parenchymal abnormality. In most cases, the uptake defects normalize during a few weeks to months after an episode of pyelonephritis. If the defects are present after 5–6 months, they usually don't disappear subsequently. Thus, if DMSA scinitigraphy is used for the evaluation of permanent parenchymal damage it should not be performed before six

months from the acute episode. Chronic changes at first evaluation can often not be separated from acute lesions. Another problem is that some patients may have dysplastic renal parenchyma with consequent uptake defects. Infants with a dilated urinary tract from grade IV reflux, found by US screening during pregnancy, may also have DMSA uptake defects in spite of no previous UTI.

MANAGEMENT OPTIONS

INVESTIGATION AND FOLLOW-UP

The early investigation is summarized in Tables 12.3 and 12.5 and the follow-up in Table 12.6.

ANTIBACTERIAL TREATMENT (Table 12.7)

Early and adequate antibacterial treatment is essential to avoid permanent renal damage, i.e. pyelonephritic scarring. The result of the urine culture may take time at many places. However, it is possible to have the result including resistance pattern within 24 hours, or 48 hours if the resistance is investigated in a second step. After urine for culture has been collected, if the child has severe symptoms,

Table 12.6 Follow-up investigation after acute pyelonephritis

Urine	Dipsticks for WBC, RBC, protein/albumin and nitrite
	Quantitative bacterial culture with resistance evaluation
	    in connection with symptoms indicating UTI
	    fever without other symptoms in the infant
	    at routine check-ups

Blood	C-reactive protein (CRP)
	
	Serum-creatinine
	Serum-urea
	    if UTI symptoms
	    follow-up of earlier pathologic information

Radiology	Micturating cystogram
	    VUR?
	    urethral obstruction (valves, strictures?)
	
	DMSA-scintigraphy
	    permanent parenchymal damage (uptake defects
	    persistent after six months)
	
	Urography
	    permanent parenchymal damage (scar)?
	    kidney size?
	    renal pelvic changes?
	    double system?
	(the extent of permanent pyelonephritic injury should not be evaluated before 12 months after the acute PN)

Table 12.7 Treatment of urinary tract infection according to location, severity, and age (Astrid Lindgren Children's Hospital, Stockholm, Sweden)

Pyelonephritis
(oral treatment for 10 days)
- Ceftibuten
- Trimethoprim-sulfamethoxazole
- Pivmecillinam
- Ciprofloxacin

Urosepsis or difficulties in giving orally
(i.v. until oral treatment possible)
- Cefotaxime (+ ampicillin)
- Gentamicin (+ ampicillin)

Cystitis (pre-school children)
(oral treatment for 5 days)
- Trimethoprim
- Cephalosporin
- Pivmecillinam
- Nitrofurantoin

Cystitis (school children)
(oral treatment for 5 days)
- Nitrofurantoin
- Pivmecillinam
- Trimethoprim
- Cephalosporin

a drug likely to cover the most common pathogens should be given without further delay. The local antibiotic resistance patterns, as well as previous cultures from the patient, should direct the choice of antibacterial treatment. Oral treatment is sufficient if the patient's clinical condition is relatively stable and they are not vomiting. Oral treatment with drugs such as co-trimazole or ceftibuten will give high serum concentrations only slightly later than after using the iv route.

Intravenous treatment has not been shown to be more effective.[10] However, local resistance and available drugs, as well as compliance, may influence the choice of treatment route. When the resistance pattern is available, oral treatment can usually be chosen.

PROPHYLAXIS

Before investigation for VUR is performed in an infant, prophylactic treatment should be given in order to reduce the risk of a new UTI. Trimethoprim may be used in countries with low or fairly low share of trimethoprim-resistant bacteria, whereas in other countries, nitrofurantoin can be used instead. Nitrofurantoin, however, very often is not accepted by the infants and smaller children, because of the taste, discomfort, and tendency to vomiting.

URINE CULTURES

Routine cultures have limited value if the child is free of symptoms. Education of parents in the symptoms and signs of UTI, and directed urine culture procedures, have a much higher value.

BLADDER DYSFUNCTION

Evaluation for residual urine and bladder dysfunction (evaluation of bladder habits and investigation of the urine flow and for residual urine) have been recognized in recent years as essential components of the evaluation of a child with a UTI. Treatment of constipation may improve bladder dysfunction to improve or normalize the bladder emptying. Encopresis may also be improved if the constipation is treated effectively. Improving voiding habits (increasing fluid intake and voiding 5–6 times/day) and avoiding bubble baths may reduce the risk of UTI in some patients.

SURGICAL TREATMENT

VESICOURETERAL REFLUX (VUR)

Dilated vesicoureteral reflux (i.e. grade III–V) predisposes patients to develop new pyelonephritic episodes and renal scarring.[1,2,4,11] However, the VUR per se, does not cause any renal scarring; renal parenchymal infection is also needed. Since VUR has a tendency to disappear with time, the first goal is to avoid new pyelonephritic episodes and initiate early and aggressive treatment in case of UTI. The VUR seems to disappear fastest during the first year of life but may happen also later, although it seems to happen very seldom after the age of 10 years. Grade III reflux disappears in 50% of the patients after five years (Fig. 12.6) and in 70% after 10 years. The International Reflux Study in Children has shown that PN episodes can be reduced by surgical anti-reflux treatment. The risk of lower UTI, however, was not influenced.

In case of recurrent PN and VUR, and especially in spite of prophylactic treatment or if such treatment is difficult to give, surgical treatment is indicated. In the 1–2 year old child, neo-implantation (Cohen's method is today the commonly used method, Fig. 12.7) is probably the method of choice, especially in cases of parenchymal reduction and failure to avoid recurrent acute pyelonephritis in spite of prophylaxis, and the need to stop this

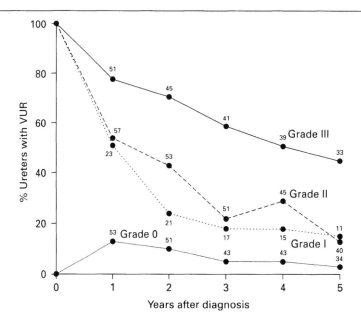

Figure 12.6 Course for VUR after diagnosis[17]

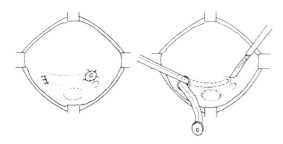

Figure 12.7 Vesico-ureteral reflux treatment by reimplantation of the ureter using Cohen's method[18]

Table 12.8 Conservative treatment (antibacterial prophylaxis) of VUR, advantages and disadvantages

- **Advantages**
  Reduces the risk of pyelonephritis and renal scarring
  No surgery
  Less worry for new infections

- **Disadvantages**
  Risk of new infections because of resistance development or poor compliance
  Side effects from drugs
  Daily medication, compliance problems
  More follow-up than after successful surgery
  Persistent VUR
  Worries from having VUR

---

pattern in order to avoid more parenchymal loss. Transurethral injection treatment with silicon or Deflux® is also commonly used at many centers, also in small children and in all degrees of VUR. However, this treatment is less effective and may need repeated treatment before the VUR has disappeared. In the older child, transurethral injection treatment probably should be the first treatment-of-choice. If the injection method is not available, neo-implantation may be used also for older children.

Tables 12.8–12.10 summarize the advantages and disadvantages of conservative treatment (prophylaxis), neo-implantation, and endoscopic injection treatment for VUR.[1,2,4,11,12]

CIRCUMCISION

Although very early circumcision reduces the risk of pyelonephritis in infant boys, the American Academy of Pediatrics does not consider that the potential benefits justify routine use of this treatment. Circumcision at older age does not significantly influence the risk of UTI. In Sweden, circumcision is only performed in patients with recurrent local infection and very thick phimosis.

LONG-TERM COURSE AND OUTCOME

The incidence of first-time UTIs is highest during the first year of life, and most infections are in the form of acute pyelonephritis.[1,2] The recurrence rate is high also in children with predisposing urologic malformation. Girls have a higher risk of new UTIs than boys. Within one year, 30% of the girls will get a new UTI, and within five years the rate is 50%. The recurrence rate in boys is 15–20%, and seldom after one year of age. Repeated infections are uncommon in boys with normal radiology. After the first year of life, lower UTI (=cystitis) will be more and more common, and in many children with a tendency for UTI the episodes of acute pyelonepritis will be followed by cystitis, and in some cases ABU. Some individuals seem to have a tendency for UTI that persists into adult life with special risk in early childhood, adolescence and young adulthood (in women often related to sexual activity), and in old age.

Most children will only have one or a few episodes of UTI, with or without fever, and most of them will not suffer any significant parenchymal loss. Slight isotope uptake defects on the DMSA scan will be seen in approximately 40% of the children after an episode of acute PN. However, most uptake defects will not correspond to a scar seen on urography. A small urography scar will probably be

Table 12.9 Neoimplantation of the ureter for treatment of VUR, advantages and disadvantages

- **Advantages**
  Definitive treatment of the VUR
  Less follow-up
  Reduced risk of pyelonephritis
  Less worry for the disease

- **Disadvantages**
  Trauma of surgery
  Complications with surgery
  Referral of patients for treatment
  Social difficulties in connection with surgery
  Psychologic trauma in connection with surgery

Table 12.10 Transurethral injection treatment of VUR, advantages and disadvantages

- **Advantages**
  Less invasive than neoimplantation
  Short hospital visit
  Short prophylaxis treatment
  Less psychologic trauma than neoimplantation

- **Disadvantages**
  Persistent VUR not uncommon
  Surgical complications (anesthesia)
  Migration of injection material; local granuloma
  Long-term follow-up limited
  Referral of patients for treatment
  Repeated micturating cysto-urethrography
  Psychologic trauma from treatment

of no significance in the absolute majority of the patients. In more severe pyelonephritic scarring, and especially if the scarring is bilateral, there is a risk of progressive scarring and deteriorating renal function. There is also an increased risk of hypertension, which may be manifest already during childhood. Pregnancy is a period of increased risk for hypertension, and new UTIs, in patients with recurrent UTI during childhood.

When small scars are seen on urography, the risk of hypertension is only marginally elevated. Most patients have normal blood pressure in early adulthood. The significance of slight uptake defects on DMSA scintigraphy is probably even less. Routine follow-up of patients with slight remaining pyelonephritic scars, normal blood pressure and no UTIs is probably not warranted. In more severe pyelonephritic scarring and recurrent UTI there is substantial risk of terminal renal failure, hypertension, and pregnancy eclampsia. After a follow-up period of 25–35 years, the patients in one study showed these complications in 10, 23, and 13%, respectively. Terminal failure from UTI has also been reported from Italy and the UK in the order of 10–15%. In children with hypertension, a substantial part is caused by pyelonephritic scarring. However, newer follow-up information from Sweden has shown much lower risk figures for renal failure from UTI. During the period 1978–1985 the incidence of chronic renal failure from UTI was about 5%,[13] and during the period 1986–1994, no patient who fits this description was found.[14] However, pyelonephritis substantially contributes to the progression of renal failure in the patients with obstructive nephropathies and reduced parenchyma from dysplasia.

SUMMARY AND THOUGHTS FOR THE FUTURE

Urinary tract infection is common in children. The majority of the children will only have one or a few infections, and there is a predisposing urologic malformation in only a minority of the patients. It is possible to prevent or reduce permanent injury (i.e. scarring) by accurate diagnosis, treatment, investigation, and follow-up. The diagnosis of PN in the febrile infant is probably most important. Without correct diagnosis the treatment may be delayed with unnecessary risk of scarring. Obstruction should be excluded in the infant with pyelonephritis, especially if the infection is severe and is not responding promptly to treatment. If no prenatal examination of the urinary tract has been performed, ultrasonography in close connection to the PN probably is a good screening test for significant anatomic abnormality predisposing to new infections.

Ultrasonography is of no or very limited value for examination or diagnosis of VUR.

It is especially important to be active in the treatment and follow-up of patients with dilated VUR, and especially grade IV–V, and reduced renal parenchyma. Investigation for infravesical obstruction is essential in boys. Surgical treatment should be considered especially in this group of patients. Neoimplantation of the ureters is the most effective treatment to avoid new PN, but transurethral injection treatment is also of value.

With time, the VUR will disappear in the majority of patients. The important thing is to avoid PN and to give early and correct treatment when the patient develops a UTI. By giving antibacterial prophylaxis many patients will have no, or few, recurrences. This approach is chosen for many children during the waiting period until they have grown out of the VUR. To find out which approach is superior for the child with grade III and IV VUR, a Swedish multi-center study has started. The effect from transurethral injection with Deflux®, prophylaxis treatment and early treatment without prophylaxis are being compared.

It is possible that the investigation and follow-up program sometimes have been too extensive in children with uncomplicated UTI. It is likely that the approach will be more individualized in the future, and focus on the high-risk patients. However, to be able to define your patients as high-risk patients or not, a first careful evaluation has to be made, and most importantly to diagnose correctly the first-time PN without delay.

SUMMARY

1. UTI is common in children.
2. Investigate for UTI in the febrile infant.
3. Perform urine cultures with evaluation of antibiotic sensitivities.
4. Investigate for obstruction and VUR.
5. Educate the families about symptoms of UTI, and also general practioners, who may use adult rules for investigation and treatment, without urinalysis and urine culture.
6. VUR is often familial and congenital, but VUR has a tendency to disappear with time.
7. VUR as such does not give renal scarring, but increases the risk of PN.
8. Keep the child free from infection until the VUR has disappeared.
9. In case of difficulties in keeping the child free from PN, in spite of prophylaxis, consider surgical treatment.
10. Progressive renal scarring may be preventable by early diagnosis and treatment.

REFERENCES

1. Hansson S, Jodal U. Urinary tract infection. In Barratt TM, Avner ED, Harmon WE, eds, Pediatric Nephrology, 4th edn. Lippincott Williams & Wilkins: Baltimore, 1999 835–850.
2. Lambert H, Coulthard M. The child with urinary tract infection. In Webb NJ, Postlethwaite, eds, Clinical Paediatric Nephrology, 3rd edn. Oxford University Press: 2003. 197–225.
3. Medical versus surgical treatment of primary vesicoureteral reflux: report of the International Reflux Study Committee. Pediatrics 1981; 67:392–400.
4. Rushton HG Jr. Vesicoureteral reflux and scarring. In Barratt TM, Avner ED, Harmon WE, eds. Paediatric Nephrology, 4th edn. Lippincott Williams & Wilkins: Baltimore. 1999. 851–871.
5. Biggi A, Dardanelli L, Pomero G et al. Acute renal cortical scintigraphy in children with a first urinary tract infection. Pediatr Nephrol 2001; 16:733–738.
6. Dick PT, Feldman W. Routine diagnostic imaging for childhood urinary tract infections: a systematic overview. J Pediatr 1996; 128:15–22.
7. Hoberman A, Charron M, Hickey RW, Baskin M, Kearney DH, Wald ER. Imaging studies after a first febrile urinary tract infection in young children. N Engl J Med 2003; 348:195–202.
8. Linné T, Fituri, O, Escobar-Billing R, Karlsson A, Wikstad I, Aperia A, Tullus K. Functional parameters and 99mTc-dimercaptosuccinic acid scan in acute pyelonephritis. Pediatr Nephrol 1994; 8:694–699.
9. Stapleton FB. Imaging studies for childhood urinary infections. N Engl J Med 2003; 348:251–252.
10. Hoberman A, Wald ER, Hickey RW et al. Oral versus initial intravenous therapy for urinary tract infections in young febrile children. Pediatrics 1999; 104:79–86.
11. Jodal U, Hansson S, Hjalmas K. Medical or surgical management for children with vesico-ureteric reflux? Acta Paediatr Suppl 1999; 88(431):53–61.
12. Jodal U, Lindberg U. Guidelines for management of children with urinary tract infection and vesico-ureteric reflux. Recommendation from a Swedish state-of-the-art conference. Swedish Medical Research Council. Acta Paediatr Suppl 1999; 88(431): 87–89.
13. Esbjorner E, Aronson S, Berg U, Jodal U, Linne T. Children with chronic renal failure in Sweden 1978–1985. Pediatr Nephrol 1990; 4:249–252.
14. Esbjorner E, Berg U, Hansson S et al. Epidemiology of chronic renal failure in children: a report from Sweden 1986–1994. Pediatr Nephrol 1997; 11:438–442.

15. Taylor, CM, Chapman, S. Handbook of Renal Investigations in Children. London: Wright, 1989.
16. Kallings LO, Sv. Lakartidningen, Suppl III 1968; 65:30.
17. Arant BS. Medical management of mild and moderate vesicoureteral reflux: follow-up studies of infants and young children. A preliminary report of the Southwest Pediatric Nephrology Study Group. J Urol 1992; 148:1683–1687.
18. Blandy J. Urology, 5th edn. Blackwell Science: Oxford, 1998.

CYBER SOURCES FOR INFORMATION

http://www.aafp.org/afp/980401ap/ahmed2.html
A fairly detailed information from American Family Physician on "Evaluation and Treatment of Urinary Tract Infections in Children"

http://www.cincinnatichildrens.org/health/info/urinary/well/urinary.htm
The advice from Cincinnati Children's Hospital Medical Center also includes some information on UTI

http://pediatrics.about.com/cs/commoninfections/l/bl_uti.htm
Gives a general presentation on urinary tract infection in children

http://www.cirp.org/library/disease/UTI/
Covers con and pro aspects of circumcision

13. Nocturnal enuresis and voiding disorders

Søren Rittig

INTRODUCTION

Failure to obtain urinary continence during the day and/or night is one of the most common disorders of childhood. Although only a minority of incontinent children have an underlying pathologic condition associated with morbidity and mortality, 'wetting' is still one of the most feared events among children – especially when school age is reached. Nevertheless, members of the medical community have been reluctant to treat children with these conditions actively, often referring to the lack of morbidity, and to the misconception that the symptoms are most often mild and short-lived. However, over the last two decades, physicians have developed a better understanding of the different subtypes of patients that constitute the heterogeneous population of children with enuresis, and this has been associated with an increasing awareness of the need for a more active treatment attitude. The improved knowledge about various subtypes of wetting has resulted in such children being carefully differentiated with respect to both their evaluation and treatment.[1] As a result, we now draw a clear distinction between isolated nighttime wetting as opposed to other forms of urinary incontinence, and between bladder reservoir problems and voiding problems. The following chapter will describe the different syndromes, their prevalence, diagnosis, and treatment options.

NOCTURNAL ENURESIS

DEFINITION AND EPIDEMIOLOGY

The term nocturnal enuresis (NE) is defined as micturition that occurs at night, although it really pertains to involuntary voiding while the child is asleep. Wetting both day and night, or isolated day wetting, is referred to as urinary incontinence. Monosymptomatic nocturnal enuresis (MNE) indicates that the child has few or no daytime symptoms that suggest a disorder of the lower urinary tract (Fig. 13.1). In primary nocturnal enuresis (PNE), the child has never been dry for a period longer than six months, whereas in secondary nocturnal enuresis there has been such a period. Physicians in most countries regard NE as pathologic when it is present after the age of 5–6 years, but in practice treatment is often not considered before the age of 6–7 years, and sometimes much later. It is the second most frequent chronic disorder in children (after asthma) with a prevalence of 5–10% at the age of 7 years and of 0.5–1% in adulthood. More boys than girls have NE, although this difference tends to diminish with increasing age. The spontaneous cure rate has been estimated

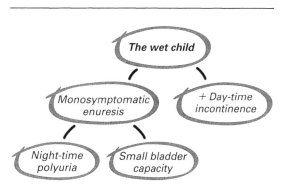

Figure 13.1 A schematic drawing illustrating the diversity of the enuresis population.

Patients with additional daytime incontinence constitute a group with a different pathophysiology, and these symptoms should be treated before the nocturnal symptoms. The monosymptomatic patient population consists of some patients with predominantly nocturnal polyuria, and some patients with predominantly low functional bladder capacity

to be approximately 15% annually after six years of age.[2]

PATHOPHYSIOLOGY

Nocturnal enuresis is a heterogeneous disorder which can be caused by one or more of several pathophysiologic mechanisms, the two most important factors being the nocturnal urine volume and the nocturnal functional bladder capacity (Fig. 13.1). A unifying pathogenic concept with important clinical implications defines NE as being caused by a mismatch between the nocturnal bladder capacity and the volume of urine produced during the night, associated with an inability to awaken when the bladder capacity is exceeded.[3]

NOCTURNAL URINE PRODUCTION

In humans, a marked circadian rhythm of urine production is developed from early childhood with a pronounced nocturnal reduction in urine production to approximately 50% of daytime levels.[4] In children, this rhythm is controlled by increased nocturnal release of hormones that regulate free water excretion (arginine vasopressin, AVP) as well as solute excretion (renin, angiotensin II, aldosterone, and atrial natriuretic peptide). Although a number of studies have now confirmed that an abnormally large nocturnal urine output is often an important pathophysiologic factor in NE, no consensus has yet been reached regarding the optimal method of measuring this variable (e.g. diaper weighing or sequential voiding) nor a clear definition of nocturnal polyuria. The recent demonstration that nocturnal urine volume is significantly larger on wet nights compared with dry nights has emphasized that nocturnal polyuria may only be evident on nights when NE occurs.[5] It has also been demonstrated that increased nocturnal urine output occurs in only a subgroup of enuretics, who generally can be characterized as having normal functional bladder capacity, and a favorable response to treatment that reduces their nocturnal urine volume.[6]

The prevalence, as well as the underlying cause of the defect in urine volume and/or solute excretion in NE is still unclear, although several factors seem to play a role. Some studies have provided evidence of an abnormal circadian rhythm of the human antidiuretic hormone arginine vasopressin (AVP). Lack of the normal nocturnal rise of this hormone seems to correlate with the occurrence of polyuria as well as the response to a synthetic form of AVP (DDAVP). The background behind the increased nocturnal excretion of solutes in some patients is so far unclear, although the role of sodium regulating hormones and prostaglandins is currently being investigated. Finally, other factors such as sleep apnea, hypercalcuria, and aquaporin 2 dysfunction may play a role in some children with nocturnal polyuria.

BLADDER FUNCTION

The function of the bladder in NE has been a focus of study for many years, but the type of dysfunction, its prevalence, and clinical importance are still unclear. Although the incidence of significant anatomic and functional bladder abnormalities is very low in primary NE it seems that adult onset nocturnal enuresis is a sign of an underlying abnormality that demands urologic investigation.[7] This may also be true for patients with severe, treatment-resistant enuresis.

In MNE, most evidence points towards a deficient development of nocturnal bladder reservoir function, at least in a subgroup of patients. Nocturnal bladder capacity in normal children is significantly larger than daytime capacity, probably due to inhibitory effects of sleep on the micturition centers. Nocturnal bladder capacity is not easy to measure in enuretic patients even with diaper weighing, as many enuresis episodes are incomplete voidings associated with significant residual urine. However, when estimated during daytime and excluding the morning void, functional bladder capacity (FBC) is also reduced in many enuretics. Clinically, an estimate of daytime FBC is relatively easy to obtain by asking a child to delay voiding for as long as possible, and then determining the volume of urine in his/her bladder following spontaneous voiding into a urinal. It has been shown to be of value when selecting a treatment modality in the individual patient. Thus, a FBC below 70% of the predicted FBC for age, (defined as age $\times$ 30) + 30 ml, is associated with a poor response to treatment with DDAVP. This contrasts with the good response in this patient subgroup to a conditioning alarm system – a treatment modality that increases nocturnal bladder capacity but has no effect on nocturnal urine production.[8]

SLEEP/PSYCHOLOGY

Regardless of the cause of the mismatch between nocturnal bladder capacity and nocturnal urine volume, it is important to emphasize that enuresis only occurs when the child fails to be aroused by his/her full bladder. This has caused many authors to conclude that sleep disturbance per se is a major pathophysiologic factor in enuresis, and it is still a general belief in the population that enuretics are deep sleepers. However, the inability to show convincing abnormalities in sleep patterns, together with the observation that a considerable proportion of non-enuretic children are also unable to wake up when polyuria is induced overnight, have questioned this hypothesis. In conclusion, although there is little doubt that a disturbance of sleep and/or arousal plays a role in the pathophysiology of NE, the clinical relevance and possible implications are still unclear and in-center sleep investigation is not a part of the routine evaluation of enuretic children.

Regarding the psychologic aspects of enuresis, it has been reported that children with this disorder have a significantly lower self-esteem than normal children. However, it has been shown that these psychologic abnormalities are secondary to the wetting problem as they normalize after successful treatment of the NE.[9] In contrast, children with secondary NE have a higher prevalence of behavioral dysfunction and obtaining a psychologic profile in such children may be indicated.

GENETICS

It has been known for many years that NE has a strong hereditary component. Thus, if one parent has a history of NE, the offspring have a 5–7-fold higher risk of having NE compared to children who have a negative family history. As a result of studies reported over the last decade, the molecular understanding of NE has increased significantly with the demonstration of linkage between enuresis and several gene loci on different chromosomes.[10] The genetic influence seems to exist in all enuresis subtypes although the specific gene products and the genotype-phenotype relationship have not yet been identified.

EVALUATION

In children with primary NE, evaluation and therapy should not be initiated before 5 to 6 years of age, in contrast to children with secondary NE where an underlying disease (e.g. diabetes mellitus, constipation, urinary tract infection [UTI]) should be sought and treated as needed when the cause of the wetting is identified. The initial evaluation should comprise a detailed history where the focus should be pointed towards duration and severity of the night wetting, but also towards any accompanying symptoms (e.g. daytime incontinence, UTI, constipation) that indicate a more complex disorder. The physical examination should include examination of external genitalia (e.g. congenital anomalies, phimosis) and lumbar region (deformations, pigmentations, and hair growth), neurologic examination (including anocutaneous and cremaster reflexes, lower extremity reflexes, muscle tone, and gait). The office investigation should include a urinalysis in a morning or spot urine sample with examination for glucose, leukocytes, nitrite, albumin, and specific gravity. In the majority of children with NE, all investigations will be normal.

A cornerstone in the further evaluation of a child or adolescent with NE is an estimation of FBC and nocturnal urine production. For this purpose, in our clinic we utilize a frequency-volume chart (registration of the time and volume of all micturitions and fluid intakes during daytime) during a weekend, and a recording of night-time urine production (weight of diaper in the morning (g) – weight of diaper before bedtime (g) + volume of morning micturition (ml)) during one week is a very useful tool, and when the purpose is explained to the parents compliance is usually good. The largest void seen on the frequency-volume chart, excluding the morning void, is a good estimate of FBC, and nocturnal polyuria (usually defined as > 130% of the expected FBC for the age) should be evaluated on wet nights. Daytime micturitions should be recorded for 2–4 days and night-time urine production during one week, for reliable estimates of FBC and nocturnal urine production.[11]

TREATMENT

Before selecting therapy for NE, it is important to treat any accompanying symptoms first, especially daytime voiding symptoms. In most developed countries today, two treatments for NE are most often prescribed: conditioning alarm and treatment with the vasopressin analog DDAVP (Fig. 13.2). It appears that the response to these two treatments in patients with NE depends to a large extent on the underlying mechanism of the disorder, i.e. patients

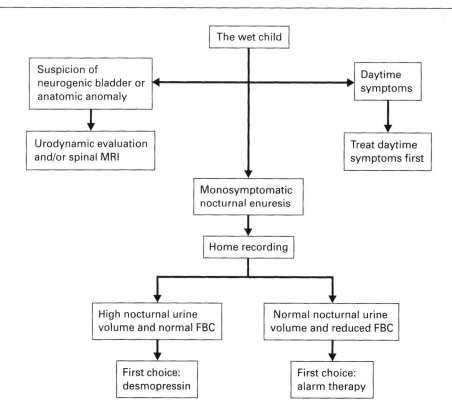

Figure 13.2 A simple flow-chart illustrating a suggestion for evaluation and treatment strategy of nocturnal enuresis.

If concomitant symptoms exist, such as daytime incontinence or constipation, these should be addressed first. In the monosymptomatic child, a home recording of nocturnal urine production (by diaper weighing) and functional bladder capacity (FBC) (by a frequency-volume chart) can identify patients with nocturnal polyuria (e.g. nocturnal urine volume on wet nights exceed 130% of predicted FBC for age) and patients with reduced FBC (less than 70% of value predicted for age, i.e. from the formula: FBC (ml) = [age (yrs) × 30] + 30). Desmopressin (DDAVP) is the first choice treatment of nocturnal polyuria, and alarm treatment is first choice for children with reduced FBC

with normal nocturnal urine production and small FBC, respond poorly to desmopressin, whereas patients with large nocturnal urine production and normal FBC respond poorly to the alarm. In general, DDAVP and alarm treatments should not be regarded as competing modalities, but as supplementary to each other and targeting different patient types. If, however, initial evaluation of the underlying enuresis mechanism is not possible, other factors such as family motivation and preferences, availability of close follow-up, costs, and frequency of enuretic episodes should all be included in the decision-making process.

CONDITIONING ALARMS

Alarm treatment has been used for many years in NE with relatively high efficacy even in unselected individuals.[12] The conditioning alarm device consists usually of a small sensor which is attached to the underwear and which activates an alarm attached to the shoulder region when it becomes wet. It is important that the treatment is continued every night for at least eight weeks and, therefore, it requires a great effort from the entire family. Frequent supportive follow-up visits and phone calls from the clinic increase the efficacy of the treatment. A positive response to the alarm is associated with an increase in bladder capacity whereas nocturnal urine production is unaffected.

DDAVP

DDAVP administered perorally or intranasally at bedtime reduces nocturnal urine production significantly provided that the child has a lack of the normal nocturnal rise in urinary concentration.[13] This treatment is especially efficient in patients with a normal functional bladder capacity and high nocturnal urine production. The dose needs to be titrated in each patient and treatment is usually necessary for long periods, interrupted by a short break every three months to see if treatment is still necessary. Provided that the child is instructed not to drink excessively after administration of the drug

to prevent water intoxication, there are very few and mild side effects.

OTHER TREATMENTS

Some tricyclic antidepressants (e.g. imipramine) can reduce enuresis symptoms probably by reducing nocturnal urine volume. However, due mainly to the risk of serious side effects by accidental overdosing, this treatment is not used as a first line treatment in most parts of the world. Anti-muscarinic therapy (e.g. oxybutynin) is not an effective mono-therapy for patients with MNE, but might play a role in the subgroup of patients with associated daytime symptoms indicating an overactive bladder, and has been used with some success as an adjunctive form of treatment in those with a low FBC who show a partial response to DDAVP. The level of evidence for this, however, is still rather weak.

OTHER FORMS OF URINARY INCONTINENCE

DEFINITION AND EPIDEMIOLOGY

Lower urinary tract symptoms are very common in childhood, especially urgency and frequency. Urinary incontinence is also relatively common with a prevalence of approximately 3% of 7-year-old children.[14] Voiding complaints per se such as dysuria and interrupted stream are far less frequent. Bladder-sphincter dysfunction is associated with recurrent UTI and vesicoureteral reflux. Furthermore, urinary incontinence is highly associated with constipation and fecal incontinence (10–15% of children with urge incontinence) and this entity has been termed dysfunctional elimination syndrome.

Urinary incontinence can be divided into separate subtypes based upon the underlying mechanism.[1] The two subtypes that pose the greatest threat to the upper urinary tract and therefore should be identified and treated as early as possible are neuropathic bladder sphincter dysfunction and structural incontinence (Fig. 13.3). These two groups comprise only a few percent of incontinent children, as most children have no underlying neurologic or anatomic cause (non-neuropathic bladder-sphincter dysfunction). Based upon voiding pattern, uroflowmetry, and investigation for residual urine, non-neuropathic bladder-sphincter dysfunction can be further divided into urge incontinence, dysfunctional voiding, and lazy bladder syndrome. Finally, two types that are not easy to include in the above definition are vaginal voiding and giggle incontinence.

VOIDING DYSFUNCTION, URINARY TRACT INFECTION, AND VESICOURETERAL REFLUX (VUR)

The triad of concomitant voiding dysfunction, recurrent UTI, and VUR is not uncommon in children and adolescents. When the components of the complex occur together, the risk of renal scarring and nephropathy increases markedly, and the entity is therefore important to identify and treat as early as possible (Fig. 13.4). Although the exact relationship between the factors is not yet fully understood, there is increasing agreement that voiding dysfunction plays a very important causal role for both VUR and recurrent UTI in children over the age of 4–5 years, and, therefore, correction of voiding dysfunction should have high priority in these patients. The value of prophylactic antibiotics and bladder-sphincter dysfunction treatment in resolving this

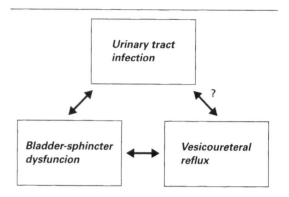

Figure 13.4 Bladder-sphincter dysfunction is often associated with and believed to cause recurrent urinary tract infections due to insufficient bladder emptying and vesicoureteral reflux, which result from increased intravesical pressures and functional obstruction.

Urinary tract infection is also thought to be a frequent cause of bladder-sphincter dysfunction. The causal interaction between urinary tract infections and vesicoureteral reflux is more uncertain. Generally, presence of the entire symptom complex is thought to increase the risk of renal damage

complex has therefore, questioned the need for early diagnosis and surgical treatment of the VUR component.

EVALUATION

If a wetting child has daytime symptoms, initial evaluation should be started from the age of 4–5 years due to the importance of excluding neurologic and structural causes (Fig. 13.5). Also at this

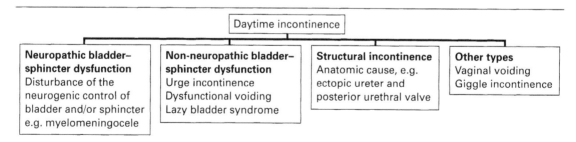

Figure 13.3 Classification of types of urinary incontinence in children based upon the underlying mechanism and clinical presentation.

Neuropathic bladder-sphincter dysfunction and structural incontinence are rare in children, but important to identify at an early age as these can be associated with renal damage. Non-neuropathic bladder-sphincter dysfunction is common in children and can be divided into three groups where urge incontinence is the most common. Vaginal voiding and giggle incontinence are less common types of incontinence that nevertheless are important to identify

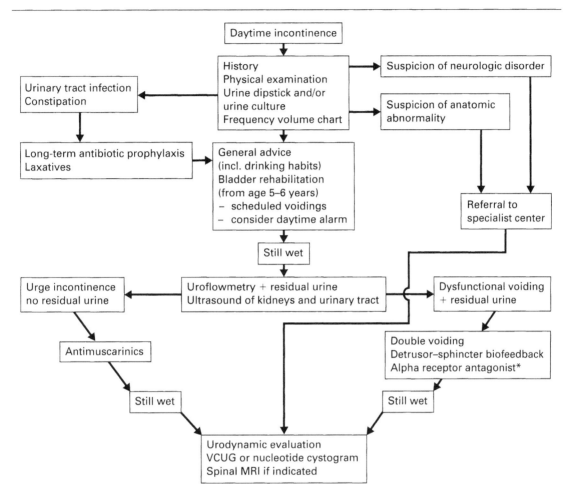

Figure 13.5 A flowchart illustrating suggestions for evaluation and treatment strategy of daytime incontinence in children

The initial evaluation should begin at age 4–5 years and should focus on complicating factors such as recurrent UTI, constipation, neurologic disorders, and anatomic abnormalities. At age 5–6 years bladder rehabilitation can be instituted with an efficacy rate of approximately 50–60%. If this treatment fails more evaluation is indicated, and referral is often necessary in order to perform ultrasound examination of the urinary tract and uroflowmetry with determination of residual urine. The subsequent treatment depends on the type of incontinence and presence of residual urine. Only if pharmacologic or biofeedback treatment fails, or if urinary tract obstruction is suspected, are more invasive investigations indicated – such as urodynamics and voiding cystourethrography (VCUG)

*Evidence level for effect on dysfunctional voiding and residual urine is low

stage, the history is very important including the psychomotor development of the child, the type of incontinence (e.g. constant dribbling indicating a structural cause), presence of recurrent UTI, constipation, and fecal incontinence. Information about the family situation, motivation, and behavioral problems should be included in a structured history. The physical examination should focus on the same areas as in a child with nocturnal enuresis, and urinalysis is also indicated. If the initial evaluation raises suspicion of an underlying disease, e.g. a neurologic disorder or anatomic anomaly, the child should be referred to a secondary or tertiary referral center. A cornerstone in the initial evaluation of an incontinent child is a frequency-volume chart with recording of all incontinence episodes as well as the time and volume of all fluid intake and voidings for two days, typically over a weekend. This tool gives highly valuable information about the severity of symptoms, drinking habits, voiding pattern, and bladder capacity. Occasionally, just filling out a frequency-volume chart enables the parents to adjust an inappropriate voiding or drinking pattern resulting in a continent child before the next visit.

If recurrent UTI is part of the history of a child, prophylactic antibiotics should be instituted and an ultrasound investigation of the urinary tract is indicated. If there is suspicion of constipation, and in all children with soiling or fecal incontinence, this should be treated aggressively. If, however, no underlying disease is suspected, further evaluation is not necessary at this stage and treatment can be reduced to general advice about good voiding habits and awareness about signs of constipation and UTI. In the motivated child, bladder rehabilitation with scheduled voidings can be commenced.

If the incontinence symptoms, however, persist after the age of 5–6 years, the initial evaluation should be supplemented with an ultrasound examination of the urinary tract, uroflowmetry, and measurement of post void residual urine, which most often requires referral to a specialist. The urodynamic tests will provide characterization of the voiding and bladder emptying, and will enable differentiation between different types of incontinence, e.g. urge syndrome and dysfunctional voiding, and may raise suspicion of a urinary tract obstruction (Fig. 13.5). More invasive evaluations such as conventional transurethral cystometry, natural fill ambulatory continuous bladder pressure monitoring, voiding cystourethrography (VCUG), and nucleotide cystography are only indicated if there is suspicion of neuropathic or structural incontinence, or if more intensive treatment approaches including pharmacologic treatment are ineffective.

NON-NEUROPATHIC BLADDER-SPHINCTER DYSFUNCTION

URGE INCONTINENCE

This type is the most common form of day-time incontinence in childhood.[15] Two to three per cent of seven-year-olds have incontinence with concomitant signs of an overactive bladder, and up to one third of seven-year-olds have urgency with increased voiding frequency. This syndrome has undergone a conceptual change over the last decade. Previously there was a clear-cut urodynamic definition of the 'unstable' bladder with bladder contractions during the filling phase of a cystometry. The urodynamic definition, however, has been widened to include bladder and urethral dysfunction, and, clinically, urge syndrome is characterized by frequent attacks of a need to void, countered by holding manoeuvres such as squatting. This eventually results in leakage of urine, usually small volumes. Because the clinical picture of this type of incontinence is so typical, the diagnosis can be made with confidence by a structured approach as described above, and no further urodynamic testing is necessary unless the child fails to respond to initial therapy (Fig. 13.5).

Treatment of urge incontinence starts with elimination of concomitant constipation and UTI followed by behavioral treatment (bladder rehabilitation). This modality will cure at least 50% of the children and can be started at the primary care level. The cornerstone in behavioral treatment is to establish the child's awareness about his or her voiding habits. Different specific strategies are used but most include a correction of fluid intake and abolishment of caffeine-containing beverages. They also include initial increase in the number of voidings followed by a gradual decrease to normality. Although not based on controlled studies, it is often helpful to use a programmable watch that gives a signal to the child when it is time for a voiding. If inappropriate postures are part of the child's voiding habits they should be corrected. At the secondary referral centers it is of paramount importance that the caretaking personnel consist of a well-educated team of doctors, specialist nurses (urotherapists), psychologists, and eventually physiotherapists. If the above treatment for a couple of months does not abolish the symptoms, pharmacotherapy with antimuscarinics should be tried.[16] There are rather few drugs with substantiated effect in children,[17] and some of them do have significant side effects, especially in children with symptoms of ADHD. The newly developed antimuscarinics seem to have less influence on cognitive function and are therefore better tolerated. Antimuscarinic therapy should not be instituted in a child with significant residual urine and many centers monitor bladder emptying 4–5 weeks after initiation of treatment.

Neuromodulation using cutaneous stimulation of either the sacral or peripheral nerves is a relatively new treatment modality whose usefulness in children should be further evaluated.[18]

DYSFUNCTIONAL VOIDING (STACCATO VOIDING)

Voiding dysfunction in children is rather rare. Approximately 1% of seven-year-olds will have a uroflowmetry clearly deviating from normal. The predominant pattern is that of staccato voiding, which consists of frequent interruptions of a detrusor initiated voiding (Fig. 13.6). Dysfunctional voiding has many names. Non-neuropathic

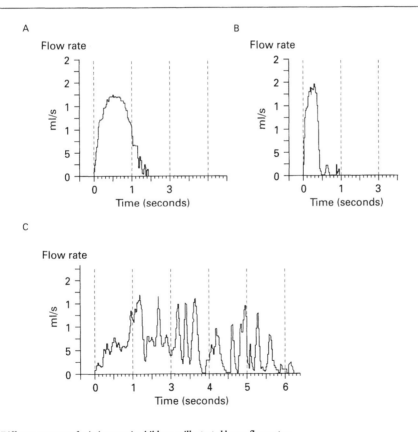

Figure 13.6 Different patterns of mictiograms in children as illustrated by uroflowmetry

The curves show the urinary flow rate (ml/s) on the abscissa and time (s) on the ordinate. The figure shows a normal bell shaped flow curve (A), a tower shaped flow curve in a child with urge incontinence (B), and a fractionated flow curve in a child with dysfunctional (staccato) voiding (C)

bladder-sphincter dyscoordination is one of the more widespread, overactive urethra another, but many adhere to the descriptive term 'staccato voiding'. The symptoms are to some extent similar to those of the urge syndrome although recurrent UTI and constipation/soiling are more prevalent in this patient group.[19] It is generally agreed that a consistent pattern of three characteristic uroflowmetries consecutively measured are prerogatives for the diagnosis. The etiology of staccato voiding is not fully elucidated. The most simple theory is that it may be a long-time effect caused by the voiding pains following a urinary tract infection, where the child learns to protect the urethra from the full urine stream by contracting the sphincter, and continues to do so after the urethral pain has disappeared, but also a long-term overtraining of the pelvic floor, and the urethral sphincter during the holding situation in children with small bladders. It is also hypothesized that it is a sign of a delayed maturation of the interaction between the detrusor and the pelvic floor or an increased nociceptive receptor response in the proximal part of the urethra.

Besides elimination of UTI and constipation, initial treatment consists of bladder rehabilitation with timed voidings and double voiding twice a day. If the response is insufficient, further pelvic floor relaxation with biofeedback training or treatment trial with an alpha-blocking agent may be tried, although the evidence level for this type of treatment is low (Fig. 13.5). In treatment resistant cases, clean intermittent catheterization for shorter or longer periods may be indicated.[20]

LAZY BLADDER SYNDROME

This entity is characterized by few (≤ 3) daily voidings with unusually large volumes, poor bladder emptying, and a very high prevalence of UTI, constipation, and vesicoureteral reflux. The child is typically straining during micturition and leakages appear secondary to overflow incontinence. The etiology is multifactorial, but one hypothesis suggests that it is the end result of sustained bladder-sphincter dyscoordination. In some of the children the syndrome has a previous infravesical obstruc-

tion as background. In order to establish the correct diagnosis, it is often necessary to perform a urodynamic examination, also to exclude an underlying neuropathy. The cystometry will show large bladder capacity, most often a weak detrusor, a negative betanechol test, and no signs of obstruction on the pressure flow examination. The treatment is similar to that described for staccato voiding, except that a larger proportion of patients end up needing a period of clean intermittent catheterization.

NEUROPATHIC INCONTINENCE

Although incontinence secondary to neuropathy is rare, it represents a series of conditions that are associated with risks of serious long-term injury to the urinary tract as well as to renal function.

This chapter will not go into details with the different types of incontinence due to neuropathic causes, but merely point to the importance of close and thorough long-term monitoring of bladder and renal function in such patients.[21] The variability of urodynamic abnormalities and their ability to change over time in children with congenital neurologic defects such as myelomeningocele, illustrates the need for life-long specialist follow-up.[22] Treatment of severe neuropathic incontinence is a specialist task and usually requires a large interdisciplinary team including pediatric nephrology, urology, neurology, neurosurgery, orthopedics, psychology, and physiotherapy. Furthermore, it is worth emphasizing that all incontinent children should be screened for neurologic defects as outlined previously. If a suspicion of neuropathy is raised, an MRI of the spinal canal should be performed together with urodynamic evaluation, cystourethrogram, and ultrasound of the urinary tract. The conservative treatment includes antimuscarinics either perorally or intravesically, clean intermittent catheterization, laxatives, and prophylactic antibiotics. The surgical treatments include bladder augmentation, vesicocutaneostomy, reflux surgery, and continence preserving surgery.[23] Intravesical injection of botulinum toxin represents a newer method of detrusor relaxant therapy.

STRUCTURAL INCONTINENCE

Anatomic abnormalities can also be associated with significant voiding symptoms and are also potentially damaging forms of incontinence.[24] Although not all are visible by physical examination, it is mandatory to inspect the genital region of the incontinent child for a possible cause of the incontinence.

SPHINCTER BYPASS

Dribbling incontinence should always be a red flag raising suspicion of a structural defect in the urinary tract, such as an ectopic ureter often arising from the upper segment of a duplex kidney. Other forms of structural incontinence with sphincter bypass are the extrophy complex and epispadia where diagnosis is much less complicated than the complex treatment which follows.

URINARY TRACT OBSTRUCTION

Voiding dysfunction and incontinence resulting from congenital forms of lower urinary tract obstruction occur more commonly in boys than girls. The classical example is a posterior urethral valve which most often arises from the colliculus and forms a membrane that obstructs urinary flow. In the severe forms, the diagnosis may be evident already by prenatal ultrasound showing a distended bladder, bilateral hydronephrosis, and hydroureter. In the milder cases, the diagnosis is often obtained by urodynamic evaluation, either by reduced flow rate on a uroflowmetry or by detrusor hyperactivity during filling and high pressures during voiding, or during invasive urodynamic investigation in a boy with treatment resistant day-time incontinence. It is characteristic for 'valve patients' to have long-lasting bladder dysfunction that often requires treatment, and should be followed to adulthood.[25] Another problem in these patients is polyuria caused by post-obstructive renal tubular dysfunction. The polyuria may result in bladder retention, especially during sleep, and a nocturnal catheter may be necessary.

OTHER TYPES OF INCONTINENCE

GIGGLE INCONTINENCE

Intense giggling, typically during pre-puberty and more commonly in girls, has for a long time been known in some individuals to be followed by partial or often complete emptying of the bladder. The etiology is more or less unknown. Physical and urodynamic examination are most often normal. It has been postulated that the giggling via central nervous system centers triggers a reflectory relaxation of the urethral sphincter, which then starts a bladder contraction and micturition. The syndrome is very often highly disturbing for the affected child, and it is of little comfort to the child that the condition generally improves in the course of time. Many different treatment modalities have been tried, but none that are well tested are very effective, and most are ineffective: sympathicomimetic agents, phenyl/phenidate and imipramine, biofeedback training for better pelvic floor control and for control of the sphincter, are some of the choices.

VAGINAL VOIDING

In a substantial number of girls, the hymen is funnel-shaped or the labia partly fused, and during voiding, part of the stream may enter the vagina so that the urine will dribble after the patient has left the toilet. Also some girls, especially obese individuals, tend to sit on the toilet with the thighs closely together which consequently will obstruct normal urine flow and direct some urine into the vagina during micturition.[26] Symptoms are diagnostic with dribbling just after leaving the toilet, and the treatment simple in most cases: the child just has to change position on the toilet to a backward position with one leg on each side of the toilet so that she will be forced to spread her legs widely.

SUMMARY

Nocturnal enuresis and voiding dysfunction are very common disorders of childhood and adolescence that despite their benign nature often are rather chronic and result in significant negative effects on the subject's wellbeing. Furthermore, although the large majority of patients have a non-organic cause for their symptoms, a few cases may be caused by an underlying structural or neurogenic anomaly that causes not only resistance to standard therapy but also poses a threat to renal function. With a structured approach based mainly upon a thorough history and physical examination, and a frequency-volume chart, it is possible to identify subjects at risk for underlying pathology and, in the majority of cases, to obtain the correct diagnosis. Only a minority of patients need invasive urodynamic investigation and imaging. In patients with nocturnal enuresis, knowledge about functional bladder capacity and nocturnal urine volume facilitate the choice of treatment modality. The initial conservative treatment of daytime incontinence is based primarily upon bladder rehabilitation, and only some patients need pharmacologic treatment, biofeedback, or more aggressive treatment. Although some advances have been obtained in our understanding of the mechanisms behind non-neuropathic bladder-sphincter dysfunction there are still many unanswered questions, and good evidence-based treatment modalities are still a hope for the future.

REFERENCES

1. Van Gool, JD et al. Conservative management in Children. In Abrams, P. Khoury, S. Wein, AJ (eds.) First International Consultation on Incontinence. World Health Organisation and International Union Against Cancer, Plymouth. 1999; 487–550.

2. Forsythe WI, Redmond A. Enuresis and spontaneous cure rate. Study of 1129 enuretics. Arch Dis Child 1974; 49.4:259–263.

3. Djurhuus JC, Rittig S. Nocturnal enuresis. Curr Opin Urol 2002; 12.4:317–320.

4. Rittig S et al. Abnormal diurnal rhythm of plasma vasopressin and urinary output in patients with enuresis. Am J Physiol 1989; 256: F664–F671.

5. Hansen AF, Jorgensen TM. A possible explanation of wet and dry nights in enuretic children. Br J Urol 1997; 80:809–811.

6. Rushton HG et al. The influence of small functional bladder capacity and other predictors on the response to desmopressin in the management of monosymptomatic nocturnal enuresis. J Urol 1996; 156:651–655.

7. Sakamoto K, Blaivas JG. Adult onset nocturnal enuresis. J Urol 2001; 165:1914–1917.

8. Oredsson AF, Jorgensen TM. Changes in nocturnal bladder capacity during treatment with the bell and pad for monosymptomatic nocturnal enuresis. J Urol 1998; 160:166–169.

9. Hagglof B et al. Self-esteem in children with nocturnal enuresis and urinary incontinence: improvement of self-esteem after treatment. Eur Urol 1998; 33 Suppl 3:16–19.

10. von Gontard A et al. The genetics of enuresis: a review. J Urol 2001; 166:2438–2443.

11. Hansen MN et al. Intra-individual variability in nighttime urine production and functional bladder capacity estimated by home recordings in patients with nocturnal enuresis. J Urol 2001; 166:2452–2455.

12. Glazener CM, Evans JH. Alarm interventions for nocturnal enuresis in children (Cochrane Review). Cochrane Database Syst Rev 2001; 1:CD002911.

13. Glazener CM, Evans JH. Desmopressin for nocturnal enuresis in children. Cochrane Database Syst Rev 2000; 2:CD002112.

14. Hellstrom AL et al. Micturition habits and incontinence in 7-year-old Swedish school entrants. Eur J Pediatr 1990; 149:434–437.

15. Bauer SB. Special considerations of the overactive bladder in children. Urology 2002; 60:43–48.

16. Nijman RJ. Role of antimuscarinics in the treatment of nonneurogenic daytime urinary incontinence in children. Urology 2004; 63:45–50.

17. Sureshkumar P et al. Treatment of daytime urinary incontinence in children: a systematic review of randomized controlled trials. J Urol 2003; 170:196–200.

18. Abrams P et al. The role of neuromodulation in the management of urinary urge incontinence. B J Urol Int 2003; 91:355–359.

19. Mayo ME, Burns MW. Urodynamic studies in children who wet. Br J Urol 1990; 65:641–645.

20. Nijman RJ. Classification and treatment of functional incontinence in children. Br J Urol Int 2000; 85:37–42.

21. Van Gool JD, Dik P, de Jong TP. Bladder-sphincter dysfunction in myelomeningocele. Eur J Pediatr 2001; 160:414–420.

22. Bauer SB et al. Predictive value of urodynamic evaluation in newborns with myelodysplasia. JAMA 1984; 252:650–652.

23. Lowe JB et al. Surgical management of the neuropathic bladder. Semin Pediatr Surg 2002; 11:120–127.

24. Parkhouse HF et al. Long-term outcome of boys with posterior urethral valves. Br J Urol 1998; 62:59–62.

25. Holmdahl G et al. Bladder dysfunction in boys with posterior urethral valves before and after puberty. J Urol 1996; 155:694–698.

26. Mattsson S, Gladh G. Urethrovaginal reflux – a common cause of daytime incontinence in girls. Pediatrics 2003; 111:136–139.

14. Renal tubular disorders

Israel Zelikovic

INTRODUCTION

Hereditary renal tubular transport disorders comprise a group of diseases that may lead to profound derangements in the homeostasis of electrolytes, minerals, or organic solutes in the body, and can be associated with significant morbidity.[1–3] On the other hand, there are some tubular disorders that are not associated with significant clinical abnormalities. It is important to distinguish between these two possibilities since the evaluation and therapy vary greatly.

For decades, the study of inherited tubular transport disorders has focused on the physiologic and metabolic alterations leading to impaired solute handling by the renal tubules. Over the past decade, breakthroughs in molecular biology and molecular genetics have provided the tools to investigate hereditary tubulopathies at both the cellular and molecular level. As a result, exciting discoveries have been made and the underlying molecular defects in many of these disorders have been defined.[1,2] The molecular study of hereditary tubulopathies has been important not only in clarifying the genetic basis of these disorders, but also in providing new and important insight into the function of specific transport proteins, and into the physiology of renal tubular reclamation of solutes. It is hoped that this will subsequently have a very significant impact on the management and outcome of the patients who are affected.

In general, renal tubular disorders are subdivided into two large groups: 1) primary isolated tubulopathies, which are mostly hereditary and involve an impairment of a single tubular function; 2) generalized tubulopathies, which are hereditary or acquired and are caused by complex tubular derangements involving more than one transport system. A variety of primary inherited tubulopathies alter specific renal epithelial transport functions.[1,2] This, in most instances, leads to the loss of an essential substance in the urine, and either impaired homeostasis of this substance in the body, or precipitation of the substance in the kidney. In some of these disorders, however, the defect in tubular function leads to accumulation of a substance in the body.

Most patients with renal tubular disorders present in the neonatal period or the first year of life. Clinical manifestations of hereditary tubulopathies are commonly non-specific and may include failure to thrive, stunted growth, poor feeding, recurrent vomiting, diarrhea, constipation, polyuria, polydipsia, or recurrent febrile episodes.[4] In some instances, however, more specific manifestations such as rickets, urolithiasis, or hypertension will aid in the diagnosis of a specific tubulopathy. In most of these disorders, the principle of therapy is replacement of the substance lost in the urine or prevention of precipitation of the substance in the kidney; as stated previously, some of the tubulopathies are benign and require no therapy (such as isolated glycosuria). In addition to a detailed history and careful examination of the child, simultaneous and accurate assessment of the serum and urine concentration of the substance involved in the tubulopathy hold the key to the correct diagnosis.[4] Renal sonography and bone radiographs are helpful studies in most tubulopathies.

This chapter summarizes the general characteristics of hereditary tubular transport disorders, reviews some aspects of the pathophysiology and genetic aspects of a few of the diseases, describes the clinical feature of the tubulopathies, and briefly summarizes the therapy of some of the disorders that are seen in children. The reader is also provided with appropriate references for details regarding the molecular pathophysiology. In Table 14.1, the disorders resulting from proximal tubule and loop of Henle defects are summarized.

PROXIMAL TUBULE DISORDERS

CLASSIC CYSTINURIA

GENERAL CHARACTERISTICS

Cystinuria is a disorder of amino acid transport characterized by excessive urinary excretion of cystine and the dibasic amino acids lysine, arginine, and ornithine.[5] The pathogenic mechanism of cystinuria is a defect in the high-affinity, low-capacity amino acid transport system shared by cystine and the dibasic amino acids which operates in the proximal tubule and the small intestine. The very low solubility of cystine in the urine results in cystine stone formation in homozygous patients. Urinary cystine calculi may produce considerable morbidity including urinary obstruction, colic, infection, and, in severe cases, loss of kidney function. Cystinuria accounts for 1–2% of all urolithiasis and 6–8% of urolithiasis in children.[7] Cystine stones are radiopaque because of the density of the sulfur molecule, and on a roentgenogram they appear smooth. Cystine also may act as nidus for calcium oxalate so that mixed stones may be found.[5]

The disease usually presents with renal colic. Occasionally, infection, hypertension, or renal failure may be the first manifestation.[6] Clinical manifestations usually occur in the second and third decades of life. Most patients have recurrent stone formation. Cystinuric patients who receive a kidney transplant have normal urinary cystine and dibasic amino acid excretion after transplantation.[5]

Table 14.1 Hereditary tubulopathies caused by primary gene defects in transporters or channels operating in the proximal tubule and the loop of Henle/distal tubule

Nephron segment disorder	Mode of inheritance	Prominent manifestations
Proximal tubule		
Classic cystinuria – Type I – Types II and III	Autosomal recessive Incomplete autosomal recessive	Urinary stones, obstruction, infection
Renal glycosuria	Autosomal recessive	None
X-linked hypercalciuric nephrolithiasis (Dent's disease)	X-linked recessive	Urinary stones, proximal tubulopathy, rickets, renal insufficiency
Proximal renal tubular acidosis	Autosomal recessive	Normal anion gap metabolic acidosis, failure to thrive, hypokalemia, polyuria, polydipsia, dehydration, muscle weakness, ocular abnormalities
Loop of Henle/distal tubule		
Bartter's syndrome – Type I (Antenatal) – Type II (Antenatal) – Type III (Classic) – Type IV (BSND) – Gitelman's syndrome	Autosomal recessive Autosomal recessive Autosomal recessive Autosomal recessive Autosomal recessive	Renal salt wasting, hypokalemic metabolic alkalosis. Failure to thrive, polyuria, dehydration, muscle weakness, hypercalciuria (in Bartter's), Hypomagnesemia and tetany (in Gitelman's)

Abbreviations: BSND, Bartter's Syndrome with deafness

Classic cystinuria is inherited in an autosomal recessive fashion. It is a common disorder with an overall prevalence of 1:7,000 to 1:15,000 and estimated gene frequency of 0.01.[6] A very high prevalence, 1:2,500, is observed in Israeli Jews of Libyan origin.[5]

Cystinuria has been classified into three phenotypes, based on the degree of intestinal uptake of cystine by homozygotes, and the level of urinary dibasic amino acids in heterozygotes.[5,8] Type I cystinuria is inherited as an autosomal recessive trait and obligate heterozygotes have normal urinary amino acid profiles. In contrast, obligate heterozygotes for type II and type III cystinuria show various degrees of hyperexcretion of cystine and dibasic amino acids in the urine. The transport defects in the 3 types of cystinuria are depicted in Figure 14.1 In addition, genetic compounds of cystinuria, such as type I/III can occur.[8] The molecular basis of cystinuria has been reviewed elsewhere.[9–11] To date, more than 100 different mutations in the genes encoding the subunits of the heteromeric dibasic amino acid transporter (Fig. 14.1) have been identified in patients with cystinuria.[5]

DIAGNOSTIC APPROACH TO CYSTINURIA

The simplest initial diagnostic test in cystinuria is provided by observing typical flat hexagonal cystine crystals via microscopic examination of the urinary sediment of a freshly voided morning urine.[6] The definitive test is measurement of cystine and the dibasic amino acid concentrations in the urine by ion exchange chromatography.

TREATMENT

The major therapeutic approaches to patients with cystinuria are designed to increase the solubility of cystine, reduce cystine excretion, and convert cystine to more soluble compounds.[6] Therapies used in the management of cystinuria include the following:

1) Increased oral fluid intake to increase urine volume and cystine solubility. Because cystinuric

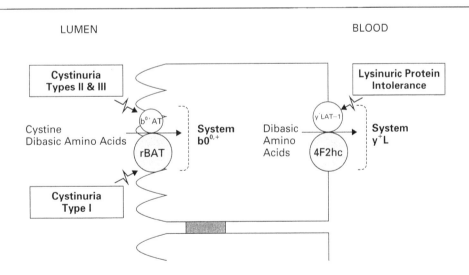

Figure 14.1 Transport pathways for cystine and dibasic amino acids at the luminal and basolateral membranes of a proximal tubular cell

Large circles represent the heavy subunits and small circles represent the light subunits of the heteromeric amino acid transporters $b^{0,+}$ and y^+L. Depicted are hereditary aminoacidurias caused by defects in these transporters

patients excrete 0.5–1.0 g cystine/day, intake of 3–4 L may be necessary to keep the urinary cystine concentration below 300 mg/L.[5,6]

2) Oral alkali in addition to high fluid intake to further increase cystine solubility in the urine.[7] A urine pH of 7.5–8.0 can be maintained by the provision of 1–2 mEq/kg/day of bicarbonate or citrate in divided doses. Because high sodium intake increases cystine excretion, potassium citrate is preferred.[7] Because urine alkalinization may result in formation of mixed Ca^{2+}-containing stones, adherence to high fluid intake is crucial.

3) Sodium (Na^+) restriction to reduce cystine excretion. Dietary Na^+ excretion is recommended in cystinuric patients because urinary excretion of cystine and dibasic amino acids correlates with urinary Na^+ excretion.[12]

4) Pharmacologic therapy to increase cystine solubility and decrease cystine excretion. A number of drugs have been used, including D-penicillamine, mercaptopropionyl glycine (MPG), and meso-1,3 dimercaptosuccinic acid (DMSA). Details of these therapeutic approaches are available elsewhere.[5,7,13,14]

5) Urologic procedures that have been used to treat cystine stones include chemolysis of stones by irrigation through a percutaneous nephrostomy, extracorporal shockwave lithotripsy, and lithotomy.

HEREDITARY ISOLATED GLYCOSURIA

GENERAL CHARACTERISTICS

Hereditary isolated glycosuria is an abnormality in which variable amounts of glucose are excreted in the urine despite normal concentrations of blood glucose.[5,15] The renal defect is specific for glucose, and there is no increase in the urinary excretion of other sugars. It is important for the primary care provider to know that renal glycosuria is a benign condition without symptoms or physical consequences except during pregnancy or prolonged starvation – when dehydration and ketosis may develop.[15] The metabolism, storage, and use of carbohydrates, as well as insulin secretion are normal. The condition exists from infancy throughout adult life, and diagnosis is usually made on routine urine

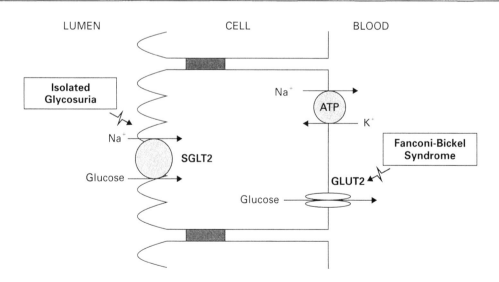

Figure 14.2 Transport pathways for glucose at the luminal and basolateral membranes of a proximal convoluted tubular cell

Depicted are hereditary tubulopathies caused by defects in these transport mechanisms

analysis. The distinction between renal glycosuria and diabetes mellitus is made with a fasting blood glucose level and a glucose tolerance test. The genetic pattern in renal glycosuria is autosomal recessive.[15]

MOLECULAR PATHOPHYSIOLOGY

Transport of glucose in the proximal convoluted tubule occurs by a low-affinity/high-capacity Na$^+$-glucose co-transporter; SGLT2, which reabsorbs the bulk (90%) of the filtered glucose (Fig. 14.2).[5,16] The residual glucose reabsorption occurs in the straight segment of the proximal tubule. To date, more than 20 different mutations in the gene encoding SGLT2 have been identified in patients with isolated glycosuria.[17,18] In some cases, the glycosuria is accompanied by aminoaciduria, the pathophysiology of which is unknown.[18]

X-LINKED HYPERCALCIURIC NEPHROLITHIASIS (DENT'S DISEASE)

GENERAL CHARACTERISTICS

X-linked hypercalciuric nephrolithiasis (XLHN) comprises several different syndromes which share many clinical and biochemical manifestations. These syndromes include X-linked recessive nephrolithiasis reported in North America,[19] Dent's disease reported in the United Kingdom,[20] X-linked recessive hypophosphatemic rickets reported in Italy,[21] and low molecular weight proteinuria with hypercalciuria and nephrocalcinosis reported in Japan.[22] All these syndromes have several features in common, including low molecular weight proteinuria (the most consistent finding), other proximal tubular defects (such as renal glycosuria, aminoaciduria, and phosphate wasting), hypercalciuria with nephrolithiasis or nephrocalcinosis, and no evidence of proximal renal tubular acidosis.[1,23] In addition, these syndromes are characterized by the presence of metabolic bone disease (hypophosphatemic rickets), progressive renal insufficiency (which usually develops by late adolescence), and

male predominance. Patients with the XLHN syndrome have decreased serum parathyroid hormone levels and elevated serum 1,25(OH)$_2$VitD levels. Most carrier females have low molecular weight proteinuria.[1,23]

MOLECULAR PATHOPHYSIOLOGY

All four syndromes described above have an X-linked recessive mode of inheritance and linkage analysis has mapped the genetic defect to the short arm of the X-chromosome.[1] Further molecular analysis has identified the CLCN5 gene as the mutated gene in all four diseases.[1,24] This gene encodes a voltage-dependent Cl$^-$ channel, ClC5, a protein which is a member of a large family of at least 10 voltage-gated Cl$^-$ channels. The ClC5 protein, which is kidney specific, is expressed throughout the renal tubule including the proximal tubule. To date, more than 70 mutations have been identified in families with XHLN.[25] These mutations inactivate the Cl$^-$ channel (Fig. 14.3).[24] It is unclear, however, why ClC5 mutations produce hypercalciuria and other related manifestations of XLHN. It has been suggested that defective proximal tubular endocytosis of calciotropic hormones could lead to impaired Ca^{2+} homeostasis and hypercalciuria.[1] Alternatively, since ClC5 is also expressed in the thick ascending limb of the loop of Henle, a major site of Ca^{2+} reabsorption, it is possible that impaired channel function in this nephron segment contributes to the hypercalciuria.

TREATMENT

Since hypercalciuria is the major cause of morbidity in XLHN leading to nephrolithiasis and contributing to the development of renal insufficiency, therapy should aim to reduce urinary calcium excretion. This may be achieved by restricting dietary intake of Na$^+$, as well as by thiazide therapy. Hypophosphatemia should be corrected using phosphate supplements.

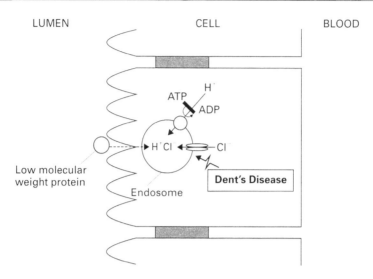

LUMEN   CELL   BLOOD

Figure 14.3 A schematic diagram showing the interplay between H^+-ATPase and ClC5 channel in the process of acidification of the endocytic vesicle in a proximal tubular cell

Defective ClC5 function in Dent's disease disrupts endosomal acidification thereby leading to impaired reabsorption of low molecular weight proteins from the tubular lumen

PROXIMAL RENAL TUBULAR ACIDOSIS

GENERAL CHARACTERISTICS

Proximal renal tubular acidosis (pRTA) is characterized by hyperchloremic metabolic acidosis that is caused by impaired capacity of the proximal tubule to reabsorb biocarbonate ions (HCO_3^-) (Fig. 14.4).[27,28] As a result, large amounts of HCO_3^- (>15% of the filtered load) escape proximal reabsorption and reach the distal tubule. This overwhelms the limited capacity of the distal tubule to reabsorb HCO_3^-, substantial bicarbonaturia occurs, and metabolic acidosis develops.[28,29] When the serum HCO_3^- level stabilizes in the acidemia range, smaller amounts of HCO_3^- are filtered and the amount that escapes reabsorption in the proximal tubule is completely reabsorbed by the distal tubule. As a result, the urine pH decreases to <5.5.[27,29] Hypokalemia usually occurs because increased delivery of Na^+ to the distal nephron results in enhanced secretion of K^+ in the collecting duct and mild volume depletion secondary to Na^+

loss results in secondary hyperaldosteronism that increases K^+ secretion.[28] pRTA may occur either as a manifestation of a generalized proximal tubular dysfunction (Fanconi syndrome), or as an isolated entity. Inheritance of isolated pRTA is autosomal recessive and occurs consistently in association with ocular abnormalities including glaucoma, band keratopathy, and cataracts.[1]

CLINICAL FEATURES

The most prominent clinical feature of pRTA is failure to thrive. Other manifestations, which are related to untreated hypokalemia, include polyuria, polydipsia, dehydration, vomiting, anorexia, constipation, and muscle weakness.[27] Hypercalciuria, nephrocalcinosis, and nephrolithiasis typically are not observed. Metabolic bone disease occurs only in patients with Fanconi syndrome, and is attributed to hypophosphatemia and impaired vitamin D metabolism.

The diagnosis of pRTA is usually straightforward and can be based on several simple laboratory

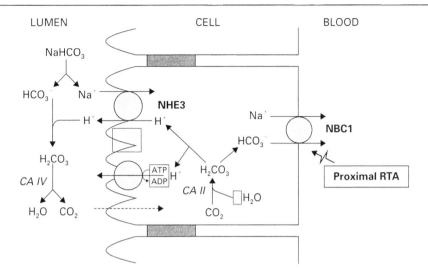

Figure 14.4 Transport mechanisms participating in acid-base handling in a proximal tubular cell

H^+ and HCO_3^- are formed in the cell as a result of carbonic anhydrase II (CAII) action. H^+ exits the cell via the apical Na^+/H^+ exchanger (NHE3) and H^+-ATPase pump. HCO_3^- exit occurs via the basolateral Na^+/HCO_3^- cotransporter (NBC1). Hereditary proximal RTA caused by a defect in NBC1 is depicted

tests. These include: (1) normal anion gap, hyperchloremic metabolic acidosis; (2) hypokalemia; (3) low urine pH during acidemia and (4) a negative urinary anion gap (calculated as $[Na^+]+[K^+]-[Cl^-]$) indicating substantial urinary ammonium concentration, in the absence of extrarenal losses of HCO_3^- such as gastroenteritis.[27] Although usually not necessary, demonstration of increased ($>15\%$) fractional excretion of HCO_3^- by HCO_3^- titration curve, can support the diagnosis. Children with pRTA require large doses of alkali, up to 20 mEq/kg/d. Hypokalemia should be treated by correcting hypovolemia and by using KCl supplements.[27]

LOOP OF HENLE/DISTAL TUBULE DISORDERS

BARTTER'S AND GITELMAN'S SYNDROMES

GENERAL CHARACTERISTICS

Bartter's syndrome is a group of closely related hereditary tubulopathies. Some of the tubular defects are shown in Figures 14.5–14.6. All variants of the syndrome share several clinical characteristics including renal salt wasting, hypokalemic metabolic alkalosis, hyperreninemic hyperaldosteronism with normal blood pressure, and hyperplasia of the juxtaglomerular apparatus.[30–32] All forms of the syndrome are transmitted as autosomal recessive traits.

Traditionally, the disease has been classified into three distinct phenotypes. Antenatal Bartter's syndrome is the most severe form of the disease. It is characterized by polyhydramnios, premature birth, life-threatening episodes of salt and water loss in the neonatal period, hypokalemic alkalosis, and failure to thrive, as well as hypercalciuria and early-onset nephrocalcinosis.[30,33] Classic Bartter's syndrome, which occurs in infancy or early childhood, is characterized by marked salt wasting and hypokalemia leading to polyuria, polydipsia, volume contraction, muscle weakness, and growth retardation. Hypercalciuria and nephrocalcinosis may also occur.[31,32] Gitelman's syndrome is characterized by a mild clinical presentation in older children or adults.[30] Patients may be asymptomatic and present with transient muscle weakness, abdominal pain, symptoms of neuromuscular irritability, or unexplained hypokalemia. Hypocalciuria and hypomagnesemia are typical.[30,31] Recently, an additional variant of antenatal Bartter's syndrome associated with sensorineural deafness, renal failure and typical appearance has been described.[30] Finally, autosomal dominant hypocalcemia associated with Bartter's syndrome has been recently reported.[30] Generally, Bartter's syndrome results from deflective transpithelial transport of Cl^- in the thick ascending limb of the loop of Henle (TAL) or the distal convoluted tubule (DCT) (Figs 14.5, 14.6).[30,31] Several genetic variants of Bartter's syndrome have been identified (Figs 14.5, 14.6).[30,34–37]

THERAPY

Treatment of all variants of Bartter's syndrome involves correction of hypovolemia as well as supplementation of lost electrolytes. This therapy includes increased oral fluid and salt intake, and KCl supplements. Occasionally, spironolactone and/or amiloride can be added to correct the hypokalemia. Indomethacin therapy should be used only in neonatal Bartter's syndrome or severe cases of Bartter's syndrome unresponsive to other therapies. However, attention should be paid to potential gastrointestinal or renal toxicity of this drug. Patients with Gitelman's syndrome should also receive supplemental magnesium in the form of $MgSO_4$ or $MgCl_2$.

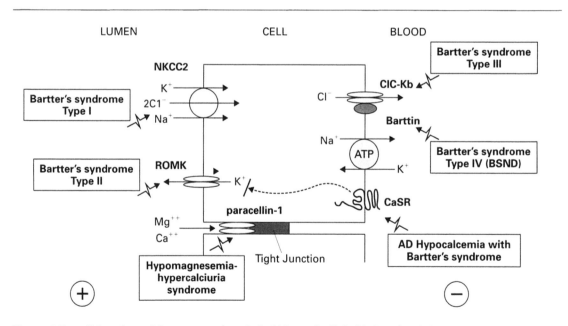

Figure 14.5 Transcellular and paracellular transport pathways in the thick ascending limb of the loop of Henle (TAL)

Cl^- reabsorption across the luminal membrane occurs via the Na^+-K^+-$2Cl^+$ cotransporter (NKCC2). This cotransporter is driven by the low intracellular Na^+ and Cl^- concentrations generated by the basolateral Na^+-K^+-ATPase and ClC-Kb, respectively. In addition, ROMK enables functioning of NKCC2 by recycling K^+ back to lumen. The lumen-positive electrical potential, which is generated by Cl^- entry into cells and K^+ exit from cells, drives paracellular Ca^{2+} and Mg^{2+} transport, via paracellin-1, from lumen to blood. Hereditary tubulopathies caused by defects in these transport mechanisms are depicted. BSND, Bartter's syndrome with deafness; AD Hypocalcemia, autosomal dominant hypocalcemia

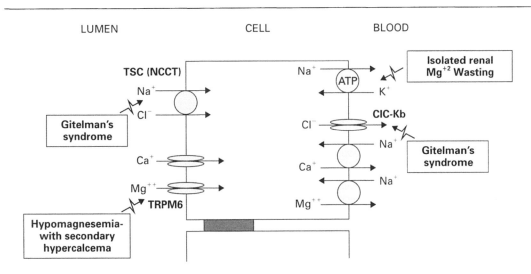

Figure 14.6 Transport mechanisms in the distal convoluted tubule

Cl^- transport occurs via the luminal, thiazide-sensitive NaCl cotransporter (TSC). Cl^- exit to blood is mediated by basolateral Cl^- channels. Ca^{2+} and Mg^{2+} enter the cell via luminal voltage-activated Ca^{2+} and Mg^{2+} channels and exit the cell via basolateral Na^+/Ca^{2+} and Na^+/Mg^{2+} exchangers. The depicted basolateral Na^+/Mg^{2+} exchanger is putative. Hereditary tubulopathies caused by defects in these transport pathways are depicted

COLLECTING DUCT DISORDERS

LIDDLE SYNDROME

GENERAL CHARACTERISTICS

Liddle syndrome is an autosomal dominant disease characterized by the early onset of severe hypertension, metabolic alkalosis, and hypokalemia[1,2] (Table 14.2). Despite the hyperaldosteronism-like picture, the patients have low plasma aldosterone and renin levels. The hypertension is spironolactone resistant but responds to salt restriction and amiloride or triamterene therapy. The disease is caused by an abnormal tendency of the kidneys to preserve Na^+ secondary to the constitutive activation of the amiloride-sensitive epithelial Na^+ channel in the terminal nephron segments.[38,39]

PATHOPHYSIOLOGY

The amiloride-sensitive epithelial Na^+ channel (ENaC), located at the apical membrane of Na^+ transporting epithelia such as kidney, colon, lung, and ducts of exocrine glands, plays an essential role in Na^+ and fluid reabsorption. In the kidney, ENaC is found primarily in the principal cells of the collecting duct, where it mediates the entry of Na^+ across the luminal membrane, a process driven by the basolateral Na^+-K^+-ATPase (Fig. 14.7).[1,40] Hence, ENac has a central role in controlling extracellular fluid homeostasis and blood pressure. The activity of ENaC is under the tight control of hormones, such as aldosterone (Fig. 14.7) and vasopressin.

ENaC is composed of a combination of three similar subunits, α, β, and γ. It has been demonstrated that mutations affecting the carboxy-terminus of either the β or the γ subunit are responsible for Liddle syndrome.[2,38] No mutations have been mapped to the α subunit. It has been shown that these mutations result in impaired ubiquitination, endocytosis and lysosomal degradation of the channel subunits.[1,2] This, in turn, leads to significantly increased channel activity.[2] These gain-of-function mutations provide the pathophysiologic basis of

Table 14.2 Hereditary tubulopathies caused by primary gene defects in transporters or channels operating in the collecting duct

Disorder	Mode of inheritance	Prominent manifestations
Liddle syndrome	Autosomal dominant	Hypokalemic metabolic alkalosis, severe hypertension, stroke
Pseudohypoaldosteronism type I	Autosomal recessive	Renal salt wasting, hyponatremia, hyperkalemia, metabolic acidosis, dehydration, hypotension, respiratory infections
Distal renal tubular acidosis – addRTA – ardRTA with deafness – ardRTA without deafness	Autosomal dominant Autosomal recessive Autosomal recessive	Normal anion gap metabolic acidosis, failure to thrive, hypokalemia, polyuria, polydipsia, dehydration, muscle weakness, nephrocalcinosis
Nephrogenic diabetes insipidus	Autosomal recessive or Autosomal dominant	Failure to thrive, polyuria, polydipsia, dehydration, enuresis, nocturia

Abbreviations: addRTA, autosomal dominant distal renal tubular acidosis; ardRTA, autosomal recessive distal renal tubular acidosis

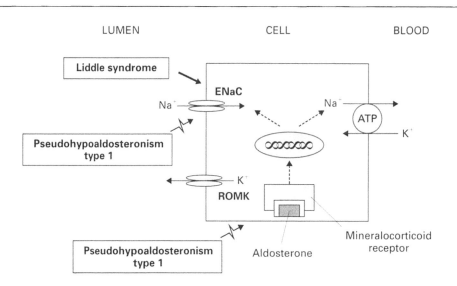

Figure 14.7 Aldosterone action and transport pathways in a principal cell of the collecting duct.

Aldosterone-mineralocorticoid receptor complex interacts with hormone-responsive elements of DNA in the nucleus. This results in production of specific proteins, which stimulate ENaC-mediated Na^+ entry (and ROMK-mediated K^+ exit) at the luminal membrane and Na^+-K^+-ATPase at the basolateral membrane. Depicted are hereditary tubulopathies caused by defects in these transport mechanisms. AR, autosomal recessive; AD, autosomal dominant

Liddle syndrome. Unregulated Na$^+$ reabsorption in the collecting duct results in volume expansion, inhibition of renin and aldosterone production, and hypertension.[1,41]

PSEUDOHYPOALDOSTERONISM TYPE I

GENERAL CHARACTERISTICS AND CLINICAL FEATURES

Pseudohypoaldosteronism type I (PHAI) is a rare inherited disorder characterized by renal salt wasting and end-organ unresponsiveness to mineralocorticoids.[1,2] The manifestations of the disease include hyponatremia, hyperkalemia, metabolic acidosis, and elevated plasma aldosterone, and plasma renin activity. The disorder is divided into two distinct forms with respect to mode of inheritance and clinical features. The autosomal dominant form is a relatively mild disease, which remits with age, is restricted to the kidney, and is caused by loss-of-function mutations in the mineralocorticoid receptor (MR) gene (Fig. 14.7).[42] The autosomal recessive form presents with severe Na$^+$ transport defects in all aldosterone target tissues including the kidney, colon, and salivary and sweat glands, as well as in lungs.[38,43] Autosomal recessive PHAI is characterized by neonatal salt wasting with dehydration, hypotension, life-threatening hyperkalemia, metabolic acidosis ('renal tubular acidosis type IV'), and failure to thrive.[2,38] The manifestations of the disease do not respond to mineralocorticoids but improve with salt supplementation. Neonatal respiratory distress syndrome and respiratory tract infections in affected children are common.[44]

PATHOPHYSIOLOGY

Autosomal recessive PHAI is caused by loss-of-function mutations, which have been described in each of the three subunits in ENaC (Fig. 14.7).[1,2] Hence, autosomal recessive PHI represents, clini-cally and pathophysiologically, the 'mirror image' of Liddle syndrome.

DISTAL RENAL TUBULAR ACIDOSIS

GENERAL CHARACTERISTICS

Distal renal tubular acidosis (dRTA) is characterized by a normal anion gap and hyperchloremic metabolic acidosis that results from deficient hydrogen ion secretion in the distal nephron.[27,45] Patients fail to lower the urine pH adequately even in the presence of systemic acidosis.[45] Urine pH usually remains above 6. The defective H$^+$ secretion results in persistent bicarbonaturia (5%–15% of filtered load in infants and children), reduced net acid secretion, and metabolic acidosis.[27,28]

The pathogenic mechanisms that are responsible for dRTA include: 1) secretory defect: a primary or secondary disorder of the transport pathways participating in acid base handling in the α intercalated cells in the collecting duct (Fig. 14.8); 2) gradient defect: a membrane permeability defect causing increased backleak of luminal H$^+$ (e.g. due to amphotericin B administration); 3) voltage-dependent defect: inability to generate an effective lumen-negative transepithelial potential difference in the distal nephron (e.g. due to impaired reabsorption of Na$^+$ or decreased distal delivery of Na$^+$)[27,28].

Untreated dRTA is characterized by renal wasting of Na$^+$ and K$^+$ as well as HCO$_3$. As in proximal RTA, the urinary K$^+$ loss in dRTA is due to extracellular fluid volume contraction and secondary hyperaldosteronism.[27]

Distal RTA in children is most commonly a primary entity that is inherited as either an autosomal dominant or autosomal recessive trait.[28,46] Patients with the autosomal dominant form usually have mild disease, whereas those with autosomal recessive dRTA may be severely affected in infancy with growth retardation and early nephrocalcinosis leading to renal failure.[45,46] Many patients with autosomal recessive dRTA also have progressive bilateral

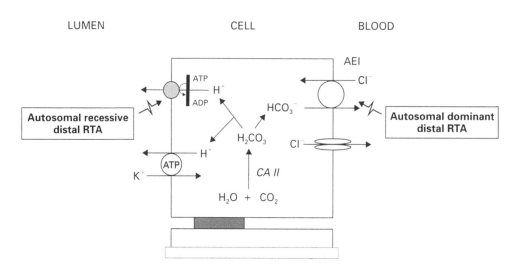

Figure 14.8 Transport pathways participating in acid-base handling in an α intercalated cell of the collecting duct

H^+ and HCO_3^- are formed in the cell as a result of intracellular carbonic anhydrase (CAII) action. H^+ is secreted into the lumen via H^+-ATPase and H^+-K^+-ATPase. HCO_3^- exit is mediated by the basolateral Cl^-/ HCO_3^- exchanger (AE1). Variants of distal RTA caused by defects in these transport mechanisms are depicted

sensorineural hearing loss.[46] The molecular basis of dRTA has been reviewed elsewhere.[1,28]

CLINICAL FEATURES

Prominent clinical manifestations of dRTA include failure to thrive, polyuria, polydipsia, constipation, vomiting, muscle weakness, nephrocalcinosis, and nephrolithiasis.[27,28] The factors promoting the nephrocalcinosis and stone formation in dRTA are hypercalciuria, hypocitraturia, and alkaline urine. The hypercalciuria probably is related to chronic accumulation of acid that is buffered by Ca^{2+} release from bone. The hypocitraturia is secondary to intracellular acidosis that promotes citrate uptake from the renal tubular lumen.[27]

The diagnosis of primary, classical dRTA can be based on: 1) normal anion gap, hyperchloremic metabolic acidosis; 2) hypokalemia (as opposed to the hyperkalemia observed in the voltage-dependent defect); 3) urine pH>5.5 during spontaneous acidosis; 4) a positive urinary anion gap (see proximal

RTA) indicating low urinary ammonium concentration.[27,28] Although usually not necessary, the diagnosis of dRTA can be substantiated by the demonstration of an inability to acidify the urine maximally after NH_4Cl loading or by the finding of urine-blood pCO_2 (U-BpCO_2) <20 mmHg after alkali loading.[27] The evaluation of dRTA should include examination of urinary Ca^{2+} and citrate levels as well as a renal sonogram to investigate for the presence of nephrocalcinosis.

TREATMENT

The goals of dRTA therapy are to improve growth, to prevent nephrocalcinosis/nephrolithiasis, and to prevent progressive renal insufficiency. Infants and young children with dRTA may require up to 10 mEq/kg/day of alkali to correct acidemia, depending on the magnitude of renal HCO_3^- wasting.[28] As renal HCO_3^- wasting decreases with age, alkali requirements decrease. Hypokalemia, which can be significant, should be corrected. Provision of

HCO_3^- by using citrate salts provides the additional advantage of exogenous citrate to prevent nephrocalcinosis/nephrolithiasis.[27]

NEPHROGENIC DIABETES INSIPIDUS

GENERAL CHARACTERISTICS

Congenital nephrogenic diabetes insipidus (NDI) is characterized by an inability of the kidney to concentrate urine in response to the antidiuretic hormone arginine vasopressin (AVP).[1,47] Polydipsia and polyuria, hyposthenuria, dehydration, constipation, and hypernatremia are the hallmarks of NDI in infants and children.[4,48] Failure to thrive is common and recurrent episodes of dehydration may cause severe neurologic sequelae. Older children can present with poor growth, nocturia, and enuresis, and learning and behavior difficulties.[4]

Clinical diagnosis of NDI can be established by a water deprivation test demonstrating inappropriate urinary concentration unresponsive to DDAVP administration. The evaluation of an infant or a child with NDI should include a renal sonogram to evaluate for NDI secondary to disorders that result in impaired ability to concentrate the urine. These include conditions such as dysplastic and polycystic kidneys, renal scars, and nephrocalcinosis.[4]

MOLECULAR PATHOPHYSIOLOGY

The movement of water across the renal tubular epithelial membrane is of central importance in maintaining water and electrolyte balance. Reabsorption of water in the renal tubule occurs mainly through aquaporin (AQP) water channels. Aquaporins are members of a large family of pore-forming intrinsic membrane proteins, the MIP family.[1,48] There are now 10 well-characterized mammalian aquaporins, AQP 0–9, of which six (AQP 1, 2, 3, 4, 6, 7) are expressed in the kidney.[49] Ultrastructural studies have shown that AQPs have a barrel-like structure and they are assembled in tetramers.[1]

AQP2 is the vasopressin-responsive AQP in the principal cells of the kidney collecting duct, where 10% of the filtered volume is reabsorbed (Fig. 14.9). AQP2 is localized to the apical side (lumen) of the principal cell (whereas AQP3 and AQP4 are expressed at the basolateral membrane).[49] Binding of AVP to the vasopressin type-2 receptor (V_2R) at the basolateral (blood) side of the principal cell increases intracellular cAMP levels, resulting in phosphorylation of AQP2 by cAMP-dependent protein kinase (Fig. 14.9). This, in turn, triggers intracellular vesicles containing AQP2 to fuse with the apical membrane, rendering the cell water permeable. Upon dissociation of AVP from its receptor, AQP2 is internalized by endocytosis and the cell returns to its water impermeable state.[1,48]

In the large majority of cases, congenital NDI is an X-linked recessive disorder caused by mutations in the $AVPV_2$ receptor gene located on chromosome Xq28.[50,51] In addition to the X-linked form of inheritance, NDI can be transmitted as an autosomal recessive or autosomal dominant trait. In these cases, the disease is caused by mutations in the AQP2 gene.[52,53] To date, more than 20 different mutations in the AQP2 gene have been reported in autosomal recessive NDI.[53] Most of these are missense mutations. The mutations lead to an impaired routing of channel proteins to the plasma membrane due to retention in the endoplasmic reticulum (ER).

Recently, NDI families with autosomal dominant inheritance have been identified. This form of NDI is caused by a single missense mutation in the AQP2 gene. This mutant, in contrast to the recessive mutants, is not retained in the ER but in the Golgi compartment.[1]

THERAPY

The hallmarks of therapy of NDI include: (1) replacement of urinary water losses by adequate supply of fluid (if necessary, via nasogastric or gastric tube); (2) reduction of dietary solute load by restricting Na^+ intake and by providing protein intake not higher than the recommended daily allowance, and (3) pharmacologic therapy including thiazide, amiloride, and if indicated, indomethacin.[54,55]

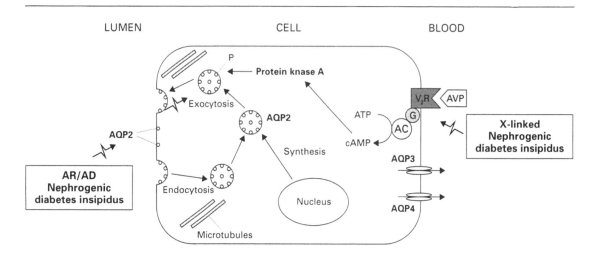

Figure 14.9 Regulation of aquaporin-2 (AQP2) recycling in a principal cell of the collecting duct

Binding of AVP2 to vasopressin type 2 receptor (V_2R) at the basolateral membrane triggers a signaling cascade, which results in protein kinase A-induced phosphorylation of AQP2 in intracellular vesicles. Following phosphorylation, AQP2-containing vesicles translocate to the apical membrane (a process that involves the microtubular machinery) thereby increasing the water permeability of the membrane. Upon dissociation of AVP from its receptor, AQP2 is retrieved endocytically from the apical membrane and the cell returns to its water impermeable state. Variants of nephrogenic diabetes insipidus caused by defects in these pathways are depicted. AR, autosomal recessive; AD, autosomal dominant

CONCLUSION

In the past decade, remarkable progress has been made in our understanding of the hereditary tubulopathies. Molecular genetics and molecular biology studies have led to the identification of numerous renal tubular disease-causing mutations, have provided important insight into the defective molecular mechanisms underlying various tubulopathies, and have greatly increased our understanding of the physiology of renal tubular transport. Nevertheless, numerous issues remain unsettled and warrant additional research. Future studies will shed more light on the molecular mechanisms and functional defects underlying the impaired transport in various tubulopathies. These studies may significantly improve our understanding of the mechanisms underlying renal salt homeostasis, urinary mineral excretion, and blood pressure regulation in health and disease. The identification of the molecular defects in inherited tubulopathies may provide a basis for future design of targeted therapeutic interventions and, possibly, strategies for gene therapy of these complex disorders.

REFERENCES

1. Zelikovic I. Molecular pathophysiology of tubular transport disorders. Pediatr Nephrol 2001; 16:919–935.
2. Scheinman SJ, Guay-Woodford LM, Thakker RV et al. Genetic disorders of renal electrolyte transport. N Engl J Med 1999; 340:1177–1187.
3. Dell KM, Guay-Woodford LM. Inherited tubular transport disorders. Semin Nephrol 1999; 19:364–373.
4. Dehoorne J, van't Hoff W. Renal tubular disorders. Curr Paed 2003; 13:478–495.
5. Zelikovic I. Aminoaciduria and glycosuria. In: Avner ED, Harmon W, Niaudet P (eds). Pediatric Nephrology, 5th Edition. Lippincott Williams & Wilkins Publishing: Philadelphia. 2004 701–728.
6. Palacin M, Goodyer P, Nunes V et al. Cystinuria. In: Scriver CR, Beaudet AL, Sly WS, et al. (eds). The Metabolic and Molecular Bases of Inherited Disease. McGraw-Hill: New York. 2001. 4909–4932.
7. Milliner DS. Cystinuria. Endocrinol Metab Clin North Am 1990; 19:889–907.

8. Goodyer P, Saadi I, Ong P et al. Cystinuria subtype and the risk of nephrolithiasis. Kidney Int 1998; 54:56–61.

9. Chillaron J, Roca R, Valencia A et al. Heteromeric amino acid transporters: biochemistry, genetics, and physiology. Am J Physiol 2001; 281:F995–F1018.

10. Palacin M, Borsani G, Sebastio G. The molecular bases of cystinuria and lysinuric protein intolerance. Curr Opin Genet Dev 2001; 11:328–335.

11. Wagner CA, Lang F, Bröer S. Function and structure of heterodimeric amino acid transporters. Am J Physiol 2001; 281:C1077–C1093.

12. Jaeger P, Portmann L, Saunders A et al. Anticystinuric effects of glutamine and of dietary sodium restriction. N Engl J Med 1986; 315:1120–1123.

13. Jaffe IA. Adverse effects profile of sulfhydryl compounds in man. Am J Med 1986; 80:471–476.

14. Pak CYC, Fuller C, Sakhaee K et al. Management of cystine nephrolithiasis with alpha-mercaptopropionylglycine. J Urol 1986; 136:1003–1008.

15. Wright E, Martin MG, Turk E. Familal glucose-galactose malabsorption and hereditary glycosuria. In: Scriver CR, Beaudet AL, Sly WS, et al. (eds.). The Metabolic and Molecular Bases of Inherited Disease. McGraw-Hill: New York, 2001. 4891–4908.

16. Wright EM. Renal Na$^+$-glucose cotransporters. Am J Physiol 2001; 280:F10–F18.

17. Santer R, Kinner M, Lassen CL et al. Molecular analysis of the SGLT2 gene in patients with renal glucosuria. J Am Soc Nephrol 2003; 14:2873–2882.

18. Magen D, Sprecher E, Zelikovic I, et al. A novel missense mutation in SLC5A2 encoding SGLT2 underlies autosomal recessive renal glucosuria and aminoaciduria. Kidney Int 2005; 67:34–41.

19. Frymoyer PA, Scheinman SJ, Dunhum PB et al. X-linked recessive nephrolithiasis with renal failure. N Engl J Med 1991; 325:681–686.

20. Dent CE, Friedman M. Hypocalciuric rickets associated with renal tubular damage. Arch Dis Child 1964; 39:240–249.

21. Bolino A, Devoto M, Enia G et al. A new form of X-linked hypophosphatemic ricket with hypercalciuria (HPDR II) maps in the Xp11 region. Eur J Hum Genet 1993; 1:269–270.

22. Lloyd SE, Pearce SH, Gunther W et al. Idiopathic low molecular weight proteinuria with hypercalciuric nephrocalcinosis in Japanese children is due to mutations of the renal chloride channel (CLCN5). J Clin Invest 1997; 99:967–974.

23. Scheinman SJ. X-linked hypercalciuric nephrolithiasis: clinical syndromes and chloride channel mutations. Kidney Int 1998; 53:3–17.

24. Lloyd SE, Pearce SHS, Fisher SE et al. A common molecular basis for three inherited kidney stone diseases. Nature 1996; 379:445–449.

25. Hoopes RR Jr, Raja KM, Koich A, et al. Evidence for genetic heterogeneity in Dent's disease. Kid Int 2004. 65:1615–1620.

26. Magen D, Adler L, Mandel H et al. Autosomal recessive renal proximal tubolopathy and hypercalciuria: A new syndrome. Am J Kid Dis 2004; 43:600–606.

27. Zelikovic I. Renal tubular acidosis. Pediatr Ann 1995; 24:48–54.

28. Rodriguez-Soriano J. New insights into the pathogenesis of renal tubular acidosis – from functional to molecular studies. Pediatr Nephrol 2000; 14:1121–1136.

29. Cogan MG, Quan AH. Renal acidification: integrated tubular responses. In: Windhager EE (ed). Renal Physiology, Oxford University Press: New York; 1992. 969–1016.

30. Zelikovic I. Hypokalemic salt-losing tubulopathies: an evolving story. Nephrol Dial Transpl 2003; 18:1696–1700.

31. Guay-Woodford LM. Bartter syndrome: unraveling the pathophysiologic enigma. Am J Med 1998; 105:151–161.

32. Rodriguez-Soriano J. Bartter and related syndromes: the puzzle is almost solved. Pediatr Nephrol 1998; 12:315–327.

33. Seyberth HW, Rascher W, Schweer H et al. Congenital hypokalemia with hypercalciuria in pre-term infants: a hyperprostaglandinuric tubular syndrome different from Bartter syndrome. J Pediatr 1985; 107:694–701.

34. Simon DB, Karet FE, Hamdan JM et al. Bartter's syndrome, hypokalemic alkalosis with hypercalciuria, is caused by mutations in the Na-K-2Cl cotransporter NKCC2. Nat Genet 1996; 13:183–188.

35. Simon DB, Karet FE, Rodriguez-Soriano J et al. Genetic heterogeneity of Bartter's syndrome revealed by mutations in the K$^+$ channel, ROMK. Nat Genet 1996; 14:152–156.

36. Simon DB, Bindra RS, Mansfield TA et al. Mutations in the chloride channel gene, CLCNKB, cause Bartter's syndrome type III. Nat Genet 1997; 17:171–178.

37. Simon DB, Nelson-Williams C, Bia MJ et al. Gitelman's variant of Bartter's syndrome, inherited hypokalemic alkalosis, is caused by mutations in the thiazide-sensitive Na-Cl cotransporter. Nat Genet 1996; 12:24–30.

38. Rossier BC. Cum grano salis: the epithelial sodium channel and the control of blood pressure. J Am Soc Nephrol 1997; 8:980–992.

39. Stokes JB. Disorders of the epithelial sodium channel: insights into the regulation of extracellular volume and blood pressure. Kidney Int 1999; 56:2318–2333.

40. Garty H, Palmer LG. Epithelial sodium channels: function, structure and regulation. Physiol Rev 1997; 77:359–396.

41. Warnock DG. Hypertension. Semin Nephrol 1999; 19:374–380.

42. Geller DS, Rodriguez-Soriano J, Vallo A et al. Mutations in the mineralocorticoid receptor gene cause autosomal dominant pseudohypoaldosteronism Type I. Nat Genet 1998; 19:279–281.

43. Bonny O, Hummler E. Dysfunction of epithelial sodium transport: from human to mouse. Kidney Int 2000; 57:1313–1318.

44. Kerem E, Bistritzer T, Hanukoglu A et al. Pulmonary epithelial sodium channel dysfunction and excess airway liquid in pseudohypoaldosteronism. N Engl J Med 1999; 341:156–162.

45. DuBose TD Jr, Alpern RJ. Renal tubular acidosis. In: Scriver CR, Beaudet AL, Sly WS, Valle D (eds). The Metabolic and Molecular Bases of Inherited Disease. McGraw-Hill: New-York. 1995; 3655–3689.

46. Shayakul C, Alper SL. Inherited renal tubular acidosis. Curr Opin Nephrol Hypertens 2000; 9:541–546.

47. Bichet DG. Nephrogenic diabetes insipidus. Am J Med 1998; 105:431–442.

48. Deen PMT, van Os CH. Epithelial aquaporins. Curr Opin Cell Biol 1998; 10:435–442.

49. Nielsen S, Kwon TH, Christensen BM et al. Physiology and pathophysiology of renal aquaporins. J Am Soc Nephrol 1999; 10:647–663.

50. Rosenthal W, Seibold A, Antaramian A et al. Molecular identification of the gene responsible for congenital nephrogenic diabetes insipidus. Nature 1992; 359:233–235.

51. Deen PMT, Verdijk MA, Knoers NVAM et al. Requirement of human renal water channel aquaporin-2 for vasopressin-dependent concentration of urine. Science 1994; 264:92–95.

52. Mulders SM, Knoers AVAM, van Leiburg AF et al. New mutations in the AQP2 gene in nephrogenic diabetes insipidus resulting in functional but misrouted water channels. J Am Soc Nephrol 1997; 8:242–248.

53. Mulders SM, Bichet DG, Rijss JP et al. An aquaporin-2 water channel mutant which causes autosomal dominant nephrogenic diabetes insipidus is retained in the Golgi complex. J Clin Invest 1998; 102:57–66.

54. Sasaki S. Nephrogenic diabetes insipidus: update of genetic and clinical aspects. Nephrol Dial Transplant 2004; 19:1351–1353.

55. Knoers NVAM, Monnens LLAH. Nephrogenic diabetes insipidus. Semin Nephrol 1999; 19:344–352.

15. Acute renal failure and hemolytic uremic syndrome

Rajendra Bhimma and Bernard Kaplan

INTRODUCTION

Acute renal failure (ARF) is the sudden loss of the kidneys' abilities to excrete wastes, concentrate urine, and reabsorb electrolytes.[1] ARF most often occurs in the absence of prior renal dysfunction, but some cases are superimposed on chronic kidney disease.

CLASSIFICATION AND ETIOLOGY OF ARF

Causes of ARF may be considered as pre-renal, intra-renal (including vascular insults), and post-renal (Tables 15.1–15.3).[2] The primary causes of ARF differ among neonates, infants, children, and adolescents. For example, acute cortical necrosis and renal venous thrombosis occur more commonly in neonates; the hemolytic uremic syndrome (HUS) is more common in young children; post-infectious glomerulonephritis occurs in children and adolescents. It is also important to note that some cases of ARF may be multifactorial, especially in hospitalized children.

DIAGNOSIS OF ARF

Oliguria is defined as urine output of < 400 to 500 ml/24 hours in an older child or urine output of < 0.5 to 1.0 ml/kg/hour in a neonate and infant. Although oliguria is an important feature of ARF many patients have non-oliguric ARF.[3] This is defined as normal or increased urine volumes despite increasing serum creatinine concentrations. The serum creatinine concentration is the easiest method of assessing renal function, but there is no precise correlation between the serum creatinine concentration and GFR because of confounding factors. This is discussed in detail in Chapter 1. In addition it should be noted that non-steady-state conditions in ARF preclude estimations of GFR using the formulae derived from patients with chronic kidney disease. It should be noted that the

---

Table 15.1 Causes of pre-renal ARF[2]

A. Intravascular volume depletion
  i. Gastrointestinal fluid loss
     • Vomiting
     • Diarrhea
     • Enterocutaneous fistula
  ii. Renal fluid loss
     • Diuretics
     • Osmotic diuresis
     • Renal salt wasting
  iii. Cutaneous losses
     • Hypothermia
     • Burns
  iv. Hemorrhage
  v. Third-space fluid loss
     • Pancreatitis
     • Severe hypoalbuminemia
     • Capillary leak syndrome
  vi. Decreased effective arterial blood volume
     • Congestive heart failure
     • Cirrhosis
     • Nephrotic syndrome
     • Sepsis
     • Anesthesia

B. Altered intrarenal hemodynamics
  i. Pre-glomerular – afferent arteriolar vasoconstriction
     • Prostaglandin inhibition
     • Non-steroidal anti-inflammatory agents
     • Cyclooxygenase-2 inhibitors
     • Hypercalcemia
     • Hepatorenal syndrome
     • Calcineurin inhibitors (cyclosporin, tacrolimus)
  ii. Postglomerular – efferent arteriolar vasodilation
     • Angiotensin-converting enzyme inhibition
     • Angiotensin receptor blockade
  iii. Abdominal compartment syndrome

Table 15.2 Causes of intrinsic ARF[2]

A. Acute tubular necrosis
  i. Ischemia
    • Hypotension
    • Hypovolemic shock
    • Sepsis
    • Cardiopulmonary arrest
    • Cardiopulmonary bypass
    • Snake venom
  ii. Nephrotoxic
    • Medications
      • Aminoglycosides, radiocontrast agents
      • Amphotericin B, cisplatin, acetaminophen
    • Poisons
      • Diethylene glycol
    • Pigment nephropathy
      • Hemolysis
      • Rhabdomyolysis
B. Acute interstitial nephritis
  i. Medication induced
    • Penicillins, cephalosporins, sulfanomides
    • Rifampin, dilantin, furosemide
    • Non-steroidal anti-inflammatory agents
  ii. Infections
    • Bacterial, viral, rickettsia
  iii. Systemic disease
    • Lupus nephritis
    • Tubulointerstitial nephritis
  iv. Malignancy
    • Tumor lysis syndrome
    • Tumor infiltration
  v. Transplantation
    • Solid organ transplants
    • Bone marrow transplantation (BMT)
  vi. Metabolic disorders
    • Wilson disease
    • Primary hyperoxaluria type 1
  vii. Idiopathic
C. Acute glomerulonephritis
  i. Post-infectious glomerulonephritis
  ii. Endocarditis-associated glomerulonephritis
  iii. IgA nephropathy
  iv. ANCA-positive glomerulonephritis
  v. Rapidly progressive glomerulonephritis (RPGN)
D. Thrombotic microangiopathy
  i. Hemolytic uremic syndrome
  ii. Thrombotic thrombocytopenic syndrome
E. Acute vascular syndromes
  i. Renal venous thrombosis

Table 15.3 Causes of post-renal ARF[3]

Upper tract obstruction (bilateral obstruction or obstruction of a single functioning kidney)
  i. Intrinsic
    • Stone
    • Papillary necrosis
    • Blood clot
  ii. Extrinsic
    • Retroperitoneal fibrosis
  iii. Lower urinary tract obstruction
    • Urethral stricture
    • Bladder stones
    • Blood clot
    • Fungus ball
    • Neurogenic bladder
    • Malpositioned urethral catheter

bleeding, and tetracyclines – which increase the BUN without changes in GFR, whereas protein-energy malnutrition or severe liver disease may dampen the increase in BUN usually associated with a declining GFR.[3]

STAGES OF ARF

A diagnosis of intrinsic renal failure is made after an indeterminate amount of time has resulted in acute renal parenchymal damage.[4] Pre-renal and post-renal causes of ARF usually do not cause intrinsic renal damage because anticipation of ARF, and early intervention to correct the cause of the decreased function enables normal renal function to be maintained.[1,5] ARF evolves through four distinct phases, although in clinical practice a patient may present to the physician after advancing beyond the first stage[5] (Table 15.4).

HISTORY AND PHYSICAL EXAMINATION

A careful medical history, including information about pre-existing conditions, medications, and family history of renal problems can provide clues as to whether the ARF is due to pre-renal, renal, or post-renal factors. Physical examination should be done to assess the total volume and effective

blood urea nitrogen (BUN), which is also commonly used to provide an estimate of renal function, is affected by many other factors including hypercatabolic states, total parenteral nutrition high in protein, glucocorticoids, gastrointestinal

Table 15.4 Stages of ARF

Stage 1 *Phase of anticipation* – time period when the risk of ARF is recognized prior to a renal insult.

Stage 2 *Initiation phase* – begins at time of renal insult and lasts minutes to hours. The decrease in renal function may be corrected if the cause is identified and eliminated.

Stage 3 *Maintenance phase* – ensues if there is no early or successful intervention; serious renal damage may occur.

Stage 4 *Recovery phase* – begins when kidneys start to heal as reflected by improving GFR. This phase ends with return of renal function and lasts weeks to months.

Adapted with permission[5]

circulating volume status of the patient, and determine which stage of ARF has been reached. Evidence of systemic diseases must be looked for, such as vasculitis, congestive cardiac failure, and liver disease. Symptoms of ARF include anorexia, fatigue, mental status changes, nausea, vomiting, seizures, and dyspnea. Signs include asterixis, myoclonus, pericardial rub, pleural rub, peripheral edema, rales, and elevated right atrial pressure. Despite a careful history and physical examination, the cause for ARF in an individual patient is sometimes not found without additional investigations.

URINE STUDIES

URINALYSIS

A dipstick test that shows ≥ 3+ proteinuria indicates intrinsic renal disease with glomerular damage; milder amounts of proteinuria (trace to 2+) may occur with prerenal ARF, obstructive uropathy, and acute tubular necrosis. Proteinuria may be quantified by a 24-hour urine collection or by determining the protein:creatinine ratio in a random urine sample. Proteinuria > 2 grams/day or a urine protein:creatinine ratio > 2 indicates that the process is more likely glomerular than interstitial or vascular. A positive dipstick test for blood usually reflects the presence of red blood cells (RBCs), but

the absence of RBCs on microscopy is a clue to myoglobinuria or hemoglobinuria. The sediment of a centrifuged urine sample must be examined. In pre-renal ARF, there are no casts, cells, or cellular debris. In post-renal ARF, depending on the cause of the obstruction, RBCs or crystals may be seen, or the urine sediment may be bland. RBCs with RBC casts characterize a glomerular lesion. White blood cells and casts are seen in pyelonephritis, acute post-infectious glomerulonephritis, and acute interstitial nephritis. The sediment in ischemic ATN typically consists of coarse, pigmented, granular casts, tubule epithelial cells and casts, and cellular debris.

URINE DIAGNOSTIC INDICES

Urine and serum diagnostic indices that may be helpful in differentiating the type of ARF are shown in Table 15.5. When these are being interpreted, it should be noted that urine electrolyte excretion and renal concentrating ability are affected by pre-existing renal disease or concurrent use of diuretics which significantly limit the utility of these indices. There are some other important caveats when using these indices. In glomerular diseases the indices more closely reflect those of pre-renal ARF than intrinsic renal disease. Early in the course of obstruction the indices may be similar to prerenal

Table 15.5 Diagnostic indices that help determine the site of the disorder

	Pre-renal	Intra-renal	Post-renal
Urine sodium concentration (mEq/L)	< 20	>20	>20
Fractional excretion of sodium (FE_{Na})	<1%	>2%	>2%
Urine osmolality m0m/kg	>500	<350	<350
Urine/serum creatinine	>40	<20	<20
Renal failure index	<1%	>2%	>2%
Urine/serum urea	>8	<3	<3
BUN/serum creatinine	>20	≅ 10	≅ 10

Adapted with permission[6]

ARF. However, with prolonged obstruction and progressive tubular function impairment, the indices are similar to those of intrinsic renal disease.

URINE SODIUM CONCENTRATION

Urinary sodium excretion reflects the avidity and ability of nephron segments to reabsorb filtered sodium. In prerenal failure, intact tubular function results in avid sodium retention as a result of increased proximal and distal reabsorption. This physiologic response may be used to differentiate between pre-renal and intrinsic ARF.[7] These distinctions are helpful except in contrast-induced ARF, pigment induced injury, and non-oliguric ARF.[7]

The other indices in the table may also be complementary to the Na indices.

BLOOD UREA NITROGEN AND SERUM CREATININE

A BUN serum creatinine ratio of > 20 suggests pre-renal ARF. The ratio is about 10 in ATN. However, this ratio is affected by many factors other than volume status (Table 15.6).

DIAGNOSTIC IMAGING STUDIES

The choice of imaging study that is most appropriate for an individual patient depends on the information needed and the risks of the procedure.

Details of many of the following studies are given in Chapter 2, but the application of a selection of radiographic studies that may be used for the evaluation of a patient with ARF will be reviewed briefly in this section.

RENAL ULTRASONOGRAPHY

This is performed easily in a patient with ARF with no side-effects. Limitations are gross obesity and the operator's skill. Ultrasonography is a sensitive test for diagnosing obstruction (93–98%).[8] It also provides information about kidney size and consistency. Chronic renal disease usually results in small kidneys (scarring, dysplasia), whereas in patients with ARF, the kidneys are often swollen. They are usually echogenic and lack corticomedullary differentiation in both instances.

COMPUTERIZED TOMOGRAPHY

This provides better delineation of anatomic detail in patients with suspected urinary tract obstruction. However, this must be balanced against the risk of contrast-induced renal failure if contrast agents are used.

RADIONUCLEOTIDE SCANS

These offer little value in the clinical evaluation and management of ARF.

ARTERIOGRAPHY, VENOGRAPHY

These are rarely indicated in ARF.

PERCUTANEOUS NEPHROSTOMY, ANTEGRADE PYELOGRAPHY

These procedures are sometimes used to determine the level of obstruction in the urinary tract.[9] Nephrostomy drainage is a safe method for relief of urinary tract obstruction.[10] The technique is simple, is done with ultrasound guidance, and does not require general anesthesia. Potential complications include vascular injury and infection.

Table 15.6 Factors that alter BUN/serum creatinine ratios

Increase ratio	Decrease ratio
Pre-renal failure	Increasing age
Hepatorenal syndrome	Decreased muscle mass
Gastrointestinal bleeding	
Tetracyclines	
Corticosteroids	
Hypercatabolism	
Hyperalimention	

Adapted with permission[6]

RENAL BIOPSY

A percutaneous renal biopsy may be indicated in children with ARF if the etiology is unknown or if there is evidence of rapidly progressive crescentic glomerulonephritis. However, this is rarely performed in children with ARF.

PATHOGENESIS OF ACUTE RENAL FAILURE

The basic pathophysiologic mechanisms of ARF involve hypoperfusion, ischemic cell damage, and nephron injury from toxins and inflammation. The eventual outcome is cellular destruction.[11] Intense intra-renal vasoconstriction occurs during the initiation phase and, to a lesser extent, during the maintenance phase in ATN caused by sepsis, ischemia, radiocontrast agents, and rhabdomyolysis.[12] Insults to tubular epithelial cells result in release of vasoactive compounds that increase cortical vascular resistance, thereby decreasing renal blood flow and perpetuating tubule injury. Release of vasoconstrictive compounds diminishes GFR by constricting the afferent and efferent arterioles and reduced GFR leads to diminished urine output.[12] Increased renin-angiotensin system activity, impairment of renal autoregulation, and enhanced adrenergic activity are implicated in renal vasoconstriction.

ARF is also associated with endothelial dysfunction resulting in an imbalance between production of endothelin, a potent vasoconstrictor, and nitric oxide (NO), a vasodilator.[13,14] Endothelin antagonists are not consistently renoprotective despite increased endothelin levels in experimental models of ARF. Although reduced, NO generation by endothelial NO synthase (eNOS), may contribute to renal vasoconstriction; increased NO production by inducible NO synthase (iNOS) may serve as a mediator of cellular injury.[15]

RENAL TUBULAR CELL INJURY

Ischemic injury results in the rapid development of structural changes in the renal epithelial cells, especially in the proximal tubule. The straight segment of the proximal tubule depends on oxidative phosphorylation for the energy required for transport functions. It is susceptible to ischemia and to nephrotoxins that disrupt energy supply or mitochondrial function.[16,17] A series of intracellular processes causes the loss of epithelial integrity and the shedding of epithelial cells into the tubular lumen. The viable and dead tubular cells form casts that cause intratubular obstruction, increase in intratubular pressure, and a fall in GFR. Loss of the epithelial-cell barrier, and the disruption of the tight junctions between viable cells, permit the back-leak of glomerular filtrate, further reducing the effective GFR.[18] Cellular mechanisms underlying these changes are incompletely understood.

SPECIFIC DISORDERS ASSOCIATED WITH INTRA-RENAL ARF

ACUTE TUBULAR NECROSIS (ATN)

ATN can evolve from prerenal failure if the insult causes sufficient vasoconstriction and tubular necrosis. However, ATN frequently develops in combination with other critical pathologic events such as sepsis, renal hypoperfusion, and nephrotoxic agents. Ischemic ATN may occur after severe volume depletion, cardiogenic shock, burns, sepsis, or following cardiac or vascular surgery. Nephrotoxic ATN results from endogenous or exogenous toxins. Hemoglobin and myoglobin are endogenous toxins that induce tubular injury in the setting of massive intravascular hemolysis or rhabdomyolysis. Exogenous toxins include aminoglycoside antibiotics, anti-neoplastic agents, amphotericin B, calcineurin inhibitors, and radiocontrast agents. When other medical illnesses exist in association with ATN, the morbidity and mortality are increased.[19]

AMINOGLYCOSIDE NEPHROTOXICITY

Aminoglycosides accumulate in high concentrations in proximal tubular cells where they are cytotoxic. Nephrotoxicity usually begins after 7–10 days of therapy in 10–15% of patients. Early toxicity may occur within a day or two of treatment and manifests itself by increased excretion of low molecular weight proteins, lysosomal enzymes, and brush-border membrane enzymes. With progression to ARF there is increased shedding of tubular epithelial cells and formation of tubular casts. There is increased fractional excretion of sodium with variable potassium, calcium, and magnesium wasting.

The dose of the aminoglycoside is a critical factor in the development of ARF. Elevated peak levels in schedules using multiple dosing correlate with toxicity and increasing trough levels reflect a decreasing GFR.[26] Once-daily dosing decreases tubular cell toxicity by reducing the percentage of the cumulative dose of the medication that is taken up by the proximal tubular cells, while taking advantage of enhanced concentration-dependent killing. Most patients recover renal function although the duration of ARF may be prolonged. Risk factors for aminoglycoside nephrotoxicity are volume depletion, prolonged use, advanced age, cardiac surgery, pre-existing renal disease, and hepatobiliary disease. Additional information regarding the use of aminoglycocide antibiotics in patients with renal disease is given in Chapter 19.

AMPHOTERICIN B NEPHROTOXICITY

Amphotericin B can injure many different nephron segments. This may result in acute renal failure, distal renal tubular acidosis from back-leak of hydrogen ions in the collecting duct, potassium and magnesium wasting. The risk for renal failure is dose dependent, with a progressive increase in the risk of ARF with increase in cumulative dose.[27] The renal dysfunction occurs as a result of direct tubular toxicity and intrarenal vasoconstriction. Risk factors for the development of amphotericin B induced ARF are male gender, maximum daily dose, duration of therapy, hospitalization in a critical care unit at initiation of therapy, and concomitant use of cyclosporine A.[27]

PIGMENT-INDUCED ARF

Hemolysis or rhabdomyolysis can result in sufficient hemoglobinuria or myoglobinuria to cause tubular injury and ARF. Rhabdomyolysis is usually subclinical and is not associated with the development of ARF. Severe rhabdomyolysis may cause severe hypovolaemia, metabolic acidosis, hyperkalemia, hyperphosphatemia, hypocalcemia, and ARF.

The mechanisms of injury include vasoconstriction, pigment precipitation in tubule lumens, and heme protein-induced oxidant stress.[28] Causes of rhabdomyolysis are viral infections, muscle compression from immobilization, medications, drugs, and seizures. Causes of hemolysis-associated ARF are incompatible transfusions, sickle cell disease, and G-6-PD-deficiency. The presenting symptoms are usually those of the primary disease with superimposed symptoms of muscle injury or ARF. Physical findings are tender, 'doughy' muscles, edema, and weakness. Rapid fluid resuscitation can prevent or limit renal injury if the rhabdomyolysis is a result of a crush injury with substantial third-space fluid losses.[28] Once intravascular volume is re-established, tubular injury may be reduced by treatment with a loop diuretic to promote flow and prevent precipitation of the heme proteins in the tubules. Urine alkalization increases hemoglobin and myoglobin solubility. Prompt treatment is required for hyperkalemia, acidosis, and other electrolyte abnormalities.

POSTOPERATIVE ARF

This may complicate vascular, cardiac, major abdominal surgery, and solid organ transplants. The pathogenesis of the ARF is multifactorial and includes hypotension, sepsis, and medications. The mortality rate of post-operative ARF is high.[29]

RADIOCONTRAST NEPHROPATHY

A mild, transient decrease in renal function is observed in most patients after contrast administration, but clinically significant renal dysfunction is uncommon.[30] Risk factors for contrast nephropathy are baseline renal insufficiency, diabetes mellitus, congestive heart failure, administration of large doses of contrast media, reduced renal perfusion from volume depletion, non-steroidal anti-inflammatory drugs (NSAIDs), and angiotensin converting enzyme inhibitors (ACE i). Radiocontrast nephropathy is uncommon in children.

ACUTE INTERSTITIAL NEPHRITIS

Acute interstitial nephritis is a cause of ARF in which inflammatory cells infiltrate the renal interstitium. Children with acute interstitial nephritis may have rash, fever, arthralgias, eosinophilia, and pyuria with or without eosinophilia. Diagnosis is difficult and can only be achieved with certainty by means of kidney biopsy. Treatment includes withdrawal of any offending medication or specific treatment of the underlying disease. Corticosteroids may aid the resolution of the interstitial nephritis in selected cases.

HEPATORENAL SYNDROME

This syndrome is characterized by the development of ARF as a result of profound renal vasoconstriction, in children with advanced liver disease, whose kidneys are histologically normal. Many features of hepatorenal syndrome resemble pre-renal ARF, the main difference being the lack of improvement in renal function with volume expansion. Hepatorenal syndrome may represent the end-stage of a disordered systemic and renal hemodynamic state associated with advanced liver disease. In the earlier stages, renal perfusion is maintained within normal or near normal levels despite the overactivity of vasoconstrictor systems. Later in this process, renal perfusion is no longer maintained because progressive splanchnic vasodilation worsens the effective arterial underfilling and maximally activates the vasoconstrictor systems. The clinical presentation is oliguric renal failure associated with a bland urine sediment and a low urine sodium concentration. Renal failure can be precipitated by an acute insult such as acute variceal bleeding, rapid diuresis, paracentesis, or spontaneous bacterial peritonitis.

HEMOLYTIC UREMIC SYNDROME (HUS)

The diagnostic criteria of HUS are acute hemolytic anemia with fragmented erythrocytes, thrombocytopenia, and acute renal failure. HUS occurs mainly in infants and children, is uncommon in blacks, and in most patients follows a prodromal illness of acute gastroenteritis, often associated with bloody diarrhea. This condition is usually caused by Shiga toxin (Stx) producing *E. coli*. Although there are other causes for HUS, this section will focus on the type associated with acute diarrheal illness, since this is the form that is most often encountered by primary care physicians and has the most well identified prodrome. It is important to anticipate the development of HUS whenever possible (Table 15.7).

ETIOLOGY AND PATHOGENESIS

E. coli 0157:H7 is the Stx producing bacterium that usually causes HUS.[20] Stx1 and Stx2 are shiga-like toxins that injure glomerular endothelial cells.[21] The toxins inhibit protein synthesis, injure the cell, and initiate local intravascular coagulation. Approximately 10% of children with *E. coli* 0157:H7 infection develop HUS.

EPIDEMIOLOGY

HUS occurs at any age but peaks between six months and four years. It occurs mainly in summer, sporadically, and in epidemics.[22] HUS usually results from the ingestion of E coli contaminated fruit, vegetables, water, apple cider, milk-containing products, and many different kinds of undercooked

---

Table 15.7 Anticipation of Stx HUS

Anticipate Stx HUS in a patient with bloody diarrhea.

Suspect Stx HUS in a patient with diarrhea whose urine volume does not increase after he/she is rehydrated.

Suspect Stx HUS in a patient who becomes pale or edematous during or after an episode of bloody diarrhea.

Suspect Stx HUS in a patient with seizures during or after bloody diarrhea.

and prepared meats, especially ground meats. It may also follow other activities that expose a child to Stx producing *E. coli* (e.g. in petting zoos).

Affected cases must be reported to the appropriate health department and contacts that develop diarrhea must be evaluated. The incubation period is one to ten days. Antibiotics do not reduce the risk of developing symptomatic *E. coli* 0157:H7 infection and may even increase the risk of HUS in patients who have the infection. In developing countries, HUS usually follows epidemics of *Shigella dysenteriae* infections.[23] This type of HUS is more severe, has a higher mortality, and more severe extra-renal manifestations. In a large series reported from South Africa, the majority of patients were black-Africans from rural backgrounds.[23]

CLINICAL FINDINGS

GASTRO-INTESTINAL FEATURES

Most patients with HUS present initially with gastrointestinal symptoms such as abdominal pain, vomiting and diarrhea, usually with bloody and/or mucoid stools. However, in rare cases, HUS occurs in the absence of diarrhea and may be associated with a urinary tract infection. Colonic symptoms resemble ulcerative colitis, appendicitis, intussusception, rectal prolapse, gastroenteritis, or acute bacterial enterocolitis. Acute colitis is usually transient but complications include toxic megacolon and bowel wall necrosis. Barium enema or sigmoidoscopy is rarely indicated. Hypoalbuminemia may result from an associated protein-losing enteropathy.

Sudden onset of pallor subsequently develops a few days after the gastrointestinal illness and often at the time of improvement of gastrointestinal symptoms. This may be followed by increasing edema and, occasionally, mild jaundice, petechiae, or seizures. Hypertension, with or without congestive heart failure and pulmonary venous congestion, may result in part from excessive fluid administration before recognition of oliguria. Pancreatic dysfunction sometimes causes marked

elevation of serum amylase and lipase levels, and islet cell necrosis occasionally results in hyperglycemia with low insulin levels.

RENAL FEATURES

Oligoanuria occurs in half the cases and some patients have non-oliguric renal failure. Microscopic hematuria is more frequent than macroscopic hematuria. Blood pressure is usually normal at the onset, but often increases after a blood transfusion or administration of excessive amounts of other intravenous fluids. Fluid overload causes edema, hypertension, and heart failure. Urinalysis shows red blood cells and various casts. Biochemical changes of renal dysfunction are increased levels of serum creatinine, potassium, phosphorus, hydrogen ion, uric acid, and BUN. The serum potassium concentration may be low initially as a result of gastroenteritis. Hyperkalemia may develop with reduced glomerular filtration rate, hemolysis, and transcellular shifts caused by acidosis. Serum concentrations of sodium, calcium, bicarbonate, and albumin are low especially in severely ill patients. Serum levels of cholesterol, triglycerides and phospholipids may be elevated. A renal biopsy is rarely indicated in patients with HUS.

HEMATOLOGIC FEATURES

Hemolytic anemia varies from slight decreases in hemoglobin concentration to levels of 3 g/dl. There is no correlation between the severity of hemolysis and of renal failure. Repeated episodes of hemolysis may occur during the first few weeks. The erythrocytes are fragmented as a result of a microangiopathic injury and/or peroxidative damage.[24] Serum levels of lactic dehydrogenase, unconjugated bilirubin, and reticulocyte count are increased. Haptoglobin levels are decreased but the Coombs' tests are usually negative. A leukocytosis often occurs during the first week. Thrombocytopenia lasts for up to two weeks and has no relationship to the course of the renal disease.

NEUROLOGIC FEATURES

Neurologic symptoms are quite variable and range from irritability, somnolence, behavioral changes, restlessness, ataxia, dizziness, tremors, seizures, and even coma in individual patients. Hyponatremia, hypocalcemia, azotemia, and accelerated hypertension may exacerbate the central nervous system disturbances. Magnetic resonance imaging is sensitive for early detection of structural lesions. Brain edema and microthrombi are found in some cases at autopsy.

CARDIOPULMONARY FEATURES

Cardiovascular abnormalities usually result from volume overload but some patients have myocarditis, or cardiogenic shock caused by microthrombi, cardiomyopathy, or aneurysms. A few patients have features of adult respiratory distress syndrome.

TREATMENT

Electrolyte and fluid balance must be managed carefully. Dehydrated patients need appropriate fluid repletion, but if oliguria does not respond to a fluid challenge, care should be taken to avoid volume overload. Hyponatremia, hyperkalemia, hyperphosphatemia, and metabolic acidosis are managed medically. If this fails, dialysis or hemodiafiltration may be required. Dialysis is generally started once it is apparent that the patient manifests clinical symptoms of uremia or is anuric.[25] Continuous hemodiafiltration can be used for patients with a precarious hemodynamic status or colonic gangrene. Packed red blood cells are transfused when the hemoglobin concentration falls below 6 g/dl. Blood is given slowly because of the danger of severe hypertension. Platelet transfusions are indicated for active bleeding or for surgery. Hypertension is treated by vasodilators and fluid removal. Adequate nutrition is maintained enterally or parenterally. There is no specific treatment for the colitis and antibiotic treatment is not recommended. Surgery is indicated if ischemic bowel lesions are suspected. Diabetes mellitus and seizures are treated by established methods. There is no evidence that antithrombotic, fibrinolytic or antiplatelet drugs provide any benefit, nor for the use of fresh frozen plasma, intravenous gamma globulin, or plasmapheresis.

OUTCOME

A poorer outcome is associated with a long and severe diarrheal phase, anuria for more than 14 days, severe neurologic impairment, and high initial neutrophil count. Patients with diffuse cortical necrosis have a worse renal outcome. The acute mortality rate is under 5% in HUS caused by *E. coli*. Complete recovery occurs in 64%, chronic renal insufficiency with hypertension in 4%, late sequelae in 12%, and end-stage renal disease in 9% of patients. Diabetes mellitus and cholelithiasis are additional complications. Recurrent episodes after recovery from Stx HUS are uncommon as are post-transplant recurrences.

NON-DIARRHEA-ASSOCIATED HUS

Non-diarrhea associated HUS is a less common condition that usually follows a respiratory tract viral infection which is often pneumococcal in type. Other causes are bone marrow transplantation, severe HIV infection, and factor H deficiency. This disorder may be inherited as autosomal recessive or dominant traits.

POST-RENAL ARF

Post-renal ARF occurs if both urinary outflow tracts are obstructed or the outflow tract of a solitary kidney is obstructed. Most patients with post-renal ARF are oliguric, although non-oliguric renal failure can occur with partial obstruction. Hydronephrosis detected by renal ultrasonography is an important finding. False negative ultrasound examinations occur if the obstruction is very early or if there is retroperitoneal fibrosis.

Treatment is directed at the underlying disease, and the potential for recovery of renal function is often inversely related to the duration of obstruction. In patients with suspected obstruction of the bladder or urethra, catheterization is mandatory, may be diagnostic, and is often therapeutic. Percutaneous nephrostomy, lithotripsy, ureteral stenting and urethral stenting, are used where appropriate.

MANAGEMENT OF ARF

The approach to the management of patients with ARF is divided into maneuvers to a) prevent or ameliorate ARF; b) treat established ARF, and c) treat patients recovering from ARF.

PREVENTION OF ARF

The events leading to ARF are often unavoidable or unpredictable thus making pre-emptive intervention to prevent ARF impractical in most cases. Even when nephrotoxic or ischemic insults can be anticipated, there is limited specific pharmacologic therapy to prevent ARF.[33]

In virtually all circumstances, renal hypoperfusion is a predisposing factor to the development of ARF. Therefore, optimizing vascular hemodynamics to ensure adequate renal perfusion is a fundamental principle in avoiding the development of ARF. In addition, avoiding or stopping medications that increase renal vasoconstriction can diminish the risk of ARF. Potential nephrotoxic drugs should be used only when absolutely necessary with specific dosing schedules and monitoring of blood levels, if drug assays are available.

PHARMACOLOGIC TREATMENT

There is no uniformly successful specific pharmacologic therapy that can be used to prevent ARF. Diuretics may increase urine output and simplify fluid management, but do not alter the clinical course or mortality in ARF.

DIURETICS

Although mannitol can reverse oliguria in some patients if given early in the course of ARF, it does not always improve renal function. Beneficial effects of pre-treatment with mannitol has been shown in pigment injury, radiocontrast nephropathy, and amphotericin B or cis-platinum nephrotoxicity. Preventive use of loop diuretics in surgical patients or nephrotoxic models of ATN showed no benefit. High doses of loop diuretics should be used cautiously because of the risk of ototoxicity. Furthermore, solute and water diuresis may result in hypovolemia and decreased renal perfusion, with worsening of ARF if fluid and solute losses are not replaced.

DOPAMINE

Dopamine may be vasodilatory or vasoconstrictive, but when infused at low doses (2 to 5 mcg/kg per minute) the vasodilatory effects on the renal vasculature predominate. At higher doses, dopamine binds to adrenergic receptors, resulting in vasoconstriction and inotropic effects. A meta-analysis of studies of dopamine for the prevention and treatment of ARF published between 1966 and 2000,[34] and the results of a randomized clinical trial of low-dose dopamine in 328 patients,[35] failed to demonstrate a beneficial effect of dopamine in the prevention of ARF. Side effects of dopamine therapy, even at low doses, include cardiac arrhythmias, myocardial ischemia, intestinal ischemia with increased risk of Gram-negative bacteremia, and suppression of pituitary secretion.[35] The use of low-dose dopamine in the management of ARF is not supported by clinical evidence.

NUTRITIONAL SUPPORT

ARF is a hypercatabolic state that can result in rapid nutritional deficiency which often leads to delayed recovery. Prompt and proper nutrition is essential to hasten recovery. If the gastrointestinal system is intact and functional, enteral feeding should be instituted as soon as possible. If enteral feeding is not possible, hyperalimentation should be instituted through a central line. A solution with a high concentration of dextrose (25%), lipids (10 to 20%), and protein (1 to 2.0 g/kg per day) is used. Dialysis is started if oliguria or anuria precludes administration of sufficient calories because of difficulty in maintaining fluid balance. In older children, a diet of high biologic value protein, low-phosphorus, and low-potassium containing foods should be given. Infants should receive at least maintenance calories (120 kcal/kg per day), and older children often need a higher calorie intake because of the malnutrition resulting from the hypercatabolism. Protein intake should be restricted to 0.6 g per kg per day in patients not on dialysis. Those on dialysis should have a protein intake of 1 to 1.5 g per kg per day.[36]

DIALYSIS

The indications for starting dialysis in ARF include volume overload unresponsive to diuretic therapy; hyperkalemia unresponsive to medical therapy, and progressive uremia with lethargy, changing mental status, pericarditis, bleeding tendency, or metabolic abnormalities (such as hyperuricemia). It is important to note that when making a decision to start dialysis this must be done in the context of the patient's overall clinical picture.

Dialysis can be performed either by hemodialysis or by peritoneal dialysis. There is increasing use of continuous renal replacement therapies (CRRT). CRRT includes arteriovenous (AV) and venovenous (VV) forms of slow continuous ultrafiltration (SCUF), continuous hemofiltration (CAVH, CVVH), continuous hemodialysis (CAVHD, CVVHD), and continuous hemodiafiltration (CAVHDF, CVVHDF).[37] There are no consistent criteria for using CRRT and practice patterns vary widely within and across geographical regions. It is postulated that the more gradual removal of solute and volume achieved using a CRRT induces less hemodynamic stress than with the rapid volume and solute removal by conventional hemodialysis. There are no specific outcome data supporting the use of CRRT compared with conventional hemodialysis for ARF, except for acute brain injury where CRRT is associated with improved stability of intracranial perfusion as compared with intermittent hemodialysis.[38]

THE RECOVERY PHASE OF ARF

Recovery of renal function is heralded by an increase in urine output, which ultimately may reach several liters per day. The excretion of urea and creatinine lag behind the increase in urine output, and serum levels may continue to increase despite increasing urine output. During the early diuretic phase it is important to monitor renal salt and water excretion accurately in order to adjust input. Management of these patients involves careful fluid replacement to keep pace with urine output. Patients may not respond adequately to changes in hydration and can easily become dehydrated. As tubule function recovers, fluid replacement can be reduced because the patient regains the ability to maintain fluid and electrolyte balance. The urine sodium content can be used to gauge sodium content in the replacement fluid. In general, 0.45% of saline solution is adequate for replacement.

PROGNOSIS

The mortality rate of children with ARF as part of multi-organ failure is much higher compared to those in whom ARF is a manifestation of intrinsic renal disease. Recovery from intrinsic renal disease also depends on the underlying cause of the ARF. Children with acute interstitial nephritis or ATN typically recover normal renal function and are at low risk for late complications. There is hyperfiltration of the remaining nephrons in patients with substantial loss of nephrons from the underlying condition (hemolytic uremic syndrome, cortical necrosis, or rapidly progressive glomerulonephritis). Glomerular hyperfiltration is a risk factor for the late development of glomerulosclerosis and progressive decline in renal function.[39] Such children need lifelong monitoring of their renal function, blood pressure, and urinalysis.

REFERENCES

1. Hand M, Mcmanus M, Harmon W. Renal disorders in pediatric intensive care. In: Rogers MC, Nichols DG., eds. Textbook of Pediatric Intensive Care 3rd ed. Baltimore: Williams & Wilkins. 1992; 2.

2. Palevsky PM. Acute Renal Failure Glassock RJ, eds. Nephrology Self-Assessment Program. 2003; 2:1–48

3. Anderson RJ, Linas SL, Berns AS et al. Non-oliguric renal failure. N Engl J Med 1977; 296:1134–1138.

4. Maxwell LG, Colombani PM, Fivush BA. Renal, metabolic and endocrine failure. In: Rogers MC, Nichols DG. eds. Textbook of Pediatric Intensive Care. 2nd ed. Baltimore: Williams & Wilkins: 1992; 1. 181–182, 224.

5. Feld LG, Springate JE. Acute renal failure. In: Barakat AY, ed. Renal Disease in Children: Clinical Evaluation and Diagnosis. New York: Springer-Verlag. 1990.

6. Corwin HL, Bonventre JV. Acute renal failure. Med Clin North Am 1986; 70 (5):1037–1054.

7. Miller TJ, Anderson RJ, Linas SL et al. Urinary diagnostic indices in acute renal failure. A prospective study. Ann Intern Med 1978; 89:47–50.

8. Ellenbogen PH, Scheible FW, Talner LB et al. Sensitivity of grey scale ultrasound in detecting urinary tract obstruction. AJR 1978 130:731–733.

9. Elyaderani MK, Kandzari SJ. Antegrade pyelography and the urethral perfusion test. In: Elyaderani MK, Kandzari SJ, Castaneda WR et al, eds: Invasive Uroradiology. Toronto: Collamore Press. 1984; 9–22.

10. Elyaderani MK, Kandzari SJ. Percutaneous nephrostomy. In: Elyaderani MK, Kandzari SJ, Castaneda WR et al, eds. Invasive Uroradiology. Toronto: Collamore Press. 1984; 23–54.

11. Seigel NJ, Gaudio KM, Van Why SK, Boydstun II, Devarjan P. Acute renal failure. In: Holliday MA, Barratt MA, Avner ED. eds. Pediatric Nephrology, 3rd ed, Baltimore: Williams & Wilkins. 1993; 1:176–1, 203.

12. Gaudio KM, Siegel NJ. Pathogenesis and treatment of acute renal failure. Pediatr Clin North Am 1987; 34:771–778.

13. Kon V, Bodi K. Biologic actions and pathophysiologic significance of endothelin. Kidney Int 1991; 40:1–12.

14. Peer G, Blum M, Iaina A. Nitric oxide and acute renal failure. Nephron 1996; 73:375–381.

15. Goligorsky MS, Noiri E. Duality of nitric oxide in acute renal injury. Semin Nephrol 1999; 19:263–271.

16. Stein JH, Lifschitz MD, Barnes LD. Currrent concepts on the pathophysiology of acute renal failure. Am J Physiol 1978; 234:F171–F181.

17. Donohoe JF, Venkatachalam MA, Bernard DB et al. Tubular leakage and obstruction after renal ischaemia: structural-functional correlations. Kidney Int 1978; 13:208–222.

18. Sutton TA, Molituris BA. Mechanisms of cellular injury in ischemic acute renal failure. Semin Nephrol 1998; 18:490–497.

19. Levy EM, Viscoli CM, Horwitz RI. The effect of acute renal failure on mortality – A cohort analysis. JAMA 1996; 275:1489–1494.

20. Remuzzi G, Ruggenenti P. The haemolytic uraemic syndrome (Perspectives in Clinical Nephrology) Kidney Int 1995; 48:2–19.

21. Scotland SM, Smith H, Rowe B. The distinct toxins active on vero cells from *Escherichia coli* O157. Lancet 1987; 885–886 II.

22. Su C, Brant LJ. *Escherichia coli* O157:H7 infections in humans. Ann Intern Med 1995; 123:698–714.

23. Bhimma R, Rollins NC, Coovadia HM, Adhikari M. Post-dysentric haemolytic uremic syndrome in children during an epidemic of Shigella dysentery in KwaZulu/Natal. Ped Nephrol 1997; 11:560–564.

24. Turi S, Nemeth I, Vargha I, Matkovic B. Oxidative damage of red blood cells in haemolytic uraemic syndrome. Pediatr Nephrol 1994; 8:26–29.

25. Mariscalco MM. Acute renal failure (Chapter 46) In: Oski, DeAngelis CD, Feign RD, Warshaw. (eds) Principles and Practice of Pediatrics. Philadelphia: Lippincott 1990; 100–1011.

26. Swan SK. Aminoglycoside nephrotoxicity. Semin Nephrol 1997; 17:27–33.

27. Bates DW, Su L, Yu DT et al. Correlates of acute renal failure in patients receiving parenteral amphotericin B. Kidney Int 2001; 60:1452–1459.

28. Better OS, Stein JH. Early management of shock and prophylaxis of acute renal failure in traumatic rhabdomyolysis. N Engl J Med 1990; 322:825–829.

29. Ascione R, Nason G, Al-Ruzsch S et al. Coronary revascularization with or without cardiopulmonary bypass in patients with preoperative nondialysis-dependent renal insufficiency. Ann Thorac Surg 2001; 72:2020–2025.

30. Murphy SW, Barrett BJ, Parfrey PS. Contrast nephropathy. J Am Soc Nephrol 2000; 11:177–182.

31. Michel DM, Kelly CI. Acute interstitial nephritis. J Am Soc Nephrol 1998; 9:506–515.

32. Gines P, Arroyo V. Hepatorenal syndrome. J Am Soc Nephrol 1999; 10:1833–1839.

33. Lamiere N, Vanholder R. Pathophysiologic features and prevention of human experimental acute tubular necrosis. J Am Soc Nephrol 2001; 12:S20–S32.

34. Kellium JA, Decker JM. Use of dopamine in acute renal failure: A meta-analysis. Crit Care Med 2001; 29:1526–1531.

35. Australian and New Zealand Intensive Care Society Clinical Trials Group. Low-dose dopamine in patients with early renal dysfunction: a placebo-controlled randomised trial. Lancet 2000; 3546:2139–2143.

36. Wolfson RM, Kopple JD. Nutritional management of acute renal failure. In: Lazarus JM, Brenner BM. eds. Acute renal failure. 3rd ed. New York: Churchill Livingstone. 1993; 467–485.

37. Kellum JA, Metha RL, Angus DC, Palevsky PM, Ronco C. The first International Consensus Conference on Continuous Renal Replacement Therapy. Kidney Int 2002; 62:1855–1863.

38. Niaudet P, Haj-Ibrahim MH, Gagnadoux MF et al. Outcome of children with acute renal failure. Kidney Int 1985; S148–S151.

39. Brenner BM, Lawler EV, Mackenzie HS. The hyperfiltration theory: a paradigm shift in nephrology. Kidney Int 1996; 49:1774–1777.

16. Chronic renal failure and dialysis options

Kai Rönnholm and Christer Holmberg

INCIDENCE

The real incidence of chronic renal failure (CRF) in children is uncertain. Most estimates are based on the number of patients accepted into dialysis and transplantation programs. However, these figures do not include patients who are excluded for technical reasons, lack of dialysis facilities or specialized centers, or for health policy reasons. Available reports reveal striking geographic differences in the incidence and recognition of renal diseases. Differences between countries are mainly related to their economic development. In developed countries, the incidence of CRF remains stable or decreases slowly owing to early diagnosis, improved conservative treatment, and prevention of genetically transmitted diseases, whereas the prevalence increases steadily as a consequence of improved replacement therapy.

The median annual incidences of CRF in developed countries vary from 4.5 to 12.5, and terminal renal failure (TRF) from 4.4 to 9.5 (Sweden, France) per million child population (pmcp).[1] In developing countries the incidence of CRF is lower, about 3.0–3.2 pmcp (Nigeria, Jamaica).

There is a male predominance among children with congenital structural diseases, whereas no such gender-related difference is noted for most other diseases. It has also been shown that in specialized pediatric centers there is a tendency for an increase in the annual incidence of TRF, and a decrease in uremia as a cause of death due to more active treatment with dialysis and transplantation. In these centers, the proportion of children below five years of age has increased to 40–50% as renal replacement therapy (RRT) has become more common in very young children.

ETIOLOGY

Chronic glomerulonephritis is the renal disorder seen in 38% of children with CRF in developing countries, a frequency twice that observed in Europe.[1] About 60–70% of CRF in children in developed countries is caused by congenital diseases (kidney malformations, urinary tract obstructions, hereditary diseases). Hereditary familial nephropathies, including nephronophthisis, polycystic kidney disease, Alport's syndrome, cystinosis, and oxalosis are reported three times more frequently in Europe than in developing countries. This contrasts sharply with the diseases that cause CRF in adults: hypertension (30%), diabetic nephropathy (20%), and glomerulonephritis (20%).

PATHOPHYSIOLOGY

The pathophysiology of renal damage in CRF is not well understood. Experimental models in animals have been utilized in order to analyze the pathogenesis of the renal injury and progression to glomerulosclerosis. Many investigations suggest that, in response to the renal insult, a group of humoral, chemical, and cellular mechanisms are trying to repair the tissue, which leads to further damage to the remaining nephrons. In various forms of glomerulonephritis, or after ischemia and reperfusion, neutrophils and the expression of adhesion molecules have been correlated with the degree of injury, and they play an important role in mediating tissue injury with subsequent renal failure. Arterionephrosclerosis and arteriolonephrosclerosis are common features in the hypertensive patient.

This leads to renal ischemia and secondary focal segmental glomerulosclerosis. Ischemia also induces renal fibrosis and atrophy. The pathophysiology is mainly involved with increased generation of angiotensin II.

Apoptosis of renal tubular cells also plays a major role in progressive renal failure. Several external and internal signals can induce apoptosis, which then is amplified via several pathways. Potential therapeutic interventions to prevent renal tubular apoptosis in chronic renal disease include angiotensin system inhibition. At present it appears that angiotensin II (AT2) receptor blockade is more promising in apoptosis inhibition than the inhibition of other subtypes.

NUTRITION

Healthy children and children with CRF need at least a minimum intake of energy to maintain adequate growth. According to the RDA recommendations, daily energy needs decrease from 108 kcal/kg body weight in infants to 30 kcal/kg in adults.[2] Adults and children with CRF tend to develop protein-calorie malnutrition because of lack of appetite and/or vomiting. Feeding difficulties of the infant

and young child with CRF are also well recognized. Refusal, reduced spontaneous oral intake, and vomiting all result in an inadequate nutritional intake and in growth failure. It has been shown in infants with CRF that some of the growth failure can be corrected with adequate nutrition. Nasogastric tube feeding or feeding via a gastrostomy tube is often needed to provide sufficient nutrition for infants. However, oral stimulation should be continued to avoid feeding dysfunction that may be associated with long-term tube-feeding. Sufficient, age-corresponding energy intake is recommended for all children with CRF. However, it is important to note that exaggerated caloric intake may induce obesity, hyperlipidemia, hyperinsulism, and arterial sclerosis in the long term.

Lowering protein intake in children with CRF reduces the amount of protein degradation products which are not adequately excreted by the diseased kidneys and cause acidosis. Acidosis is one main reason for catabolism in uremic patients. It also impairs growth. Phosphorus intake usually is reduced in parallel with protein intake. When acidosis, high plasma phosphate, or high BUN concentrations develop in patients with CRF, protein restriction should be started (Table 16.1). Earlier lowering of protein intake does not reduce the progression of renal

---

Table 16.1 Treatment of CRF in children (CKD Stages 2–5)*

GFR, ml/min/1.73 m²	Symptoms	Treatment	Drugs and dosage
60–90 (CKD Stage 2)	– decreased renal reserve	avoid UTI and hypertension	ACE-inhibitor, e.g. enalapril 0.05–0.25 mg/kg 1–2 times/day
30–60 (CKD Stage 3)	– elevation of BUN and serum creatinine – secondary hyper-parathyroidism – mild anemia	diet, phosphate binders vitamin-D EPO	25(OH)D₃: 10–25 µg/day and/or calcitriol or alfacalcidiol: 0.1–075 µg/day 100 IU/kg/wk
15–30 (CKD Stage 4)	– higher BUN and serum creatinine – acidosis – hyperkalemia – severe anemia – growth retardation	protein restriction alkali therapy p.o. diet EPO rhGH	0.7–2.0 g/kg/day (age-dependent) 2–5 mEq/kg/day 100-300 IU/kg/wk 0.048 mg/kg/day s.c.
<15 (CKD Stage 5)	– nausea, vomiting	dialysis/transplantation	

*See Chapter 1 for further definition and description of CKD stages
Abbreviation: GFR, Glomerular filtration rate

damage, and is often accompanied by a drop in energy intake. The protein intake should never be lower than RDA and reduction of protein intake must be compensated by increased energy intake to avoid malnutrition and growth failure.

Patients with CRF tend to have dyslipidemia, dyslipoproteinemia, and high serum lipids. Approximately 60% of children aged 2–18 years, with GFRs between 15 and 60 ml/min/1.73 m^2 (CKD Stages 3 and 4), exhibit lipid levels above the 95th centile for healthy children. Hyperlipidemia is correlated with the degree of renal damage and proteinuria. Therapeutic options to lower serum lipids are low fat diets and lipid lowering drugs like statins, which also have been used in children, although there are no well designed controlled trials of these medications in children with CRF in the United States. It is important to note, however, that fat has a high calorie density and is an important factor for the palatability of food. Therefore, a very strict reduction of fat intake is not advisable for renal patients, who suffer from lack of appetite and malnutrition. Fat composition should be optimal, and a good mix from animal and vegetable origin is preferred. Because of poor nutrition, a multivitamin preparation without vitamin A is recommended for children with CRF to avoid vitamin deficiency.

Nutritional assessment and dietetic support is an essential part of the multidisciplinary team approach for children with CRF and their families. All nutritional advice should be directed towards individualized nutritional requirements of each patient to maintain his or her nutritional status and promote growth. They should prevent the accumulation of waste products and metabolic abnormalities, but satisfy individual psychosocial needs. Regular assessment by a pediatric renal dietitian is crucial for close and frequent supervision in order to monitor and maintain qualitative standards of care for each child, because of the changing needs for growth and development.

RENAL OSTEODYSTOPHY

Renal osteodystrophy is a well-recognized complication of chronic renal failure. The spectrum of skeletal disorders ranges from high-turnover lesions of secondary hyperparathyroidism, which is the most common histologic lesion in pediatric patients with end-stage renal disease, to low-turnover lesions of adynamic renal osteodystrophy, which is often the result of treatment with large intermittent doses of vitamin D metabolites that are given to control secondary hyperparathyroidism.[3]

PATHOPHYSIOLOGY

CALCIUM

In children with CRF, hypocalcemia results from hyperphosphatemia, diminished calcium absorption due to calcitriol deficiency, and decreased response to parathyroid hormone (PTH). Short-term hypocalcemia reduces calcium-sensing receptor (CaR) activity in the parathyroid gland and stimulates PTH secretion. The set point for calcium regulated PTH release was found to be normal in mild and moderate secondary hyperparathyroidism. Thus, maintaining serum calcium concentrations within the normal range should be sufficient to eliminate any calcium-dependent stimulus to PTH secretion. However, in patients with severe secondary hyperparathyroidism, a higher set point was found. Sustained hypocalcemia increases PTH gene transcription and parathyroid cell proliferation. Calcium suppresses PTH gene transcription by negative regulatory elements in the PTH gene. In addition, serum calcium regulates PTH mRNA levels by a post-transcriptional mechanism, which determines PTH mRNA stability and levels.

PHOSPHATE

Phosphate retention develops when renal function falls below 25–30% of normal. Hyperphosphatemia contributes to excess PTH secretion and parathyroid hyperplasia. Studies have also shown that phosphorus directly influences parathyroid gland function. The effect on the PTH gene appears to be post-transcriptional by stabilizing PTH mRNA and enhancing PTH synthesis. It is not known yet whether there is a specific receptor for phosphorus. Hyperphosphatemia accelerates parathyroid cell proliferation, which can result in nodular hyperplasia and severe hyperparathyroid bone disease and may even necessitate parathyroidectomy in some patients.

CALCITRIOL

Calcitriol (1,25-dihydroxyvitamin D_3) is the most potent metabolite of vitamin D. It is produced by 1-α-hydroxylation of 25(OH)D_3 in the proximal tubules of the kidney. PTH, hypocalcemia, and hypophosphatemia stimulate renal 1-α-hydroxylase activity, while increased levels of calcium, phosphorus, and calcitriol inhibit enzyme activity. In children with CRF, the synthesis of calcitriol is impaired.

Calcitriol influences PTH synthesis indirectly by increasing serum calcium through increased intestinal calcium absorption. In addition, calcitriol regulates PTH synthesis via the vitamin D receptor (VDR) by inhibition of PTH gene transcription. Moreover, calcitriol reduces pulsatile PTH secretion at baseline and during hypocalcemia by genomic actions.

PARATHYROID GLAND HYPERPLASIA

Parathyroid gland hyperplasia is a significant feature of secondary hyperparathyroidism. The mechanisms whereby parathyroid cell proliferation is regulated in CRF are poorly understood. In early CRF, parathyroid cell proliferation is often diffuse and polyclonal (non-neoplastic), while the nodular (neoplastic) type of growth is found frequently in patients with ESRD and in more advanced secondary hyperparathyroidism.

SKELETAL LESIONS OF RENAL OSTEODYSTROPHY

Children with ESRD, who have plasma levels of PTH that are 2–3 times above the upper limit of normal, show evidence of osteitis fibrosa or secondary hyperparathyroidism in their bone biopsies. On the other hand, children who have lower PTH levels may have signs of adynamic renal osteodystrophy in their biopsies. Adynamic bone is characterized histopathologically by an overall reduction in cellular activity. Both the number of osteoblasts and osteoclasts are reduced. Adynamic renal osteodystrophy has been connected with poor growth, especially in children with ESRD who have received calcitriol pulse therapy.

TREATMENT OF RENAL OSTEODYSTROPHY

HYPERPHOSPHATEMIA

The serum phosphate level should be kept within the normal age-specific range. If serum phosphate is elevated, phosphate intake should be limited to 400 mg/day (child) to 1000 mg/day (adolescent). On the other hand, the protein intake should not fall below the recommended levels.

Phosphate binders are often necessary to reduce phosphate absorption from the gut in children with CRF. Calcium-containing phosphate binders, e.g. calcium carbonate or calcium acetate, should be used first line. Dosing in children ranges from 1–10 g/day. The higher doses must be used with caution and with careful monitoring of serum calcium levels. Calcium carbonate can be crushed to a fine powder for administration in infants or given via a feeding tube. Phosphate binders should be taken with meals, because fecal excretion of phosphate is higher when taken with meals instead of between meals. Compliance with the intake of phosphate binders is often poor. Correct dosing requires repeated evaluation by an experienced dietician.

Hyperphosphatemia, hypercalcemia, and/or a high calcium x phosphorus product may cause soft tissue and vascular calcification. Calcification of vascular smooth muscle through extensive calcification of the tunica media is quite distinct from atherosclerosis due to factors other than end-stage renal disease. Vascular calcification increases the risk of cardiovascular mortality.

If hypercalcemia, the most common side effect of calcium-containing phosphate binder therapy, occurs, or the calcium x phosphorus product exceeds 5.0 mmol^2/l^2 (= 60 mg^2/dl^2) with the use of calcium-containing phosphate-binders, there is a risk of vascular calcification; the doses should be reduced or calcium-free phosphate binders used. Aluminum-containing phosphate binders should be avoided in pediatric patients. The only commercially available aluminum- and calcium-free phosphate binder is sevelamer (poly-allyl-amine hydrochloride), which is an ion exchange resin that effectively binds phosphorus in the gastrointestinal tract and prevents its absorption. Sevelamer is not yet licensed for children. However, there is some experience with its use in children with CRF.

HYPOCALCEMIA

Dietary calcium intake is usually far less than the amount recommended in children with CRF. In addition, intestinal calcium absorption is compromised in most of these patients because of reduced renal calcitriol production and vitamin D-dependent intestinal calcium transport.

Serum calcium concentration should be kept in the normal range to satisfy nutritional requirements and to avoid hyperparathyroidism. Calcium-containing phosphate binders increase serum calcium concentration and serve as calcium supplements. As stated previously, if patients develop hypercalcemia, or elevated calcium x phosphorus product above 5.0 mmol^2/l^2 (= 60 mg^2/dl^2), calcium-containing phosphate binders and active vitamin D metabolites should be decreased or stopped temporarily.

PTH SECRETION

Maintaining serum calcium concentration within the normal range should be sufficient to eliminate any calcium-dependent stimulus to PTH secretion. In mild CRF, the increase of PTH correlates positively with 25(OH)-vitamin D$_3$ levels. It could be shown that supplementation with vitamin D$_3$, to keep 25(OH)-vitamin D$_3$ levels between 20 and 50 pg/ml, decreases PTH concentration. Furthermore, 25(OH)-vitamin D$_3$, but not 1,25(OH)$_2$D$_3$ improved muscular function and phosphate content. Therefore 10–25 µg (400–1000 IU) of vitamin D$_3$ should be given daily (Table 16.1).

Serum PTH levels should be kept at 2–3 times the upper limit of the normal range in advanced CRF or on dialyisis to avoid low turnover bone disease with risks for poor growth and hypercalcemia, tissue and vascular calcifications. This higher PTH concentration is needed to stimulate bone turnover due to the skeletal resistance to PTH in uremia. If serum PTH is elevated more than 2–3 times normal in the presence of a normal serum phosphate concentration, active vitamin D metabolites (calcitriol or alfacalcidiol) should be administered (Table 16.1). The oral route is preferred and the daily doses (0.1–0.75 µg/d) should be given in the evening, because fewer episodes of hypercalcemia have been reported when comparing it to vitamin D metabolite intake in the morning. Intermittent high-dose vitamin D therapy should be avoided, because it has not been shown to be more effective in suppressing PTH levels and the intermittent mode might influence bone turnover and chondrocyte activity more, resulting in low turnover bone disease and reduced growth.

Severe hyperparathyroidism may no longer react to even high doses of 1,25(OH)$_2$ vitamin D$_3$ and a reduction of phosphate levels. Parathyroidectomy has to be considered in severe, therapy-resistant hyperparathyroidism with radiologic signs of severe renal osteodystrophy in combination with hypercalcemia and/or an elevated calcium x phosphorus product.

Calcimimetic agents are new small organic molecules that activate the calcium receptor in the membrane of the parathyroid cell, thereby inhibiting PTH release. In contrast to treatment with vitamin D analogs, serum calcium concentrations remain unchanged or decrease modestly during calcimimetic therapy. Safety and efficacy of calcimimetics has not been studied in children.

Because serum calcium and phosphorus concentrations often rise during treatment with calcitriol, new vitamin D analogs (paricalcitol, doxercalciferol,

22-oxacalcitriol) have been developed. These compounds lower the PTH concentration effectively, but it is uncertain whether the frequency of episodes of hypercalcemia and/or hyperphosphatemia is less. However, in the near future both calcimimetics and these new vitamin D analogs can help us to treat secondary hyperparathyroidism more individually and prevent severe hyperparathyroidism, and thus modify our approach to the management of this condition.

RENAL ANEMIA

Erythropoietin (EPO), the main promoter of erythropoiesis, is inadequately produced if the kidneys fail, leading to anemia in patients with CRF. EPO is mainly produced in the proximal tubular cells of the kidneys, and in small amounts in the liver. Renal anemia develops when EPO production decreases in the kidney. In addition, the response to EPO in erythroid progenitor cells is decreased in uremia. The renal anemia is normocytic and normocromic and develops usually when the average GFR falls to less than 35 ml/min/1.73 m², although in patients with nephronophthisis often it occurs earlier.

In children, the normal levels of hemoglobin, hematocrit, ferritin, transferrin, and iron are age-dependent. In children with CRF, normal hemoglobin levels should be the goal. After a thorough diagnostic work-up, excluding other causes of anemia, treatment with erythropoietin should be initiated in children with anemia and CRF. Correction of anemia leads to better appetite, improvement in exercise tolerance, improved school performance or even IQ, and reduction in the patient's blood transfusion requirements.

EPO is available as erythropoietin alpha and beta. Erythropoietin alpha must be given by injection and hence its use before or during peritoneal dialysis is problematic. The starting dose of EPO is usually 50–100 IU/kg subcutaneously 1–3 times per week (Table 16.1). If the increase in hematocrit after initiation of the therapy is less than 2% over a 2–4-week period, the dose should be increased by 50%. If the increase in hematocrit after initiation or after

a dose increase exceeds 8% per month, the weekly dose should be reduced by 25%. The hematocrit should be kept within normal age-dependent limits. Maintenance recommendations of EPO vary from 300 IU/kg/week for a child with a weight of < 20 kg to 120 IU/kg/week for a child with a weight of > 30 kg.[4]

Recently, an erythropoietin analog was developed (darbepoietin alpha), a hyperglycosylated erythropoiesis-stimulating protein with a presumed threefold-longer half-life than erythropoietin in man. The pharmacokinetics after intravenous or subcutaneous administration appears to be the same in adult and pediatric patients. Because of its longer half-life, darbepoietin can be administered once a week or once every other week, which decreases the number of injections in children. However, at the time of writing, darbepoietin has been approved only for children over eleven years of age.

Side effects of erythropoietin therapy are rare; increased clotting tendency, hypertension, and seizures are consequences of the therapeutic effect rather than an adverse effect of the preparation. However, blood pressure should be carefully monitored because about 30% of patients have been reported to get hypertension during EPO therapy. Recently, attention was drawn to a new severe side effect, pure red blood cell aplasia due to the occurrence of neutralizing antierythropoietin antibodies, which are most frequently associated with subcutaneously administered erythropoietin alpha.

Iron supplementation is indicated in all pediatric patients with renal anemia, who are treated with erythropoietin. Transferrin saturation should be maintained above 20% and the serum ferritin concentration above 100 ng/ml. Iron should preferably be prescribed as an oral preparation. A dosage of 2–3 mg/kg body weight per day is recommended and administered in two to three divided doses either 1 h before or 2 h after meals. In children responding poorly to erythropoietin therapy, special emphasis should be put on the possible contribution of inflammation or hyperparathyroidism. Other causes of erythropoietin resistance may be malnutrition, hemolytic disorders, folate or vitamin B_{12} deficiency, vitamin C deficiency, ACE inhibitors, or anti-erythropoietin antibodies.

HYPERTENSION

Hypertension is a common problem in children with CRF. Ambulatory blood pressure monitoring (ABPM) has shown that hypertension may develop even before serum creatinine levels are increased. The incidence of hypertension in renal parenchymal disease of the young is very high, varying from 38–78%. The two main pathomechanisms of hypertension, both before and after initiation of dialysis treatment, are hypervolemia and vasoconstriction. Volume overload is related to fluid and salt retention because of diminished sodium excretory capacity. Vasoconstriction may result from activation of the renin-angiotensin system, caused by the sympathetic nervous system, or result from endothelium-derived vasoconstrictors (e.g. endothelin-1), which lead to elevation of systemic vascular resistance. Other possible mechanisms include reduced production of vasodilators (e.g. nitric oxide), vascular rigidity by altered glycosylation of collagen, causing reduced compliance of elastic arteries, elevated intracellular calcium ions (e.g. hyperparathyroidism), administration of erythropoietin, and genetic factors.

Hypertension accelerates progression of CRF by glomerular hyperfiltration or ischemia. Intraglomerular hypertension promotes proteinuria, which further activates the renin-angiotensin system. Angiotensin II also stimulates local pro-inflammatory and pro-fibrotic signaling molecules resulting in renal scarring. Other consequences of chronic hypertension are LV hypertrophy, LV diastolic and systolic dysfunction, congestive heart failure, and vascular disease.

Ambulatory blood pressure monitoring assesses hypertension in children with CRF better than casual blood pressure measurements. This methodology is discussed in more detail in Chapter 10. Daytime diastolic hypertension is detected using ABPM, and nighttime systolic as well diastolic hypertension has been documented in 40% of all children with CRF. In addition 30–60% of children have reduced systolic and/or diastolic blood pressure dipping during the night. ABPM may better predict end-organ damage in children with CRF than casual blood pressure measurements. The primary goal of antihypertensive therapy is to normalize blood pressure below the height- and sex-related 95th percentile.

Control of hypervolemia is achieved by dietary restriction of salt and fluid intake. It may be enhanced by the administration of loop diuretics (e.g. furosemide) as long as there is sufficient renal function. In advanced CRF these agents no longer are effective, and may even be toxic.

The choice of antihypertensive drugs in CRF should consider their specific action and possible side effects. ACE inhibitors (e.g. enalapril 0.05–0.25 mg/kg 1–2 times/day) are particularly effective in patients with heart failure due to systolic dysfunction (Table 16.1). However, initiation of treatment with an ACE inhibitor can cause an exaggerated fall in intraglomerular pressure and fall in GFR with increase in serum creatinine and potassium concentrations. If the potassium concentration increases to > 5.6 mEq/l or serum creatinine > 30%, the drug should be discontinued and another antihypertensive agent started. Calcium channel blockers (e.g. nifedipine 0.25–0.5 mg/kg 4–6 times/day) are usually well tolerated, even in the presence of volume expansion. The combination of an ACE inhibitor, a calcium blocking agent, and eventually a loop diuretic may have the advantage that the side effects of very high doses of monotherapy are reduced. The use of beta-blockers is somewhat limited in CRF by their tendency for bradycardia and worsening of cardiac failure. With most antihypertensive agents, the dosage must be lowered in advanced CRF. Hypotensive episodes must be avoided by frequent blood pressure monitoring.[5]

GROWTH

CRF in childhood is associated with growth retardation characterized by retarded bone maturation, delayed pubertal development, and a final adult height deficiency. Delayed diagnosis and institution of treatment of CRF, age, duration of dialysis, metabolic disorders, nutritional deficits, fluid, electrolyte, acid-base, and calcium balance disorders, all increase the growth deficit. Growth rate decreases significantly when GFR is lower than 30 ml/min/1.73 m². High circulating growth hormone (GH), low GH-binding protein, low-normal insulin-like growth factor-I (IGF-I), high IGF-binding protein (IGFBP) levels, and reduced free IGF-I levels have all been reported in children with CRF. Growth retardation is partly due to an inhibition of IGF-I activity by an excess of high affinity IGFBP and also IGH-I resistance in the end-organ.

Supraphysiologic doses of recombinant human growth hormone (rhGH) increases serum IGF-I and partially overrides the GH/IGF-I-resistant state and improves growth. Daily GH treatment with a dose of 0.048 mg/kg sc, induces catch-up growth of height and all body segments without signs of disproportionate growth, and also improves bone mineralization during the first year of treatment. In prepubertal children, during the first year of treatment, the height velocity is two-fold higher than the pre-treatment value and remains higher during the second year. rhGH treatment has a beneficial effect on final height,[6] but the efficacy of rhGH during puberty is less evident. rhGH treatment has also been reported to improve growth in infants. Catch-up growth is slightly lower in dialyzed and transplanted children, and discontinuation of rhGH treatment results in catch-down growth in 75% of the patients. Thus, if nutrition is adequate and the biochemical parameters are in control and the height of the child is more than 2.0 SD below the normal growth curve for their age and gender, rhGH treatment should be initiated (Table 16.1). The available evidence suggests that treatment should start in early childhood and early in the course of renal failure, and should be continued until renal transplantation.

Side effects of rhGH treatment are limited to a stimulation of insulin secretion, which is not associated with changes in glucose tolerance, and occa-sional cases of benign intracranial hypertension. In terms of renal function, there is no proof that GH treatment can produce significant deterioration in the GFR.

PROGNOSIS

In children with CRF, mortality has dramatically decreased in developed countries during the last decades, being, for example, in Italy only 1.41%. However, in developing countries, it is still high (Nigeria 65%, Jamaica 46.7%). Morbidity has also decreased, and growth and development are today under strict control. However, it is important to institute optimal nutrition aggressively, and careful monitoring and correction of all biochemical variables from the beginning and early diagnosis of CRF is extremely important. Even newborns with renal failure, who often grow poorly during the first three months when hospitalized for diagnostic and therapeutic purposes, subsequently grow well if nutrition and biochemical parameters are adequately monitored and treated as needed. It is also important to motivate and stimulate the parents by offering support by the whole team, especially the dietitian and a feeding therapist.

DIALYSIS OPTIONS

The indication to initiate ESRF treatment in children is based on a combination of clinical, biochemical, and psychosocial assessments that are different for each patient. Dialysis should be initiated when the glomerular filtration rate is between 10 and 15 ml/min/1.73 m², unless the child remains asymptomatic and growth is well maintained. Symptoms such as nausea, vomiting, and lethargy are common with a fall in height velocity, and fluid restriction may compromise adequate nutrition. Hypertension and hyperkalemia, hyperphosphat-emia, and acidosis may contribute to these symptoms. Suboptimal school performance and restriction of daily activities are important additional indications in children.[7]

The patient and his/her family should be actively involved in the choice of therapy. This also has to take into account possible difficulties with vascular access in small children, a long distance to the tertiary-care center, co-morbidity factors, and the psychosocial situation. If peritoneal dialysis is chosen, automated peritoneal dialysis (APD) rather than continuous ambulatory peritoneal dialysis (CAPD) is generally advocated for children, as APD gives more freedom during the day for school and social activities.

RENAL TRANSPLANTATION

Since successful renal transplantation is always the goal for children with ESRF, an increasing number of units offer pre-emptive transplantation for children with progressive decline in renal function. A complete description of this mode of therapy for children with CRF is provided in Chapter 21.

SUMMARY

It is apparent that children with CRF develop clinical and laboratory abnormalities that can involve multiple organ systems. It is therefore important that primary care physicians and pediatric nephrologists develop a comprehensive treatment plan for these children in order to provide optimal care.

REFERENCES

1. Gusmano R, Perfumo F. Worldwide dermographic aspects of chronic renal failure in children, Kidney Int 1993 43(Suppl. 41):S31–S35.
2. Wingen A-M, Mehls O. Nutrition in children with preterminal chronic renal failure. Myth or important therapeutic aid? Pediatr Nephrol 2002; 17:111–120.
3. Kuizon BD, Salusky IB. Cell biology of renal osteodystrophy. Pediatr Nephrol 2002; 17:777–789.
4. Schröder CH. The European Paediatric Peritoneal Dialysis Working Group. The management of anemia in pediatric dialysis patients. Guidelines by ad hoc European Committee. Pediatr Nephrol 2003; 18:805–809.
5. Schärer K, Schmidt KG, Soergel M. Cardiac function and structure in patients with chronic renal failure. Pediatr Nephrol 1999; 13:951–965.
6. Haffner D, Schaefer F, Nissel R et al. Effect of growth hormone treatment on the adult height of children with chronic renal failure. German Study Group for Growth Hormone Treatment in Chronic Renal Failure. N Engl J Med 2000; 343:923–930.
7. Watson AR, Gartland C. On behalf of the European Paediatric Peritoneal Dialysis Working Group. Guidelines by an ad hoc European committee for elective chronic peritoneal dialysis in pediatric patients. Perit Dial Int 2001; 21:240–244.

17. The effects of kidney disorders on the endocrine system

Franz Schaefer and Otto Mehls

MECHANISMS OF ENDOCRINE ABNORMALITIES

Chronic renal failure (CRF) interferes with the metabolism and regulation of many hormones by various mechanisms. In principle, disturbed endocrine function may arise either from inappropriate circulating hormone concentrations or from changed hormonal action at the target tissue level. Both conditions can occur in the uremic state.

INCREASED PLASMA HORMONE CONCENTRATIONS

Renal catabolism accounts for a major part of the metabolic clearance rates of many peptide hormones. Most polypeptide hormones are filtered quite freely across the glomerulus, followed by degradation in tubular cells. Any reduction of glomerular filtration rate (GFR) will necessarily result in accumulation of the plasma levels of such hormones, provided the distribution space and the rate of production and release remain unchanged. If catabolic mechanisms differ for individual isoforms or subunits of a hormone, an imbalance of these constituents may arise, altering the relation between biologically active and inactive hormone fragments. Besides renal metabolic clearance, extrarenal hormone elimination may be reduced in renal failure, e.g., degradation of insulin in skeletal muscle tissue is diminished, and hepatic catabolism of biologically active PTH is reduced in uremia.

Apart from reductions in hormone clearance, hypersecretion of various hormones or hormone binding proteins may occur in patients with CRF, either as an appropriate response to secretory stimuli (e.g., PTH) or without an apparent homeostatic signal (e.g., prolactin).

DECREASED PLASMA HORMONE CONCENTRATIONS

The reduction in functional renal mass in patients with CRF is assumed to be the main cause for decreased levels of hormones produced by the kidney (erythropoietin,$1,25(OH_2)$ Vitamin D_3). In addition, the uremic milieu may suppress the production of these hormones. Levels of extrarenal hormones may be decreased when the hormone-producing gland is the final effector-organ of complex hormonal axis (e.g., testis–testosterone, ovary–estradiol). In these cases, insufficient production of hormones may result either from direct toxic damage to the endocrine gland, from insufficient stimulatory input from the superior part of the hormonal axis or from hyporesponsiveness of the gland.

DISORDERS OF HORMONE ACTION

DISTURBED CONVERSION OF PROHORMONES TO HORMONES

Concentrations of certain prohormones are elevated in CRF, e.g. pro-IGF1A, a precursor of insulin-like growth factor 1 (IGF1), which is not detectable in normal serum, or proinsulin, which is not converted appropriately to insulin or C-peptide in patients with end-stage renal disease (ESRD). Peripheral conversion of T4 to tissue-active T3 is impaired. Some prohormones may block hormone action by competitively inhibiting receptor binding at the tissue level.

SHIFTS IN ISOHORMONE SPECTRUM

Some polypeptide hormones circulate in plasma in multiple isoforms characterized by varying composition of their carbohydrate side chains. In uremia, certain low-molecular weight degradation products of low bioactivity accumulate (e.g., glucagon). In addition, altered glycosylation and sialization may shift the isohormone spectrum towards less bioactive forms (e.g., LH).

ALTERATIONS OF HORMONE-BINDING PLASMA PROTEINS

Altered concentrations of and/or affinity to circulating binding proteins explain part of the alterations of the somatotropic hormone actions in uremia. Whereas low circulating GH binding protein is believed to reflect downregulation of GH receptor expression in the target tissue, increased levels of some of the IGF-1 binding proteins probably result in reduced bioavailability of IGF-1.

ALTERATIONS OF TARGET TISSUE SENSITIVITY

Reduced responsiveness of the target tissues to endocrine signals, exemplified by the disturbed stimulation of hepatic IGF-1 production by GH, or by the Leydig cell's resistance to human chorionic gonadotropin, may be explained by reduced receptor density and abnormal hormone-receptor interaction, due to the presence of competitive or non-competitive inhibitory substances and/or structural changes of either the hormone or its receptor. Alternatively, impaired responsiveness of target tissues may result from alterations of hormone-dependent intracellular (post-receptor) processes (e.g., insulin; Fig. 17.1).

GONADOTROPIC HORMONE AXIS

GONADAL HORMONES

The testicular response to supraphysiologic stimulation by human chorionic gonadotropin (HCG) is universally impaired in males with CRF. In pubertal, and even prepubertal boys with CRF, low or low-normal plasma concentrations of testosterone

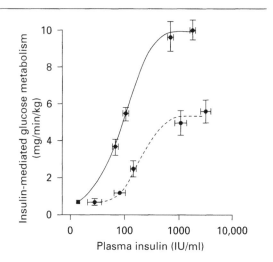

Figure 17.1 Dose-response relationship between the plasma insulin concentration and insulin-mediated glucose metabolism in patients with CRF (dashed line) and controls (uninterrupted line)

Diminished maximal insulin-mediated glucose metabolism suggests insulin resistance by postreceptor defect. (From Smith & De Fronzo)

(T) may partially explain the sparse development of secondary sexual characteristics. Testicular insufficiency is most prominent in boys on hemodialysis. Leydig cell resistance is caused by a cAMP-dependent mechanism, and may be caused by an endogenous LH inhibitor accumulating in uremic serum (Fig. 17.2). This alteration is reversible after renal transplantation.

In children with ERSD at any age, sex-hormone binding globulin concentrations are higher and unbound T fractions lower than in normal children. The increase of sex-hormone binding globulin may be due to accumulation in ERSD, since a normal fraction of free T has been reported in prepubertal children receiving conservative treatment.

Estradiol plasma concentrations in the low–normal range are observed in women and pubertal girls with CRF. An inverse correlation between serum creatinine levels and estradiol concentrations was found in patients with predialytic CRF. Longitudinal analysis revealed an insufficient increase in estradiol during puberty in those patients whose renal function deteriorated, whereas following renal transplantation, even after

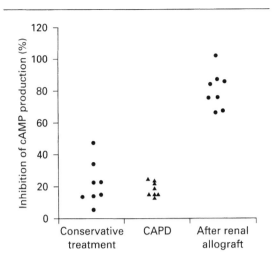

Figure 17.2 Evidence for circulating LH inhibitor in sera of boys with CRF

HCG-induced cAMP production by cell line expressing human LH/HCG receptor is suppressed in presence of serum of patients on conservative or CAPD treatment. (Adapted from Dunkel et al.)

several years of dialysis, estradiol concentrations increased.

GONADOTROPINS

Plasma luteinizing hormone (LH) levels are usually high–normal or elevated in adult men and women, as well as in prepubertal and pubertal boys and girls with CRF. Follicle-stimulating hormone (FSH) concentrations are also universally elevated in adults and children with CRF. After transplantation, LH levels usually return to normal, whereas FSH plasma levels frequently remain elevated. The combination of elevated gonadotropins with decreased or low–normal gonadal hormone levels has been taken as evidence for a state of compensated hypergonadotropic hypogonadism. However, the degree of hypergonadotropism in CRF is usually inadequate for the prevailing degree of hypogonadism, suggesting an additional defect of hypophyseal gonadotropin secretion.

LH is released from the pituitary in episodic (pulsatile) bursts occurring every 90 to 120 min. The plasma LH concentration peaks reflect inter-mittent secretion of hypothalamic gonadotrophin releasing hormone (GnRH) into the hypophyseal-portal blood stream. Hence, the analysis of plasma LH pulses gives indirect information about the functional state of the hypothalamic GnRH 'pacemaker'. Plasma half-life of LH is inversely correlated with GFR. In contrast, actual pituitary LH secretion rates are decreased in CRF; pubertal dialysis patients secrete three times less immunoreactive LH and 2.5 times less bioactive LH in episodic nocturnal peaks than normal adolescents. This abnormality, which has been reproduced in experimental uremia, gives strong evidence for a dysregulation of the gonadotropic axis at the hypothalamo-pituitary level. After transplantation, a regular pattern of LH pulses is re-established.

As the onset of puberty is heralded by the emergence of a nocturnal pattern of pulsatile LH secretion, the observed disturbance of pulsatile LH secretion suggests that the delayed pubertal development in CRF is caused by a primary hypothalamic defect. Clinical and experimental evidence indicates that the neuroendocrine control of pulsatile LH secretion is altered in patients with CRF. Although overt hypogonadotropism is masked by a simultaneous reduction in the metabolic clearance rates, deficient physiologic pulsatile GnRH-LH signal may be the key abnormality underlying the delayed onset of puberty in children with CRF.

Besides the quantitative insufficiency of the hypothalamo-pituitary unit, the biologic quality of the circulating gonadotropins is also altered in uremia. LH bioactivity, measured by the potency of a plasma sample to induce testosterone production in a Leydig cell culture, depends on the degree of glycosylation and sialization of this glycoprotein hormone. During normal puberty, the relative bioactivity of LH gradually increases. In pubertal and adult patients on dialysis, the ratio of bioactive to immunoreactive plasma LH is reduced, suggesting that the spectrum of circulating LH molecules is shifted towards bioinactive forms. This may be attributed to altered glycosylation of plasma proteins in uremia. The physiologic increase in hormone bioactivity during puberty is absent in dialysis patients. The recently characterized inhibitor of

LH action circulating in the serum of uremic boys may represent an accumulating LH fragment (Fig. 17.2). After successful renal transplantation, LH biopotency tends to normalize.

SOMATOTROPIC HORMONE AXIS

During normal childhood, the somatotropic hormone axis plays a key role in the regulation of body growth. In addition, growth hormone is part of a complex system of counter-regulatory hormones maintaining the homeostasis of carbohydrate metabolism.

GROWTH HORMONE (GH)

SERUM CONCENTRATIONS AND KINETICS

The kidney is a major site of GH degradation. In patients with end-stage renal failure, the metabolic clearance rate of GH is reduced by approximately 50% (Fig. 17.3). Fasting GH serum concentrations are variably elevated in uremic children. The increase in plasma GH concentrations is mainly due to an increased plasma half-life of the hormone,

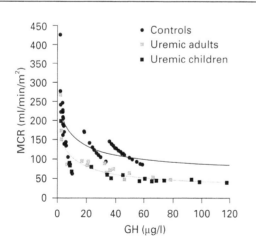

Figure 17.3 Total metabolic clearance rate (MCR) of GH as a function of steady-state plasma GH concentrations in controls and CRF patients

MCR is reduced in children and adults with CRF at any prevailing plasma GH level. (From Haffner et al.)

whereas the actual pituitary GH secretion rate varies between patients and studies. GH secretion rate is high-normal in prepubertal children with ESRD, and increased in adult patients on hemodialysis, possibly as a result of attenuated bioactive IGF-I feedback of the hypothalamo-pituitary unit. In pubertal patients with advanced CRF, GH secretion rates are reduced, indicating an altered sensitivity of the somatotropic hormone axis to the stimulatory effect of sex steroids during this stage of development.

The variability of plasma GH levels in CRF may in part be due to associated conditions such as acidosis and malnutrition, which independently affect GH secretion. Metabolic acidosis suppresses GH release in both rodents and humans.

NEUROENDOCRINE CONTROL OF GH RELEASE

Dysregulation of GH secretion may be related to abnormalities of central neuroendocrine control mechanisms. Evidence for this is provided by several hypothalamo-pituitary function tests. The GH response to intravenous administration of GH-releasing hormone (GHRH) is augmented and prolonged in children. Exogenous thyrotrophin-releasing hormone (TRH), which does not affect GH release in healthy subjects, markedly enhances GH secretion in subjects with CRF. Also, CRF patients respond to acute hyperglycemia by a paradoxical increase of GH secretion. Stimulation tests such as arginine infusion and insulin-induced hypoglycemia lead to a sustained, exaggerated increase of GH. However, the altered metabolic clearance rates of GH as well as of the provocative agents in renal failure make a meaningful clinical interpretation of such tests virtually impossible.

GH RECEPTOR SIGNALING AND TISSUE ACTION

Growth failure despite elevated circulating GH concentrations suggests a state of GH resistance in children with CRF. Indeed, GH-induced hepatic IGF-I synthesis is markedly reduced in experimental uremia. This GH insensitivity may in part be due to deficient GH receptor expression, although this is controversial. Discrepancies between studies may be related to the effect of reduced nutritional intake in uremia, which independently downregulates GH receptor expression. On the other hand, reduced GH receptor protein expression was observed in the growth cartilage of rats with CRF even though nutritional intake was controlled. In humans, serum levels of GH binding protein, putatively reflecting hepatic GH receptor status, were decreased in some studies, but normal in others. Another mechanism accounting for the resistance to GH in uremia is provided by a marked post-receptor GH signaling defect recently observed in chronically uremic rats.

INSULIN-LIKE GROWTH FACTORS

As most metabolic effects of GH are mediated by IGF-I, GH insensitivity in uremia may also be due to IGF resistance. Indeed, numerous studies in the rat as well as in humans have clearly documented marked IGF-I resistance in CRF.

IGF SERUM CONCENTRATIONS

The effect of GH on longitudinal growth is partially mediated by stimulating the production of somatomedins, the two most important of which are the insulin-like growth factors (IGF) I and II. Serum IGF-I and IGF-II levels in children with preterminal CRF are in the normal range, whereas in patients with ESRD mean age-related serum IGF-I levels are slightly decreased and IGF-II levels moderately elevated. Hence, total immunoreactive IGF levels in CRF serum are normal. In contrast, IGF bioactivity is markedly reduced, and the level of free IGF-I is reduced by 50% in relation to the degree of renal dysfunction.

IGF PLASMA BINDING AND TISSUE ACTION

The discrepancy between low somatomedin activity by bioassay and normal or elevated insulin-like growth factor by radioimmunossay or radio-receptor assay, suggests the presence of circulating somatomedin inhibitors in uremia. The most likely explanation for the inhibition of somatomedin

action in uremia has emerged from the identification of six insulin-like growth factor-binding proteins (IGFBP-1 to -6) of which IGFBP-3 appears to be the most abundant in humans, constituting more than 95% of total circulating IGFBP. In children with CRF, the serum concentrations of IGFBP-1, IGFBP-2, IGFBP-4 and IGFBP-6 are increased in a manner inversely related to glomerular filtration rate (Fig. 17.4). IGFBP-1, IGFBP-2 and IGFBP-6 inhibit somatomedin bioactivity in vitro. Somatomedin bioactivity in uremic serum can be returned to normal by removing unsaturated IGFBP. Experimental evidence suggests that the increase of IGFBP-1 and IGFBP-2 is not only due to reduced renal metabolic clearance, but also to increased hepatic synthesis. An important question is whether the imbalance between normal total IGF and the excess of unsaturated IGFBPs contributes to growth failure in children with CRF. Serum levels of IGFBP-1, IGFBP-2 and IGFBP-4 correlate inversely with standardized height in CRF children. While it is tempting to speculate that these IGFBPs could contribute to growth failure in these children, it is difficult to prove causality since IGFBP levels and height SDS are all correlated with GFR.

Apart from the increased plasma IGF-I binding capacity, a post-receptor IGF-I signaling defect may also contribute to IGF-1 resistance in CRF.

GH-IGF-1 HOMEOSTASIS IN CRF

The pattern of elevated GH, normal total IGF, and markedly elevated IGFBP plasma concentrations in uremia has interesting implications with respect to the estimated IGF production rate. In a functioning homeostatic system, the diminished free IGF-1 levels would be expected to stimulate IGF production in order to restore the steady-state between bound and unbound hormone at a higher level. In uremia, however, total IGF concentrations are normal rather than increased. Kinetic modeling suggests that the metabolic half-life of IGFs is markedly elevated, and the IGF production rate is decreased 10- to 100-fold in uremia. Taken together, the markedly deficient IGF1 synthesis and the modest elevation of plasma GH levels, which is mainly due to

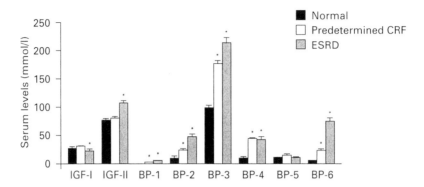

Figure 17.4 Molar concentrations of IGFs and IGF binding protein concentrations in children with pre end-stage CRF and on dialysis in comparison to age-matched healthy children

(From Ulinski T, Mohon S, Kiepe D et al.)

impaired metabolic clearance, in the presence of increased IGF binding capacity strongly support the notion of a multilevel homeostatic failure of the GH-IGF-1 system in uremia: pituitary GH secretion is insufficiently feedback-stimulated by reduced free IGF-1 levels, and marked tissue GH resistance prevents an increase in total IGF-1 levels in the presence of elevated GH.

THYROID HORMONE AXIS

CLINICAL FINDINGS

The thyroid hormone axis plays an important role in the regulation of tissue metabolism. Throughout childhood, thyroid hormone is involved in growth and skeletal maturation, stimulating both cartilage proliferation and epiphyseal differentiation.

Epidemiologic data on the incidence of thyroid disorders in children with CRF are not available. The prevalence of goiter in patients with ESRD is increased compared with patients with non-renal disease. The prevalence of hypothyroidism ranges between 0 and 9.5% in adults with ESRD. Primary hypothyroidism was observed 2½-times more frequently in dialysis patients than in patients with other chronic non-renal disease; the prevalence of

hyperthyroidism was not different. In children, the prevalence of hypothyroidism may be higher due to the greater proportion of patients treated for cystinosis and nephrotic syndrome. In cystinotic patients, deposition of cystine crystals in the thyroid can lead to destruction of the gland and frank hypothyroidism. Children with severe nephrotic syndrome, particularly with the congenital form, may become hypothyroid due to the renal loss of thyroid-hormone binding globulin.

As some manifestations of hypothyroidism, such as hypothermia, pallor, and dry skin also occur in uremia, the exclusion of the diagnosis of hypothyroidism on clinical grounds may be difficult in a uremic child. Therefore, exploration of the hormonal status of a patient is essential for the recognition of an accompanying thyroid disorder.

THYROID HORMONES

The plasma levels of total T4 (thyroxine) and T3 (triiodothyronine) are decreased in patients with CRF. Significant depression of T4 and T3 levels usually occurs once the glomerular filtration rate falls below 50%. Thyroid hormone production rates are normal in CRF, whereas metabolic clearance may or may not be increased. Due to impaired peripheral deiodination of T4 to T3, there is a more distinct suppression of T3 than of T4 levels. In ESRD, diminished T4 levels are found in a third, and diminished T3 levels in 50% of patients, including children.

The more pronounced decrease of plasma T3 compared to T4 levels in CRF resembles the thyroid hormone pattern observed in other states of chronic non-thyroidal diseases (sick euthyroid or low T3 syndrome). However, whereas in the sick euthyroid syndrome the plasma levels of rT3, the inactive metabolite of T4, are elevated as a result of impaired peripheral conversion of T4 to T3, rT3 concentrations are in the low normal range in patients with CRF due to redistribution of rT3 into an increased extravascular compartment in uremia.

BINDING PROTEINS

Circulating thyroid hormones are bound to thyroid hormone binding globulin (TBG), albumin, and prealbumin. TBG levels are usually normal in hemodialysis patients, but tend to be low in patients treated with peritoneal dialysis because of the loss of TBG into the dialysate. Patients with severe nephrotic syndrome may have markedly low plasma TBG levels due to urinary protein loss. Only the unbound (free) T4 (fT4) and T3 (fT3) fractions are biologically active. Plasma fT4 and fT3 are low, and dissociation constants for specific T4 and T3 binding are normal.

THYROID-STIMULATING HORMONE (TSH)

Despite low plasma total and free T4 and T3 levels, TSH concentrations are usually normal in adults and children with CRF. Only patients with congenital nephrotic syndrome and nephropathic cystinosis show elevated TSH levels. TSH is secreted in a pulsatile fashion. In CRF patients, the frequency of TSH pulses is increased, but the amplitudes are reduced, and the regularity of occurrence of the TSH bursts is lost. The erratic pattern of small, frequent hormone pulses is associated with a loss of the physiologic circadian rhythm.

TRH administration elicits a delayed and blunted, but prolonged increase of TSH plasma levels both in adults and children with CRF. In most of these patients, the response to TRH is inversely related to the duration of renal impairment. An exception to this rule involves children with nephropathic cystinosis, who exhibit an exaggerated TSH response to TRH because of the destruction of the thyroid gland.

The mechanism for the relative TRH insensitivity of the pituitary in CRF is not clear. The physiologic amplification of TSH release by dopaminergic blockade (metoclopramide test) is lacking in patients with CRF, arguing against hyperactivity of dopaminergic inhibitory neurons. Experimental evidence suggests an increased sensitivity of the thyrotroph cell to feedback inhibition by thyroid hormones. Moreover, the altered pattern of spontaneous pulsatile TSH secretion suggests an additional dysregulation of hypothalamic TRH release.

In summary, chronic renal failure is associated with alterations of hormone secretion and clearance at multiple levels of the hypothalamo-pituitary-thyroid axis. These are compatible with a resetting of the central thyrostat towards lower levels of circulating thyroid hormones.

The lacking upregulation of spontaneous TSH secretion, despite low thyroid hormone levels, may be interpreted as a pathologic inability of the thyrotroph to respond to the physiologic stimulus of low thyroid hormone concentrations; alternatively, the reduced responsiveness of the hypothalamo-pituitary axis may reflect a physiologic adaptation resulting from a reduced demand for thyroid hormone in the specific state of metabolism caused by uremia.

THYROID HORMONE ACTION

Patients with CRF usually appear clinically euthyroid. Measurements of basal metabolic rate and rough clinical indices yield normal results. Experimental data on thyroid hormone actions on the tissue level are controversial. Whereas the T3 content of uremic rat livers is decreased, and the activities of certain thyroid hormone-dependent liver enzymes are low in uremic rats, hepatocyte mRNA concentrations of various T3-dependent proteins are normal. T3 receptor expression is elevated in patients with CRF; this may represent a compensatory mechanism to preserve tissue euthyroidism.

Although the efficacy of thyroid hormones appears to be conserved on the nuclear level, other actions are compromised. Patients with CRF show marked resistance against thyroid hormones with regard to thermogenesis. Oxygen uptake is neither stimulated by administration of T3 nor suppressed by its antagonist sodium ipodate (Fig. 17.5). Leukocyte ouabain binding capacity and Na/K-ATPase, which are low both in CRF and hypothyroid subjects, are restored by thyroid hormone treatment in hypothyroid, but not in CRF patients.

Nitrogen balance studies of uremic patients receiving T3 supplements show hypersensitivity to the catabolic effects of thyroid hormones. Hence, the low T3 syndrome of uremia may be beneficial by lowering protein breakdown. Similar phenomena are observed in patients with chronic illness or malnutrition. Therefore, the changes of the thyroid axis in uremia may in part be interpreted as a physiologic adaptation to conserve energy in an adverse metabolic environment. Thyroid hormone supplementation might therefore be not only useless, but also even harmful.

DIAGNOSIS AND CLINICAL MANAGEMENT OF THYROID DISORDERS IN CRF

Since the clinical features of uremia and hypothyroidism may be indistinguishable, all patients with ESRD should be screened for potential hypothyroidism. In a uremic patient, hypothyroidism should only be diagnosed if total and free T4 levels are distinctly low, the TBG concentrations normal, and basal TSH levels elevated. A normal plasma TSH is probably a valid indicator of tissue euthyroidism. Treatment with thyroid hormones should be limited to patients with clinical hypothyroidism and elevated plasma TSH. The increased risk for induction of tissue catabolism by thyroid hormone substitution needs to be recognized.

In hemodialysis patients, heparin may interfere with the thyroid hormone status. Heparin competes

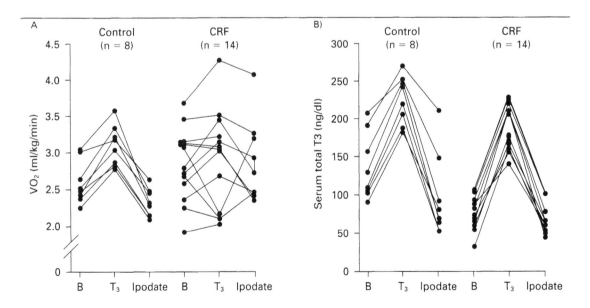

Figure 17.5 Failure of thyroxin administration to stimulate, and of thyroid suppression to reduce, oxygen consumption (VO_2, panel A) despite adequate changes in plasma T3 levels (panel B) in patients with CRF

(From Lim VS, Zavala DC, Flanigan MJ, Freeman RM)

with T4 at intra- and extravascular binding sites, thus increasing total and free T4 serum levels for at least 24 hours post-dialysis. Therefore, strict standardization of the timing of investigations relative to dialysis is essential.

Patients with CRF who undergo repeated radiologic investigations with iodinated contrast agents may be at increased risk of developing iodine-induced hyperthyroidism because of reduced iodine clearance.

ADRENAL HORMONE AXIS

CLINICAL FINDINGS

Analogous to thyroid disorders, dysfunction of the pituitary-adrenal axis may be difficult to diagnose in patients with CRF. Uremia shares certain clinical signs and symptoms with Cushing's syndrome, such as osteopenia, proximal muscle weakness with atrophy, glucose intolerance, negative nitrogen balance, and hypertension; therefore, Cushing's syndrome may easily be missed if it occurs concomitantly with renal failure. Similarly, adrenal insufficiency may present with symptoms which are not uncommon in renal failure, e.g. hypotension, weakness, and hyperkalemia. To confirm or reject the diagnosis of Cushing's syndrome or adrenal failure, the clinician has to rely on the evaluation of the patient's hormonal status under basal and stimulated conditions. For a comprehensive interpretation of the endocrine status, the changes of the hypothalamo-pituitary-adrenal axis induced by CRF per se must be kept in mind.

CORTISOL

Cortisol is conjugated in the liver to water-soluble metabolites, which are predominantly excreted by the kidney and accumulate in renal failure. While normal morning fasting cortisol levels are found in the majority of adult patients with CRF, 24-hour profiles clearly show elevated integrated mean total and free cortisol levels.

The degree of renal dysfunction and/or the treatment modality may affect plasma cortisol levels. Whereas normal basal plasma cortisol levels and no correlation between cortisol levels and GFR were found in children over a GFR range of 2 to 44 ml/min/1.73 m^2, hypercortisolism was observed in 15 out of 26 children on hemodialysis. The diurnal rhythm and the pulsatile mode of cortisol secretion are conserved in renal failure; however, the half-life of the endogenous secretory peaks is prolonged. Elevated baseline concentrations may therefore either represent increased hormone secretion, e.g. due to an endocrine state of chronic stress, or be related to deficient clearance of the hormone from the circulation. Compatible with the stress hypothesis, the secretory activity is shifted in hemodialysis patients towards the dialysis hours, whereas a normal pattern is observed on days off dialysis.

Stimulation of the zona fasciculata with exogenous ACTH in uremic patients yields a normal cortisol response, irrespective of whether supraphysiologic or low doses of ACTH are used. Zona glomerulosa steroids (aldosterone, 18-OH-corticosterone) are stimulated normally in CAPD but not in hemodialysis patients. Transient hyporesponsiveness to ACTH was observed in the majority of patients who returned to dialysis after transplant failure.

ADRENAL ANDROGENS

Adrenarche marks an important milestone in endocrine maturation. Adrenarche occurs about two years before the initiation of puberty and is independent of it. Low plasma levels of dehydroepiandrosterone (DHEA) and DHEA-sulfate, the marker hormones of the zona reticularis, are observed in adult men as well as in pre- and mid-pubertal boys on hemodialysis, whereas normal levels are found in patients on conservative treatment. Conversely, androstendione, an adrenal androgen produced by the ACTH-dependent zona fasciculata, is elevated in patients on conservative treatment, and normal or elevated in hemodialysis patients. A similar elevation of androstendione is observed in girls with CRF. In renal allograft recipients, glucocorticoid treatment invariably lowers adrenal androgen production to almost undetectable levels.

ADRENOCORTICOTROPIC HORMONE (ACTH)

Basal ACTH levels are normal or elevated in patients with CRF. The occasional finding of increased ACTH with normal cortisol levels has raised the speculation that the bioactivity of ACTH may be reduced, but this has not been substantiated. The functional status of pituitary corticotrophs in uremia is still under discussion. ACTH secretion is not suppressible by standard oral doses of dexamethasone. Oral absorption of dexamethasone is, however, reduced in uremia, and suppression of ACTH can be achieved with higher doses. After intravenous administration of dexamethasone, only incomplete suppression of plasma cortisol levels is observed; however, the metabolic clearance of dexamethasone is possibly increased in uremia. The responsiveness of the corticotroph to stimulation by metapirone may or may not be reduced in uremia. The ACTH release after administration of corticotropin-releasing hormone (CRH) occurs early, but is blunted. In normal subjects acute hypoglycemia elicits a counter-regulatory stimulation of the CRH-ACTH-cortisol axis. In patients with CRF this stress reaction is markedly suppressed. The increase of ACTH and cortisol following insulin-induced hypoglycemia is blunted in patients on hemodialysis, providing further evidence of a disordered hypothalamo-pituitary regulation of the corticotropic axis in patients with CRF.

DIAGNOSIS AND MANAGEMENT OF PITUITARY-ADRENAL DISORDERS

The most frequent circumstance for a nephrologist to encounter adrenocortical failure is upon discontinuation of glucocorticoids in patients returning to dialysis after transplant failure. Accidental adrenectomies can occur during nephrectomy particularly in young infants, and adrenal hemorrhage leading to functional disorders is not uncommon in the perinatal period, in children with coagulation disorders and as a side effect of therapeutic anticoagulation. Also adrenal insufficiency is occasionally seen as a complication of amyloidosis also comprising renal function, as typically seen in patients with severe chronic vasculitis or familial Mediterranean fever. Demonstration of low cortisol levels and insufficient cortisol response to ACTH is required to confirm the diagnosis.

In transplant recipients, adrenal responsiveness is suppressed by steroid treatment. This poses the risk of acute adrenal insufficiency during severe stress, e.g. surgical procedures or after abrupt steroid withdrawal.

The diagnosis of Cushing's syndrome in a patient with CRF requires elevated plasma cortisol levels, measured by a radioimmunoassay in extracted serum. While a single measurement of cortisol may be misleading, loss of diurnal rhythm (24-hour cortisol profile) is a characteristic of Cushing's syndrome not seen in uremia-related adrenal dysfunction. Failure of high-dose dexamethasone po (0.11 mg/kg) or iv (0.03 mg/kg) to suppress ACTH and cortisol levels is confirmatory evidence.

FURTHER READING

Daschner M, Philippin B, Nguyen T et al. Circulating inhibitor of gonadotropin releasing hormone secretion by hypothalamic neurons in uremia. Kidney Int 2002; 62:1582–1590.

Dunkel L, Raivio T, Laine J et al. Circulating luteinizing hormone receptor inhibitor(s) in boys with chronic renal failure. Kidney Int 1997; 51:777–784.

Emmanouel DS, Lindheimer MD, Katz AI. Pathogenesis of endocrine abnormalities in uremia. Endocr Rev 1980; 1:28–44.

Feneberg R, Schaefer F, Veldhuis JD. Neuroendocrine adaptations in renal disease. Pediatr Nephrol 2003; 18:492–497.

Haffner D, Schaefer F, Girard J, Ritz E, Mehls O. Metabolic clearance of recombinant human growth hormone in health and chronic renal failure. J Clin Invest 1994; 93:1163–1171.

Handelsman DJ, Dong Q. Hypothalamo-pituitary gonadal axis in chronic renal failure. Endocrinol Metab Clin North Am 1993; 22:145–161.

Holdsworth S, Atkins RC, de Kretser DM. The pituitary-testicular axis in men with chronic renal failure. N Engl J Med 1977; 296:1245–1249.

Kaptein EM. Thyroid hormone metabolism and thyroid diseases in chronic renal failure. Endocr Rev 1996; 17:45–63.

Lim VS. Thyroid function in patients with chronic renal failure. Am J Kid Dis, 2001; 38:S80–S84.

Lim VS, Zavala DC, Flanigan MJ, Freeman RM. Blunted peripheral tissue responsiveness to thyroid hormone in uremic patients. Kidney Int. 1987; 31:808–814.

Luger A, Lang I, Kovarik J et al. Abnormalities in the hypothalamic-pituitary-adrenocortical axis in patients with chronic renal failure. Am J Kidney Dis 1987; 9:51–54.

Mooradian AD, Morley JE. Endocrine dysfunction in chronic renal failure. Arch Intern Med 1984; 144:351–353.

Powell DR, Liu F, Baker BK et al. Effect of chronic renal failure and growth hormone therapy on the insulin-like growth factors and their binding proteins. Pediatr Nephrol 2000; 14:579–583.

Schaefer F. Endorine and growth disorders in chronic renal failure. In: Avner ED, Niaudet P, Harmon W (eds): Pediatric Nephrology, 5th edn. Lippincott Williams & Wilkins, 2004, 1313–1345.

Schaefer F, Baumann G, Haffner D et al. Multifactorial control of the elimination kinetics of unbound (free) growth hormone (GH) in the human: regulation by age, adiposity, renal function, and steady state concentrations of GH in plasma. J Clin Endocrinol Metab 1996; 81:22–31.

Schaefer F, Chen Y, Tsao T, Nouri P, Rabkin R. Impaired JAK-STAT signal transduction contributes to growth hormone resistance in chronic uremia. J Clin Invest 2001; 108:467–475

Schaefer F, Daschner M, Veldhuis JD et al. In vivo alterations in the gonadotropin-releasing hormone pulse generator and the secretion and clearance of luteinizing hormone in the castrate uremic rat. Neuroendocrinology 1994; 59:285–296.

Schaefer F, Rabkin R. IGF-1 and the kidney. In: LeRoith D, Zumkeller W, Baxter RC. Insulin-like Growth Factors. Kluwer Academic/Plenum Publishers, 2003, 244–261.

Schaefer F, Veldhuis JD, Robertson WR, Dunger D, Scharer K. Immunoreactive and bioactive luteinizing hormone in pubertal patients with chronic renal failure. Cooperative Study Group on Pubertal Development in Chronic Renal Failure. Kidney Int 1994; 45:1465–1476.

Schaefer F, Veldhuis JD, Stanhope R, Jones J, Scharer K, Cooperative Study Group on Pubertal Development in Chronic Renal Failure. Alterations in growth hormone secretion and clearance in peripubertal boys with chronic renal failure and after renal transplantation. J Clin Endocrinol Metab 1994; 78:1298–1306.

Schaefer F, Vogel M, Kerkhoff G et al. Experimental uremia affects hypothalamic amino acid neurotransmitter milieu. J Am Soc Nephrol 2001; 12:1218–1227.

Smith D, DeFronzo RA. Insulin resistance in uraemia mediated by postbinding defects. Kidney Int 1982; 22:54–62.

Tönshoff B, Blum WF, Wingen AM et al. Serum insulin-like growth factors (IGFs) and IGF binding proteins 1, 2 and 3 in children with chronic renal failure: relationship to height and glomerular filtration rate. J Clin Endocrinol Metab 1995; 80:2684–2691.

Tönshoff B, Cronin MJ, Reichert M. Reduced concentration of serum growth hormone (GH)-binding protein in children with chronic renal failure: correlation with GH insensitivity. J Clin Endocrinol Metab 1997; 82:1007–1013.

Tönshoff B, Eden S, Weiser E et al. Reduced hepatic growth hormone (GH) receptor gene expression and increase in plasma GH binding protein in experimental uremia. Kidney Int 1994; 45:1085–1092.

Tönshoff B, Powell DR, Zhao D et al. Decreased hepatic insulin-like growth factor (IGF)-I and increased IGF binding protein-1 and -2 gene expression in experimental uremia. Endocrinol 1997; 138:938–946.

Ulunski T, Mohan S, Kiepe D, et al. Serum insulin-like growth factor binding protein (IGFBP)-4 and IGFBP-5 in children with chronic renal failure: relationship to growth and glomerular filtration rate. The European Study Group for Nutritional Treatment of Chronic Renal Failure in Childhood. German Study Group for Growth Hormone Treatment in Chronic Renal Failure. Pediatr Nephrol. 2000; 14(7):589–597.

18. Nutritional and growth aspects of the care of children with kidney disease

Constantinos J Stefanidis

INTRODUCTION

The progressive decline of GFR in some children with chronic kidney disease (CKD) results in metabolic abnormalities, which have a negative impact on their nutritional status and growth. It has long been recognized that chronic renal failure (CRF) in children is associated with growth delay.[1] Recently this problem became more prevalent, because progress in conservative and renal replacement therapy has greatly improved the prognosis of such patients. Still today diminished growth of children with CRF remains a frequent problem in all age groups (Fig. 18.1).[2] This diminished growth frequently results in diminished final adult height. Only 50% of 376 young adults, who started dialysis before the age of 15 years, reached a normal final height.[3]

This decrease of the final height might be related with a poor body image resulting in low self-esteem and greater emotional distress.[4] Children with extreme short stature face a disability that may affect their physical, psychologic, and social well-being.[5] Therefore, children with CRF might be particularly vulnerable to these problems and extreme short stature could be a major impediment to their full rehabilitation.[5] However, in a recent literature review, concerning psychosocial consequences of short stature, it was demonstrated that short people regularly adapt well to their height and have a good self-esteem.[6] In another study, children with CRF and their parents were interviewed to evaluate their concerns about growth. Fifty per cent of patients had additional non-renal complications. Growth was a major concern for 30% of parents and 28% of children.[7] It is therefore highly likely that the psychosocial problems of children with CRF are not only dependent on their short stature, but are also related to other disabilities.

Children with poor growth should be regarded as being at high-risk. In a recent study, of 1,112 children the relationship between their growth during one year with five-year hospitalization and death rates was examined.[8] There was an increased risk of death and hospitalization for patients with poor rates of growth. Patients in the most severe growth failure category demonstrated an almost threefold increased risk of death.[8] Poor growth is unlikely to be directly responsible for this increased morbidity and mortality. The poor nutritional status of these patients was possibly related to an increased risk of infections and a high morbidity and mortality rate.

Malnutrition, renal osteodystrophy, anemia, salt wasting, metabolic acidosis, and resistance to hormones mediating growth have been shown to be significant determinants of poor linear growth in children with CRF.[9] Their importance will be discussed in the next section. Even though the management of these problems is possible, many

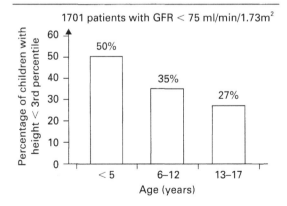

Figure 18.1 Percentage of children with height < 3rd percentile (SDS < −1.88)[2]

children with long-term renal insufficiency still have poor linear growth. It was hoped that these patients would have normal growth or even catch-up growth after renal transplantation. However, although normal growth may be seen after trans-plantation, catch-up growth is rare.[10] For these patients, the administration of recombinant human growth hormone (rhGH) is recommended. A sig-nificant improvement of growth in children receiv-ing conservative treatment, dialysis, and after renal transplantation has been documented in various multicenter studies with the administration of rhGH.[11–15] In addition, long-term rhGH treatment of children with CRF resulted in catch-up growth, and the majority of these patients achieved normal adult height.[16] The beneficial effect of the current management of growth retardation children with CRF is well documented in the 2002 report of the North American Pediatric Renal Transplant Cooperative Study (NAPRTCS). In 1987, patients receiving their initial transplant were an average of −2.4 standard deviations (SDS) below average. This has improved in the 2001 annual cohorts to −1.6 SDS.

ASSESSMENT AND INTERPRETATION OF GROWTH AND NUTRITIONAL STATUS

The reliable assessment of growth requires staff who have received training in the use of appropri-ate measuring techniques and equipment.[17] There is no single measure that provides a compre-hensive indication of protein-energy nutritional status.[18] The most valid measures of protein and energy nutrition status in children treated with maintenance dialysis include:[18]

1. Dietary interview/diary.
2. Biochemical parameters (serum albumin).
3. Anthropometric measurements:
   a. Height or length, standard deviation score (SDS or Z score) for height, estimated dry weight, weight/height index, head circumfer-ence (three years or less).
   b. Mid-arm circumference, muscle circumfer-ence or area, and skinfold thickness.

Regular dietary assessment by three-day dietary diaries, or dietary recall in the clinic by an experi-enced dietician, can provide valuable data. All nutri-ents should be computer analyzed and compared with recommended intakes for children of the same sex and chronologic age. If the child falls below the normal percentile ranges, the child's height age may be used to determine acceptable baseline energy and micronutrient requirements.[17] Using the information from the dietary assessment, early stages of malnutrition can be identified (Fig. 18.2).

Anthropometric parameters, such as weight, height (or supine length for patients up to 2 years of age), and head circumference (for children up to 2 years of age) should be measured regularly and plotted so that growth can be monitored.[17] A stan-dardized height and weight calculator is available via the internet.[19] There are two methods to stan-dardize the growth data for age and sex: percentile values and SDS. The use of SDS (or Z-scores) is more appropriate for the interpretation of growth data in children with values outside the normal range. SDS is defined as the difference between the child's height and the mean height for normal children of the same sex and chronologic age divided by the height standard deviation of this population.

The development of anthropometric measure-ments came as the result of investigations for devel-oping simpler and less expensive methods for

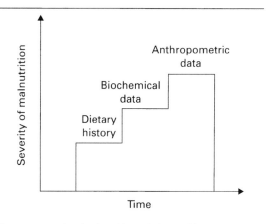

Figure 18.2 Severity of malnutrition and abnormal findings from dietary assessment, biochemical, and anthropometric data

estimating body composition. These measurements are best used for monitoring changes over time. One of the most commonly used measurements is triceps skinfold thickness. Along with mid-upper arm circumference, this measurement can be used to estimate arm fat and arm muscle area. Despite the limited precision of a single skinfold thickness assessment, acceptable reproducibility can be achieved when skinfold thickness measurements from many sites are used in calculations of the percentage of fat mass with validated prediction equations.[20]

The high technical precision of bioelectrical impedance (BIA), the lack of invasiveness and the low cost of the method, make it a very attractive tool for the routine assessment of the state of hydration and whole-body percentage fat mass in clinical practice.[20] BIA is the conductive resistance of a biologic tissue exposed to an alternating electrical current. Since only electrolyte-containing fluids, but not adipocytes, conduct electrical currents, BIA is inversely related to the total body water (TBW) content. Fat-free mass (FFM) can also be calculated from BIA, since the percentage of water of the FFM is stable (73%). However, in acute and chronic disease states, the hydration of FFM may be altered. Therefore while TBW itself may be measured correctly with BIA by use of appropriate prediction equations, the large individual variability of the TBW-FFM relationship renders FFM prediction extremely problematic in children with CRF.[20]

Serum albumin concentration is frequently used as a reliable biochemical marker for patients' nutritional status. However, the presence of acute or chronic inflammation limits the specificity of serum albumin as a nutritional marker.[18] Albumin is synthesized in the liver and is catabolized by the vascular endothelium. Serum albumin is a measure of visceral protein pool size. In a recent study, over a third of children with ESRD maintained on chronic PD had low serum albumin concentrations (below 2.9 g/dl). These patients are at risk for a number of co-morbid conditions, including infections, and they will often fail to grow.[21] Once hypoalbuminemia is identified, aggressive use of nutritional supplements should be considered to attenuate or prevent the associated complications.

Recently a nutritional score was developed based on nine parameters. Anthropometry (height, weight, BMI, midarm muscle circumference, arm muscle area and arm fat area) and BIA (reactance, phase angle and distance) parameters were given scores of 1 to 5. The anthropometry-BIA nutrition score (ABN) corresponding to the 3rd percentile in the population of healthy children was 10.3. The values of all nine parameters, as well as serum albumin levels, were significantly higher in patients with an ABN score > 10.3. This ABN score seems to be a simple and objective method of assessing, in clinical practice, the nutritional status of children on chronic peritoneal dialysis.[22]

EFFECT OF THE DEVELOPMENTAL STAGE ON GROWTH IN CHILDREN WITH CRF

The regulation of statural growth has significant differences in childhood during the following three periods: infancy, childhood, and puberty (Fig. 18.3).

a. During the first two years of life, nutrition is the most important factor for growth. Approximately 30% (40 cm) of the total postnatal statural growth occurs during this period.
b. During childhood, the role of the somatotropic hormone axis becomes more important; thyroid hormone and nutrition have roles of lesser importance. Height velocity is decelerating in this period (Fig. 18.3) to an almost constant rate of approximately of 5–6 cm/year.
c. In puberty, the gonadotropic hormone axis plays a major role. On average, the growth rate doubles during puberty (approximately 10 cm/year). The growth spurt lasts between 2.5 and 3 years; it starts in girls at approximately 11 years and in boys about two years later.

The extent of growth retardation depends on when progressive CRF manifests itself. Onset of CRF in utero or during infancy is associated with significantly diminished final height.[23,24] Growth impairment was seen in 50% of children who had CRF during the first two years of life.[23] Anorexia,

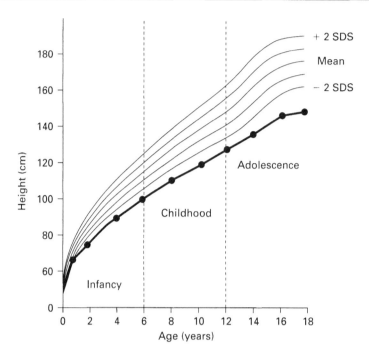

Figure 18.3 Height curve of a boy with CRF from infancy

recurrent vomiting, water, and electrolyte imbalances, and the catabolic effect of metabolic acidosis and secondary hyperparathyroidism, are the main responsible factors for growth failure in this period. This growth impairment might be prevented with early and appropriate management that is focused especially on aggressive enteral feeding.[25]

During childhood these patients usually have a growth pattern that is parallel to the normal percentile curve (Fig. 18.3).[26] However, significant deceleration of growth velocity might occur in these patients if there is not appropriate management of factors that might participate in the continued development of growth failure. This percentile-parallel growth pattern has been interpreted as 'normal' growth, but this underestimates the growth problem. A child with an SDS of −3 has a height deficit of 7.6 cm at one year of life. However, the same SDS deficit increases in absolute terms to 12.5 cm, 16.5 cm, and 18.6 cm at the 4th, 8th,

and 12th year of age. Therefore early management of growth retardation is crucial to avoid further permanent reduction of height.

Finally, pubertal height gain of CRF patients is only 50% of that observed in healthy children. In addition, on average, the onset of puberty in these children is delayed by two years. This growth impairment results in a decrease of final height. This was confirmed in a recent long-term study. Patients who were not treated with rhGH had a significant decrease of their height from an average of −2.1 SDS to −2.7 SDS.[16]

ETIOLOGY OF GROWTH FAILURE IN CHILDREN WITH CRF

Growth retardation is the consequence of a combination of several inter-related processes, which are partially understood (Fig. 18.4). The major con-

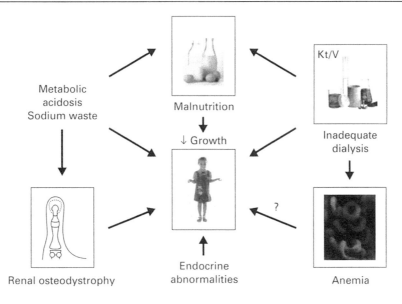

Figure 18.4 Etiology of growth failure in children with chronic renal failure. (See color plate section)

tributing factors include malnutrition, metabolic bone disease, anemia, disturbances of water and electrolyte metabolism, metabolic acidosis, and endocrine abnormalities (Fig. 18.4). There is a positive correlation between solute clearance and growth in children on chronic peritoneal dialysis, with residual renal function exerting a significant influence on that outcome.[27] This negative effect of inadequate dialysis on growth has significant clinical importance.

MALNUTRITION

Children with CRF tend to develop malnutrition, usually because of lack of appetite. Their energy intake is related to the degree of renal failure.[28] A minimum energy intake of more than 80% of the recommended daily allowance (RDA) is generally accepted as a prerequisite for normal growth velocity.[29] However, calorie intake above 80% of RDA is not associated with further improvement in growth. Although a sufficient energy intake is recommended for children with CRF, an exaggerated

calorie intake may induce hyperlipidemia, hyperinsulinism, and arterial sclerosis in the long term.[30] In addition an exaggerated calorie intake may induce hypertension[31] and high leptin levels.[32] It is also documented that children with progressive renal disease have high leptin levels,[33] which may contribute to lack of appetite[27] and progression of renal failure.

The negative effect of malnutrition on growth is well established in infants.[34] However, no correlation was found between energy intake and growth rate in patients with an age beyond two years.[35] Attempts to improve growth in older children with high-energy diets were generally disappointing.[29] In such patients, energy intake is usually considered low for their age, although it is normal when adjusted for their weight.[36] In a recent multicenter study, it was found that energy intake was low ($< 70\%$ of RDA) in 20% of children. However, only 4% of patients lost weight in relation to height during their follow-up period.[37] Obviously the majority of these patients had adequate energy intake and their poor growth was a result of different factors.

A moderate protein and phosphorus intake is advisable, for children with advanced CRF, in order to control metabolic acidosis and the accumulation of toxic nitrogen waste products. An interesting finding of a large multicenter European trial in children with CRF, was that no impairment of weight or length gain was seen following three years of a diet with protein restriction to 0.8–1.1 g/kg/day and a calorie intake of at least 85% of RDA.[38] The utilization of protein is correlated with the amount of energy intake. Therefore, a low protein intake must be accompanied by high energy intake in order to avoid malnutrition.

In all children with growth failure, aggressive nutritional intervention should be started prior to rhGH treatment. An increase in resting energy expenditure has been described in children treated with rhGH, possibly related to increased protein turnover. Therefore meticulous nutritional care should be provided during the period of rhGH treatment in order to achieve an energy intake of 100% of recommended daily allowance and administer the appropriate amount of protein.[39]

RENAL OSTEODYSTROPHY

Renal bone disease, also called renal osteodystrophy, is caused by a combination of disturbed vitamin D metabolism and secondary hyperparathyroidism. In the 1980s it was documented that daily oral calcitriol therapy was an effective treatment for secondary hyperparathyroidism and prevented the development of skeletal deformities in children with CRF.[40] These gross skeletal deformities obviously might contribute to the growth retardation. However, the effect of secondary hyperparathyroidism on the development of growth failure it is not known.

Intermittent high-dose calcitriol therapy and use of large doses of calcium-containing phosphate-binding agents effectively treated advanced secondary hyperparathyroidism, but recent evidence has demonstrated that the prevalence of adynamic bone with this management has been increasing. The prevention of this problem is crucial, since a marked reduction in linear growth has been demonstrated in children who developed adynamic bone lesions after 12 months of intermittent calcitriol therapy.[41] These findings suggest that the antiproliferative effects of calcitriol on chondrocyte proliferation may affect the epiphyseal growth plate and be responsible for a reduction in linear growth.

ANEMIA

Anemia was a consistent finding in children with CRF before the introduction of recombinant erythropoietin (EPO) treatment. It was speculated that anemia could be responsible for growth retardation. Children with thalassemia major have diminished growth rates, which usually improve when their anemia is corrected with high-frequency transfusions.[42] Therefore it was speculated that anemia could be responsible for growth retardation in children with CRF. Anemia was also considered as a cause of poor appetite, malnutrition, and infections in these patients. However, it was observed in children with CRF on EPO treatment that despite the subjective increase of their appetite, there was no consistent improvement in dietary intake or persistent growth improvement.[43,44]

DISTURBANCES OF WATER AND ELECTROLYTE METABOLISM

An increased loss of electrolytes and water occurs in young children with obstructive uropathy, renal hypoplasia, and other congenital renal diseases. Sodium depletion is known to affect not only extracellular volume, but also bone mineralization, nitrogen retention, and growth.[45] It was also found from experimental studies that plasma volume expansion appears to be required for growth, and salt deprivation may impair growth.[46] In a recent study, a dilute, high-volume sodium supplemented feeding regimen was administered to children with polyuric, salt-wasting CRF.[47] The stabilization of their growth is evidence of the benefit that may be seen with appropriate sodium and water supplementation.[47]

METABOLIC ACIDOSIS

Metabolic acidosis is manifested in children with even moderate CRF and is responsible for increased protein catabolism.[48,49] This is the effect of the activation of branched chain ketoacid catabolism[50] and the ubiquitin-proteasome pathway.[51] In addition, there is evidence that hyperleptinemia in patients with CRF may be masked by metabolic acidosis and that metabolic acidosis may inhibit leptin synthesis or secretion.[52] In young children with CRF, plasma bicarbonate was highly correlated with protein breakdown suggesting that acidosis-related protein wasting could contribute to growth retardation.[49] In addition, metabolic acidosis might be responsible for a diminished growth hormone response by down-regulating GH receptor.[53] Metabolic acidosis should be controlled by medication as soon as the serum bicarbonate falls below 22 mmol/l.[18]

ENDOCRINE ABNORMALITIES

Various hormonal alterations occur in children with CRF. Of particular importance for statural growth is GH and IGF-I resistance, which was described in chapter 17.

THE MANAGEMENT OF GROWTH FAILURE IN CHILDREN WITH CRF

The management of growth delay in children with CRF remains a stimulating challenge for the pediatric nephrologist. Before the administration of rhGH the following recommendations should always be considered:

1. Aggressive nutritional intervention should be planned (especially when the weight for height standard deviation score (SDS) is −2 or worse).
2. Anemia should be corrected with recombinant human erythropoietin and iron administration.
3. Renal osteodystrophy should be treated and adynamic bone disease should be prevented.
4. Sodium losses in the urine should be replaced.

5. Metabolic acidosis should be corrected to reduce protein catabolism.
6. Appropriate dose of dialysis should be provided in cases where ERSD has developed.

However, some children with CRF continue to grow poorly despite the appropriate management and rhGH should be administered. The current indications for rhGH treatment in children with CRF are:

1. Height for chronologic age less than − 2 SDs or height velocity for chronologic age less than − 2 SDs.
2. Growth potential shown by open epiphyses.
3. No known contraindication for recombinant human growth hormone use.[18]

In some cases, growth failure might be the result of late referral and/or suboptimal clinical care[54] and children with CRF with growth failure should be regarded as being at high-risk.[8] In the last decade, significant improvement in the management of patients with this problem has been achieved. This was the result of the early referral, modern dialysis, aggressive nutritional management, use of recombinant human erythropoietin, calcitriol, and finally the administration of recombinant human growth hormone.

REFERENCES

1. Goodhart JF. Two clinical lectures on albuminuria. BMJ 1890; 1:1183–1185.
2. Fivush BA, Jabs K, Neu AM, Sullivan EK, Feld L, Kohaut E, Fine R. Chronic renal insufficiency in children and adolescents: the 1996 annual report of NAPRTCS. Pediatr Nephrol 1998; 12:328–337.
3. Selwood NH, Wing AJ, Balas EA. Combined report on regular dialysis and transplantation of children in Europe, XIII, 1983. Proc Eur Dial Transplant Assoc Eur Ren Assoc 1985; 21:2–65.
4. Zimet GD, Owens R, Dahms W, Cutler M, Litvene M, Cuttler L. Psychosocial outcome of children evaluated for short stature. Arch Pediatr Adolesc Med 1997; 151(10):1017–1023.
5. Law CM. The disability of short stature. Arch Dis Child 1987; 62:855–859.
6. Wygold T. Psychosocial adaptation to short stature – an indication for growth hormone therapy? Horm Res 2002; 58 Suppl 3:20–23.
7. Reynolds JM, Wood AJ, Eminson DM, Postlethwaite RJ. Short stature and chronic renal failure: what concerns children and parents? Arch Dis Child 1995; 73:36–42.

8. Furth SL, Hwang W, Yang C, Neu AM, Fivush BA, Power NR. Growth failure, risk of hospitalization and death for children with end-stage renal disease. Pediatr Nephrol 2002; 17(6):450–455.

9. Warady BA, Alexander SR, Watkins S, Kohaut E, Harmon WE. Optimal care of the pediatric end-stage renal disease patient on dialysis. Am J Kidney Dis 1999; 33:567–583.

10. Kohaut EC. Chronic renal disease and growth in childhood. Curr Opin Pediatr 1995; 7(2):171–175

11. Van Es A. Growth hormone treatment in short children with chronic renal failure and after renal transplantation: combined data from European clinical trials. The European Study Group. Acta Paediatr Scand Suppl 1991; 379:42–48.

12. Tonshoff B, Tonshoff C, Mehls O, Pinkowski J, Blum WF, Heinrich U, Stover B, Gretz N. Growth hormone treatment in children with preterminal chronic renal failure: no adverse effect on glomerular filtration rate. Eur J Pediatr 1992; 151:601–607.

13. Mehls O, Broyer M. Growth response to recombinant human growth hormone in short prepubertal children with chronic renal failure with or without dialysis. The European/Australian Study Group. Acta Paediatr Suppl 1994; 399:81–87.

14. Fine RN, Kohaut EC, Brown D, Perlman AJ. Growth after recombinant human growth hormone treatment in children with chronic renal failure: report of a multicenter randomized double-blind placebo-controlled study. Genentech Cooperative Study Group. J Pediatr 1994; 124:374–382

15. Benfield MR, Parker KL, Waldo FB, Overstreet SL, Kohaut EC. Growth hormone in the treatment of growth failure in children after renal transplantation. Kidney Int Suppl 1993; 43:S62–64.

16. Haffner D, Schaefer F, Nissel R, Wuhl E, Tonshoff B, Mehls O. Effect of growth hormone treatment on the adult height of children with chronic renal failure. German Study Group for Growth Hormone Treatment in Chronic Renal Failure. N Engl J Med 2000; 28; 343(13):923–930.

17. Coleman J, Edefonti A, Watson AR on behalf of the European Paediatric Peritoneal Dialysis Working Group. Guidelines for the assessment and maintenance of nutritional status on chronic peritoneal dialysis http://www.ispd.org/guidelines/hoc.pdf

18. Kopple JD. National Kidney Foundation K/DOQI Work Group. The National Kidney Foundation K/DOQI clinical practice guidelines for dietary protein intake for chronic dialysis patients. Am J Kidney Dis 2001; 38(4 Suppl 1):S68–73.

19. Standardized Height and Weight Calculator: http://spitfire.emmes.com/study/ped/resources/htwtcalc.htm

20. Schaefer F, Wühl E, Feneberg R, Mehls O, Schärer K. Assessment of body composition in children with chronic renal failure. Pediatr Nephrol 2000; 14:673–678.

21. Brem AS, Lambert C, Hill C, Kitsen J, Shemin DG. Prevalence of protein malnutrition in children maintained on peritoneal dialysis. Pediatr Nephrol 2002; 17(7):527–530.

22. Edefonti A, Picca M, Paglialonga F, Loi S, Grassi MR, Ardissino G, Marra G, Ghio L, Fossali E. A novel objective nutritional score for children on chronic peritoneal dialysis. Perit Dial Int 2002; 22(5):602–607.

23. Karlberg J, Schaefer F, Hennicke M et al. Early age-dependent growth impairment in chronic renal failure. European Study Group for Nutritional Treatment of Chronic Renal Failure in Childhood. Pediatr Nephrol 1996; 10:283–287.

24. Jones RWA, Rigden SP, Barratt TM et al. The effects of chronic renal failure in infancy on growth, nutritional status and body composition. Pediatr Res 1982; 16:784–791.

25. Kari JA, Gonzalez C, Lederman SE et al. Outcome and growth of infants with severe chronic renal failure. Kidney Int 2000; 57:1681–1687.

26. Schaefer F, Wingen AM, Hennicke M et al. Growth charts for pre-pubertal children with chronic renal failure due to congenital renal disorders. European Study Group for Nutritional Treatment of Chronic Renal Failure in Childhood. Pediatr Nephrol 1996; 10:288–293.

27. Schaefer F, Klaus G, Mehls O. Peritoneal transport properties and dialysis dose affect growth and nutritional status in children on chronic peritoneal dialysis. Mid-European Pediatric Peritoneal Dialysis Study Group. J Am Soc Nephrol 1999 ; 10(8):1786–1792.

28. Norman LJ, Coleman JE, Macdonald IA et al. Nutrition and growth in relation to severity of renal disease in children. Pediatr Nephrol 2000; 15:259–265.

29. Arnold WC, Danford D, Holliday MA. Effects of calorie supplementation on growth in uremia. Kidney Int 1983; 24:205–209.

30. Wingen AM, Mehls O. Nutrition in children with preterminal chronic renal failure. Myth or important therapeutic aid? Pediatr Nephrol 2002; 17:111–120.

31. Barton M, Carmona R, Morawietz H et al. Obesity is associated with tissue-specific activation of renal angiotensin-converting enzyme in vivo. Hypertension 2000; 35:329–336.

32. Ballermann BJ. A role for leptin in glomerulosclerosis? Kidney Int 1999; 56:1154–1155.

33. Daschner M, Tönshoff B, Blum WF et al. Inappropriate elevation of serum leptin levels in children with chronic renal failure. European Study Group for Nutritional Treatment of Chronic Renal Failure in Childhood. J Am Soc Nephrol 1998; 9:1074–1079

34. Rees L, Rigden SPA, Ward GM. Chronic renal failure and growth. Arch Dis Child 1989; 64:573–577.

35. Betts PR, Magrath G, White RHR. Role of dietary energy supplementation in growth of children with chronic renal insufficiency. Brit Med J 1977; I:416–420

36. Foreman JW, Abitbol CL, Trachtman H et al. Nutritional intake in children with renal insufficiency: a report of the Growth Failure in Children with Renal Diseases Study. J Am Coll Nutr 1996; 15:579–585.

37. Wingen AM, Fabian-Bach C and Mehls O. Evaluation of protein intake by dietary diaries and urea-N excretion in children with chronic renal failure. Clin Nephrol 1993; 4:208–215

38. Wingen AM, Fabian-Bach C, Schaefer F et al. Randomised multi-centre study of a low-protein diet on the progression of chronic renal failure in children. European Study Group of Nutritional Treatment of Chronic Renal Failure in Childhood. Lancet 1997; 349:1117–1123.

39. Stefanidis CJ. Chronic renal insufficiency and recombinant human growth hormone treatment. Pediatr Nephrol 1998; 12 (4):340.

40. Chesney RW, Moorthy A, V, Eisman JA et al. Increased growth after long-term oral 1-alpha-25-vitamin D_3 in childhood renal osteo-dystrophy. N Engl J Med 1978; 298:238–242.

41. Kuizon BD, Goodman WG, Jüppner H et al. Diminished linear growth during intermittent calcitriol therapy in children undergoing CCPD. Kidney Int 1998; 53:205–211.

42. Kattamis CA, Kattamis AC. Management of thalassemias: growth and development, hormone substitution, vitamin supplementation, and vaccination. Semin Hematol 1995; 32:269–279.

43. Stefanidis CJ, Koulieri A, Siapera D, Kapogiannis A, Mitsioni A, Michelis K. Effect of the correction of anemia with recombinant human erythropoietin on growth of children treated with CAPD. Adv Perit Dial 1992; 8:460–463

44. Schaefer F, André JL, Krug C et al. Growth and skeletal maturation in dialysed children treated with recombinant human erythropoietin (rhEPO) – a multicenter study. Pediatr Nephrol 1991; 5:C61.

45. Wassner S. Altered growth and protein turnover in rats fed sodium-deficient diets. Pediatr Res 1989; 26:608–613.

46. Ray PE, Lyon RC, Ruley EJ, Holliday MA. Sodium or chloride deficiency lowers muscle intracellular pH in growing rats. Pediatr Nephrol 1996; 10:33–37.

47. Parekh RS, Flynn JT, Smoyer WE, Milne JL, Kershaw DB, Bunchman TE, Sedman AB. Improved growth in young children with severe chronic renal insufficiency who use specified nutritional therapy. J Am Soc Nephrol 2001; 12:2418–2426.

48. Papadoyannakis NJ, Stefanidis CJ, McGeown M. The effect of the correction of metabolic acidosis on nitrogen and potassium balance of patients with chronic renal failure. Am J Clin Nutr 1984; 40(3):623–627.

49. Boirie Y, Broyer M, Gagnadoux MF et al. Alterations of protein metabolism by metabolic acidosis in children with chronic renal failure. Kidney Int 2000; 58:236–283.

50. May RC, Hara Y, Kelly RA et al. Branched-chain amino acid metabolism in rat muscle: abnormal regulation in acidosis. Am J Physiol 1987; 252:E712–E718.

51. Bailey JL, Wang X, England BK et al. The acidosis of chronic renal failure activates muscle proteolysis in rats by augmenting transcription of genes encoding proteins of the ATP-dependent ubiquitin-proteasome pathway. J Clin Invest 1996; 97:1447–1453.

52. Zheng F, Qiu X, Yin S, Li Y. Changes in serum leptin levels in chronic renal failure patients with metabolic acidosis. J Ren Nutr 2001; 11(4):207–211.

53. Challa A, Chan W, Krieg RJ, Jr. et al. Effect of metabolic acidosis on the expression of insulin-like growth factor and growth hormone receptor. Kidney Int 1993; 44:1224–1227.

54. Furth SL, Alexander DC, Neu AM, Hwang W, Powe NR, Fivush BA. Does growth retardation indicate suboptimal clinical care in children with chronic renal disease and those undergoing dialysis? Semin Nephrol 2001; 21(5):463–469.

19. Immunization and anti-microbial therapy for children with chronic kidney disease

Ching-Yuang Lin and Yee-Hsuan Chiou

INTRODUCTION

The prevention and management of systemic bacterial and viral infections by the provision of appropriate vaccines and anti-microbial therapy are essential components of the pediatrician's daily practice. This task is often complicated by questions about safety and efficacy in children with chronic kidney disease (CKD). In this chapter, we will review current approaches to healthy children and discuss recommendations for immunization and antibiotic choices for children with CKD.

CURRENT RECOMMENDATIONS FOR IMMUNIZATION IN HEALTHY CHILDREN

In 2003, the Advisory Committee on Immunization Practices (ACIP) of the Centers for Disease Control and Prevention (CDC), and the American Academy of Pediatrics (AAP), published the latest series of immunization schedules for healthy children,[1,2] which incorporates the administration of heptavalent pneumococcal conjugated vaccine (PVC) for children aged 2–23 months and for certain children aged 24–59 months.[3,4] Varicella vaccine has been recommended for susceptible children after 12 months of age.[1,2] The recent development and release of several new combination vaccines will simplify the delivery of multiple recommended vaccines.

CURRENT RECOMMENDATIONS FOR IMMUNIZATION IN CHILDREN WITH CKD

According to the AAP recommendations, children who have CKD, including those on dialysis, should receive all age-appropriate vaccines.[5] However, patients who are on immunosuppressive medications, including renal transplant patients and patients with various forms of chronic glomerulonephritis, should not be given live viral vaccines. In discussing the immunization of children with CKD, it is important to consider the potential for different vaccine responses in children who are pre-dialysis, as compared to those on dialysis or post renal transplantation.

It is recommended that influenza vaccine be given annually to CKD children in early fall since there is increased susceptibility to influenza-related morbidity and mortality in these patients.[6-9] Therefore, the influenza vaccine is recommended for children with chronic renal disease. In addition, since the response to standard influenza vaccination doses might be suboptimal in children with CKD,[10] higher doses or increasing number of doses have been recommended for some vaccinations. Possible reasons for reduced protection include lower seroconversion rate, and lower peak titers to various immunizations. Furthermore, an unusual decline of antibody levels may occur in pediatric patients with nephrotic range proteinuria or those on peritoneal dialysis.[8,9,11]

CURRENT RECOMMENDATIONS FOR PATIENTS WITH CKD WHO ARE PRE-TRANSPLANT

As stated previously, all children with CKD who are not on immunosuppressive drugs should receive age-appropriate recommended standard and special vaccines. Evaluation of vaccine responses in patients on dialysis is complicated since they might receive their initial immunizations before starting dialysis therapy, and receive a booster dose while on dialysis. Low seroconversion rates following vaccination, low peak antibody titers, and a rapid decline of antibody levels have been reported in patients with CKD.

There are limited data on antibody responses to MMR and DTP vaccines in CKD patients.[12,13] According to Neu et al., children on chronic peritoneal dialysis can produce protective antibody titers to diphtheria, tetanus, and rubella vaccines.[12] The authors argued that infants with earlier stages of CKD will also have a good response to these vaccines. Since MMR is not recommended for use in immunocompromised patients, it is better to check the antibody level in patients with CKD before proceeding to renal transplantation. If this shows a low serum antibody titer, the patients should be reimmunized.

According to the report published by Watkins et al. for the Southwest Pediatric Nephrology Study Group (SPNSG), children with CKD showed a good response to the hepatitis B vaccine.[14] Similar responses were observed by Vazquez et al., who showed 100% seroconversion rate to this vaccine in CKD patients.[15]

Whenever possible, patients on dialysis should receive three doses of hepatitis B vaccine, as recommended for healthy children by ACIP and AAP. Watkins et al. evaluated the response to double the recommended dose of vaccine in 22 peritoneal dialysis and 16 hemodialysis patients and reported 97% of seroconversion rates.[14] From these results, response to hepatitis B vaccine may be improved by receiving the vaccination before dialysis or using higher vaccine doses. The ACIP recommends postvaccination anti-HBs testing for dialysis patients 1–2 months after vaccination is completed, and annually thereafter. A booster dose is recommended if the anti-HBs titer falls below 10 mU/ml.

Inactivated poliovirus vaccine (IPV) is the only polio vaccine that should be administered to children and adolescents, according to the 2003 recommendations by ACIP and AAP.[1,2] In children, four doses of poliovaccine are given at the age of 2, 4, 16–18 months, and 4–6 years. A fourfold increase in antibody levels in response to this vaccine is seen in

86% of children on dialysis.[16] Measles, mumps, and rubella vaccine (MMR) should be given to children on dialysis between 12 and 15 months, with a booster dose between four and six years of age. For healthy children, the seroconversion rate for one dose of MMR vaccine is more than 90%.

The H. influenza type b (Hib) vaccine is recommended for children on dialysis. There are limited data on using Hib vaccine in children on dialysis. ACIP recommends the vaccine be given at 2, 4, 6, and 12 to 15 months. Neu et al. reported in her study of children on dialysis, a seroconversion rate of 90% with persistence of immunity for at least one month after vaccination.[17] Fivush et al. reported that patients on peritoneal dialysis could produce protected antibody titers after Hib vaccination.[18]

Varicella vaccination is recommended for CKD children age one year or older if they have not had chickenpox previously. Susceptible adolescents older than 13 years of age should receive two doses given at least four weeks apart. Data on the immunogenicity of varicella vaccine among children with CKD are limited.[19–21] Since this vaccine is not recommended in severely immunocompromised patients, CKD patients should receive this vaccine before transplantation. Furth et al. reported a 98% seroconversion rate in 50 children with CKD after a two-dose regimen.[20]

The pneumococcal vaccine is also recommended for patients on dialysis.[22,23] The heptavalent pneumococcal conjugated vaccine (PCV) is recommended for children aged 2–23 months and for certain children aged 24–50 months. A single dose of the 23-valent pneumococcal polysaccharide vaccine is recommended for all dialysis patients two years of age or older. More than 75% of dialysis patients have an adequate response to this vaccine, but the antibody levels are often lower than those seen in healthy individuals. However, Furth et al. reported adequate responses to the vaccine and protective serum antibody levels for patients with CKD.[23] Unfortunately, a rapid decline in antibody levels has been reported in some children and adults with chronic renal disease. Revaccination with PCV is recommended 3–5 years after the first dose.

CURRENT RECOMMENDATION FOR PATIENTS POST RENAL TRANSPLANTATION

Patients after renal transplantation should receive standard and special vaccinations recommended by the AAP, with the exception of live viral vaccines, such as MMR and varicella. DTP vaccine can be administered post-transplantation. In Ghio's study,[13] 35 dialysis and 54 transplanted patients who had been vaccinated with DTP previously were evaluated for antibody titers to diphtheria and tetanus. Based on their data, Shio et al. concluded that primary vaccination to diphtheria and tetanus ensured long-lasting immunity in chronic dialysis patients, but not in children with renal transplantations. In the same study, renal transplant recipients received a booster dose of DT. All transplant recipients developed protective antibody titers to tetanus and 94% to diphtheria. MMR is not recommended in this population and it is better to establish protective antibody titers before renal transplantation, with reimmunization if necessary. Hepatitis B vaccine can be given safely after renal transplantation. However, in the study by Watkins et al., the vaccine was more efficacious when administered before renal transplantation.[14] Varicella vaccine is not routinely recommended in post transplant patients. However, Zamora et al. studied the use of live viral varicella vaccine in such patients.[22] The majority of the patients developed protective antibody varicella titers and the adverse reactions to this vaccine were minimal.

SUMMARY

To reduce the risk of vaccine preventable diseases, pediatric patients with CKD should receive all the standard and special vaccines currently recommended by the ACIP and AAP for healthy children. However live viral vaccines should be avoided in transplant patients. It is important that pediatricians collaborate with nephrologists monitoring the immunization status of patients with CKD. We hope that the morbidity and mortality associated with the vaccine preventable diseases could be reduced by the practice of regular immunizations in children with CKD.

ANTIBIOTIC USE IN RENAL DISEASE

This section will review a problem that often confronts physicians who are involved in the care of a child with renal disease. When such patients develop acute infections, and the clinical and laboratory features suggest that the infection is bacterial in origin, the physician must decide on a suitable antibiotic and the optimal dosing schedule for not only the type and severity of the infection – but also the type and severity of the kidney disorder. We will first consider some general aspects of antibiotic therapy, followed by some specific comments regarding children who have varying stages of CKD.

PHARMACOKINETIC BASIS OF OPTIMAL ANTIBIOTIC USE

The choice of antibiotics in patients with bacterial infections is empiric in many clinical conditions. This is especially true in children with kidney diseases because only a small fraction of the published pharmacokinetic (PK) data has been obtained in such patients. However, knowledge of the PK properties of antibiotics in normal individuals will help clinicians determine the optimal usage of antibiotics in patients with CKD.

BASIC CONCEPTS OF CLINICAL PHARMACOKINETICS

Pharmacokinetics describes the time course of drug movement in the body. The three main steps involved in the delivery of drugs to the site(s) where they are needed are: absorption, distribution, and elimination. Each of these steps will be considered.

Absorption: When a drug is given extravascularly, it must be absorbed into the systemic circulation from its site of administration (e.g. gastrointestinal tract or muscle). Bioavailability estimates the amount of a drug administered extravascularly that is absorbed into the circulatory system.

A drug's peak plasma concentration (Cp) is also influenced by its rate of absorption. The higher the rate of absorption, the higher the Cp that will be achieved. This is most relevant for concentration-dependent antibiotics since a high Cp is vital for these drugs to achieve good therapeutic efficacy. Hence, it is important to give such antibiotics on an empty stomach since gastric contents often delay the rate of absorption, causing a blunted Cp and a diminished therapeutic effect.

Distribution: The volume of distribution of a drug after it has been absorbed into the systemic circulation is determined by several characteristics of the drug. One of the characteristics that is of particular significance for children with kidney disease is the extent to which a drug binds to plasma proteins. Acidic drugs bind mostly to plasma albumin, whereas basic drugs bind to α1-acid glycoprotein. Plasma protein binding of a drug is affected by the following diseases:

a. Liver dysfunction (reduces albumin synthesis).
b. Nephrotic syndrome (causes albumin wasting).
c. Uremia (changes the affinity of binding).

The volume of distribution (Vd) of a drug varies considerably as a result of the factors listed above. In general it is apparent that a drug with a very small Vd (e.g., 0.2 l/kg) is confined to extracellular fluid. A drug with a large Vd (e.g., $\geq$ 0.7 l/kg) has extensive tissue binding and intracellular distribution. It should be noted that the loading dose of a drug that should be given to a child with kidney disease is independent of the type and extent of the individual's disease.

Elimination: Clearance (Cl) estimates the volume of body fluid cleared of drug per unit time. Cl is important to determine the proper timing of subsequent doses to maintain desired drug concentration. When the systems for elimination of drugs are not saturated, the rate of elimination of most drugs follows a linear function of plasma drug concentra-

tion (first-order kinetics). Once the mechanisms of drug elimination are saturated, a constant amount of drug is eliminated per unit (zero-order kinetics). The clearance thus becomes more complicated. Elimination half life (T$\frac{1}{2}$) reflects the time required for a drug concentration to decrease by 50%. T$\frac{1}{2}$ can be estimated from the measured fall in plasma drug concentration after a dose.

ELIMINATION OF DRUGS BY THE KIDNEYS

The kidneys are the most important organs for the excretion of many drugs. The two factors that contribute to the excretion of drugs are: renal plasma flow (RPF) and delivery of drugs to the kidney.

Glomerular filtration rate (GFR)
The glomeruli offer very little resistance to the filtration of the unbound fraction of most drugs and allow passage of molecules up to molecular weights of about 65,000 daltons. The majority of antibiotics are approximately two orders of magnitude smaller than this. For drugs such as aminoglycosides that are freely filtered at the glomerulus, renal elimination is quite rapid if the RPF and GFR are normal.

Fractional protein binding
The most important barrier to glomerular filtration of many drugs is usually not the glomerular barrier but the degree of binding of the drug to macromolecules that are too large for filtration, since only the free fraction of the drug can be filtered into the tubular lumen.

Transtubular reabsorption and secretion
The kidneys are capable of both active and passive reabsorption of many drugs. Aminoglycoside antibiotics are taken up by the brush border of the proximal tubular cells via at least two different mechanisms: a carrier-mediated system and pinocytotic uptake leading to lysosomal accumulation. The proportion of back diffusion of drugs is decreased by increasing the flow rate of tubular fluid (e.g., after mannitol administration).

Examples of organic acid antibiotics with active renal secretion are most cephalosporins and most penicillins.

ANTIBIOTIC USAGE IN PATIENTS WITH ABNORMAL KIDNEY FUNCTION

Patients with CKD often display physiologic changes that profoundly alter the pharmacology of many drugs. Decreasing kidney function will alter the absorption, distribution, metabolism and elimination of drugs, as detailed in Table 19.1. This section will discuss antibiotic therapy for patients with CKD as well as those with more acute kidney disorders.

PHARMACOKINETIC CONSIDERATIONS

Several pathophysiologic and pharmacokinetic features are changed by renal function impairment (see Table 19.1). For example, patients with more severe stages of CKD frequently have symptoms of nausea, vomiting, and gastroparesis which may discourage them from taking oral medications, and both altered intestinal motility and decreased absorptive capacity may decrease the rate of drug

absorption. Antacids, which are used frequently in patients with CKD, will chelate some drugs and decrease their bioavailability.

ANTIBIOTIC DOSING FOR PATIENTS WITH ABNORMAL KIDNEY FUNCTION

The process to determine the proper drug dosing of patients with kidney disease is illustrated in Figure 19.1. Two main factors to consider whether drug dosing should be adjusted for patients with renal insufficiency are 1) the therapeutic index of the drug, and 2) the normal elimination pathway of the drug. Generally speaking, when the therapeutic index of a drug is wide, patients can tolerate a several-fold increase of the normal serum level without toxicity. Examples include many penicillin derivatives and cephalosporins. On the other hand, if a drug has a narrow therapeutic index and more than 40% of the drug is normally excreted in urine, it is necessary to consider dosing adjustment. This even applies to some drugs which are excreted less than 40% by the kidneys, such as antibiotics with active metabolites that are mainly excreted by the kidney. Examples of antibiotics with active metabolites are shown in Table 19.2.

Table 19.1 Changes of pharmacology in patients with renal function impairment

	Events	Effects
Absorption	Nausea, vomiting, gastroparesis	Decreased absorption
	Decreased intestinal motility	Decreased absorption
	Decreased gastric acid	Decreased absorption of drugs requiring acid hydrolysis
	Antacids	Decreased absorption
	Decreased gastrointestinal absorptive function	Decreased absorption
Distribution	Lower systemic pH	Increased free form of weak acid drugs
	Decreased protein binding (from decreased albumin level and binding ability)	Increased free drug available for drug effect and elimination
	Edema	Increased Vd of water-soluble drugs
	Dehydration	Decreased Vd of water-soluble drugs
Elimination	Decreased both renal and non-renal elimination	Accumulation of drugs or metabolite

Table 19.2 Antibiotics with active metabolites that are normally excreted by the kidney

Drug	Active metabolite
Cephalosporins	
Cefotaxime	Desacetylcefotaxime
Cefoxitin	Decarbamoylcefoxitin
Cephalothin	Desacetylcephalothin
Macrolides	
Clarithromycin	14-hydroxy (R)-clarithromycin
Quinolones	
Ciprofloxacin	Four different metabolites
Fleroxacin	N-demethylfleroxacin
Norfloxacin	Six different metabolites
Pefloxacin	N-desmethylpefloxacin and norfloxacin
Sulfonamindes	
Sulfamethoxazole	Acetyl metabolite

DRUG DOSING CALCULATIONS

Loading dose. As noted previously, the loading dose of an antibiotic is independent of the patients' kidney function, unless there are significant changes in the drug's volume of distribution (e.g. pronounced edema, ascites, or dehydration). The loading dose can be calculated from the following equation:

Loading dose $= Vd \times IBW \times C$

VD: volume of distribution
IBW: ideal body weight
C: desired steady-state plasma drug
    concentration

Maintenance dose. Methods that may be used to determine the maintenance dose of antibiotic for a patient with CKD are listed in Table 19.3. For most of the drugs, any of the methods can be used. The choice depends on the ease of the regimen for the patients.

1. Dose reduction regimen
This method gives patients a maintenance dose of drugs without change of drug interval. Maintenance dose can be calculated as follows:

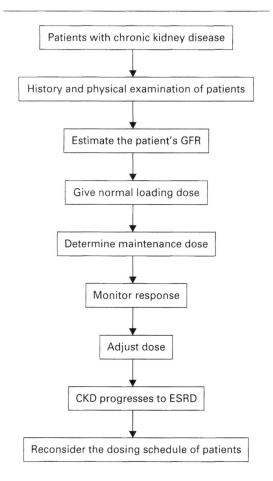

Figure 19.1 Algorithm to determine appropriate dosing of antibiotics for patients with kidney disease

Dose in renal insufficiency = normal dose × normal elimination half-life / half-life in patients with renal insufficiency.

This method is effective for drugs with a narrow therapeutic range and short elimination half-life. However, the steady state drug serum levels are subtherapeutic. Therefore, this method is not suitable for time-dependent antibiotics. The trough levels are higher than normal and the toxicity of aminoglycoside is increased.

Table 19.3 Approaches to maintenance dose adjustment in patients with renal diseases

Methods	Applications
1. Dose reduction	Drugs with narrow therapeutic index and short plasma half-life To keep trough level is important
2. Modified dose reduction	Keep normal peak level at same interval with very high trough level
3. Interval prolongation	Drugs with wide therapeutic index and long plasma half-life
4. Kunin method	Similar to modified dose reduction half the dose is given every half-life
5. Combine (1) and (3)	When keeping peak level and avoiding high trough level are important

2. Modified dose reduction regimen

This regimen gives patients a higher maintenance dose thus keeping normal peak drug plasma levels with very high trough levels. This method is suitable for time-dependent antibiotics such as penicillin and cephalosporin. It is important to maintain the peak level of such antibiotics and there is less concern about maintaining higher trough level.

3. Interval prolongation regimen

The same dose for patients with normal renal function is administered to patients with CKD at wider drug intervals. This method is suitable for drugs with a wide therapeutic window and a long elimination half-life. This method may result in prolonged periods of time with subtherapeutic drug levels and breakthrough bacteremia.

4. Kunin method

Half the normal maintenance dose is administered to patients with renal insufficiency at every half-life. It also results in higher trough drug levels and thus is not suitable for aminoglycosides.

5. Combined dose reduction and interval prolongation regimen

For aminoglycosides it is important to achieve peak plasma drug levels to kill bacteria efficiently, while avoiding high trough levels to reduce drug toxicity. This method with a lower drug dose administered at longer intervals results in a minor decrease in peak

levels and modest increases in trough levels. Thus this is the preferred method for aminoglycosides.

ANTIBIOTIC USAGE FOR PATIENTS ON DIALYSIS

When renal function impairment progresses to renal failure, most patients will begin hemodialysis or peritoneal dialysis. Since some drugs are removed during either form of dialysis, physicians should reconsider the drug dosage in such patients. Specific details regarding this topic are beyond the scope of this text.

ANTIBIOTIC USAGE IN PATIENTS WITH SPECIAL CLINICAL CONDITIONS AND UTI

The decision to choose an antibiotic regimen for the treatment of patients with urinary tract infection (UTI) during the acute phase is dependent on whether the infection is upper or lower (i.e. acute pyelonephritis or acute cystitis). When a lower UTI is suspected, antibiotics with a short serum half-life but highly concentrated in the urine can be selected. When upper UTI is suspected, bacteremia is always a concern. Oral or parenteral antibiotics with a longer half-life should be used. The need for several imaging studies as well as the need for long-term management of patients with UTI, are most influenced by the diagnosis of complicated UTI (e.g. vesicoureteral reflux or obstructed nephropathy). These issues, and appropriate references for further reading, are discussed in detail in Chapter 12.

NEONATE WITH UTI

When the diagnosis of UTI is suspected in a neonate, the physician must assume that bacteremia may also be present. A penicillin and aminoglycoside with dosage for bacteremia are necessary. The course of therapy should be 10–14 days; this includes 5–7 days of parenteral therapy. Poor response to antibiotic therapy warrants up to three weeks of antibiotic treatment. Neonates with complicated UTI require prophylaxis antibiotics. The most commonly used antibiotic in this age range is amoxicillin (20 mg/kg/day q 12 h).

TWO-MONTH TO TWO-YEAR OLD CHILDREN WITH UTI

When patients of this age period with suspected UTI appear toxic and have poor appetite, antibiotics should be administered parenterally, usually in the hospital. Otherwise they can be treated safely with an oral third-generation cephalosporin (e.g. cefixime 16 mg/day for 1 day, then 8 mg/day q 24 h for 13 days, at home. Prophylactic antibiotics should then be given until a complicated UTI is ruled out by an imaging study. Although the evidence of the efficacy of prophylactic antibiotics to prevent UTI is not strongly established, there are some clinical conditions for which long-term prophylactic antibiotics are recommended (Table 19.4). See Chapter 12 for further details.

Table 19.4 Conditions which may require prophylactic antibiotics for prevention of UTIs

Vesicoureteral reflux
Reflux nephropathy
Obstructive uropathy
Recurrent UTI
Urosepsis
Awaiting radiologic evaluation after UTI
Urethral instrumentation
Immunosuppressed or immunocompromised patients
Infants with first UTI before 8–12 weeks of age

Abbreviation: UTI, urinary tract infection

REFERENCES:

1. Centers for Disease Control and Prevention. Recommended Childhood and Adolescent Immunization Schedule – United States, 20003. MMWR 2003; 52:Q1–4.

2. American Academy of Pediatrics, Committee on Infectious Diseases. Recommended Childhood and Adolescent Immunization Schedule – United States, 2003. Pediatrics 2003; 111(1):212–216.

3. Overturf GD, and the American Academy of Pediatrics, Committee on Infectious Diseases. Technical report: prevention of pneumococcal infections, including the use of pneumococcal conjugate and polysaccharide vaccines and antibiotics prophylaxis. Pediatrics 2000; 106(2):367–376.

4. American Academy of Pediatrics, Committee on Infectious Diseases. Policy statement: prevention of pneumococcal infections, including the use of pneumococcal conjugate vaccine (Prevnar), and pneumococcal polysaccharide vaccine, and antibiotics prophylaxis. Pediatrics 2000; 106(2):362–366.

5. American Academy of Pediatrics: Immunization in Special Circumstances. In Pickering LK (ed): 2000 Red Book: Report of the Committee on Infectious Diseases, 25th edn. Grove Village, IL, American Academy of Pediatrics 2000, 59–69.

6. American Academy of Pediatrics: Influenza. In Pickering LK (ed): 2000 Red Book: Report of the Committee on Infectious Diseases, 25th ed. Grove Village, IL, American Academy of Pediatrics 2000, 351–359.

7. Centers for Disease Control and Prevention. Prevention and Control of influenza: recommendations of the Advisory Committee on Immunization Practices (ACIP). MMWR Morb Mortal Wkly Rep 2002; 51(No. RR-3):1–31.

8. Fivush BA, Furth SL, Neu AM. Immunizations in children on PD: Current guidelines and recommendations. Adv Perit Dial 1995; 11:270–273.

9. Fivush BA, Neu AM. Immunization Guidelines for Pediatric Renal Disease. Seminars in Nephrology 1998; 18(3):256–263.

10. Furth SL, Neu AM, McColley SA et al. Immune response to influenza vaccination in children with renal disease. Pediatr Nephrol 1995; 9:566–568.

11. Johnson DW, Fleming SJ. The use of vaccines in renal failure. Clin Pharmacokinet 1992; 22:434–436.

12. Neu AM, Warady BA, Furth SL, et al. Antibody levels to diphtheria, tetanus and rubella in infants vaccinated while on peritoneal dialysis: A study of The Pediatric Peritoneal Dialysis Study Consortium. Adv Perit Dial 1997; 13:296–298.

13. Ghio L, Pedrazi C, Assael BM et al. Immunity to diphtheria and tetanus in children with end-stage renal disease. J Am Soc Nephrol 1996; 7:1908.

14. Watkins SL, Hogg RJ, Alexander S et al. Response to recombinant hepatitis B vaccine (Recombivax HB) in children with chronic renal failure. J Am Soc Nephrol 1994; 5:344.

15. Vazquez G, Alvarez T, Mendoza L et al. Comparison in the response to recombinant hepatitis B virus vaccine in children with chronic renal failure, with and without dialysis. Perit Dial Int 1997; 17 (Suppl 1):S90.

16. Schulman SL, Deforest A, Kaiser BA et al. Response to measles-mumps-rubella vaccine in children on dialysis. Pediatr Nephrol 1992; 6:187–189.

17. Neu AM, Lederman HM, Warady et al. Hemophilus influenza type b immunization in infants maintained on peritoneal dialysis. Pediatr Nephrol 1996; 10:84–85.

18. Fivush B, Case B, Warady B et al. Defective antibody response to hemophilus influenza type b immunization in pediatric peritoneal dialysis patients. Pediatr Nephrol 1993; 7:548–550.

19. Zamora I, Simon JM, Da Silva ME et al. Attenuated varicella virus vaccine in children with renal transplants. Pediatr Nephrol 1994; 8:190–192.

20. Furth SL, Hogg RJ, Tarver J et al. Varicella vaccination in children with chronic renal failure. A report of the Southwest Pediatric Nephrology Study Group. Pediatr Nephrol 2003; 18:33–38.

21. Furth SL, Arbus GS, Hogg R et al. Varicella vaccination in children with nephrotic syndrome. A report of the Southwest Pediatric Nephrology Study Group. Pediatr 2003; 142:145–148.

22. Fuchshuber A, Kuhnemund O, Keuth B et al. Pneumococcal vaccine in children and young adults with chronic renal disease. Neprol Dial Transplant 1996; 11:468–473.

23. Furth SL, Neu AM, Case B et al. Pneumococcal polysaccharide vaccine in children with chronic renal disease: A prospective study of antibody response and duration. J Pediatr 1996; 128:99–101.

20. Social and developmental consequences of chronic kidney disease in children

Ken Jureidini and Paul Henning

INTRODUCTION

The kidneys are responsible for fine-tuning the body's internal environment.[1] Patients with chronic kidney disease (CKD) often develop widespread metabolic disorders, including water and salt imbalance, metabolic acidosis, a variety of other electrolyte disturbance, toxin retention, secondary hyperparathyroidism, reduced effective vitamin D production, deficient erythropoietin response to anemia, and inhibition of growth hormone activity. As a result, the clinical picture in children with CKD is characterized by severe malaise, appetite suppression, anemia, major bone disorder, and reduced growth velocity. CKD, although not usually reversible, may have varying rates of progression. In each case, as described elsewhere in Chapters 16 and 18, optimal treatment will minimize the ill effects. However, even with the best available treatment, in the most well equipped centers, there is usually a significant degree of uncertainty about long- and short-term outcome.[2]

Physical development is affected to varying degrees in children with renal disease. When CKD is inadequately treated, for any reason, growth is reduced to a very significant degree. Bones are weakened and may be markedly deformed. Energy is sapped by the accompanying anemia and the cachexia of the uremic state. These factors, compounded by the nausea and other signs of toxicity, create a child with decreased energy and reduced physical ability to partake in normal activities of siblings and peers. In addition to the potentially debilitating physical effects of CKD, there is mounting evidence that CKD has a significant effect on mental and social development. The severity of this problem is greater in those patients who developed CKD at a young age. The treatment of such patients

is often invasive and traumatic. There are also frequent financial consequences, with disruption of work and other family activities. Although chronic dialysis and/or kidney transplantation are frequently available as reasonable therapies in children of all ages, their accessibility adds to some of the uncertainties that complicate renal failure management. This is often compounded by the fact that, in less wealthy societies, when such therapies are unavailable, medical professionals and many affected subjects and their families are frustrated, knowing such treatments are available in richer countries.

Historically, in all societies and socio-economic groups, significant renal impairment from birth or early childhood often remained unrecognized until the typical presentation of marked growth retardation, obvious bone disease, and anemia in sickly, lethargic children. Almost invariably, they showed significantly slowed developmental milestones. A review in 1985 found that in twelve children who had chronic renal failure since birth, head circumference had dropped to 2 SD below the mean in the majority of children and eight had significant developmental delay.[3] It was concluded that it was impossible to determine whether this resulted from the toxic effects of uremia, malnutrition, or the associated psychosocial and experiential deprivation related to chronic, severe disease.

Children with end-stage renal disease (ESRD) are at increased risk for lower IQ and academic achievement; this is especially so in younger children, in children who have ESRD for longer periods, and in children whose caregivers have lower educational levels.[4] It would appear from these observations that, even when care is provided in major centers in an advanced industrial society, children with severe renal disease suffer intellectual disadvantages. Psychologic and social problems also appear to be highly probable in such children.

It is clear that non-treatment of children with CKD is associated with significant physical and developmental delay. In more industrially developed countries in the 1970s and, more recently in less wealthy countries, pediatric nephrologists have been faced with a dilemma. They encountered children with long established renal failure, who were miserable, cachexic, extremely short, often mentally delayed, with crippling bone and joint deformities. During the 1970s, dialysis and transplantation became commonplace in children. However, it soon became apparent that, even with a successful renal transplant resulting in improved metabolic state, bones and general health, learning difficulties often remained.[5] Catch up growth was limited and the small size of the subjects tended to exaggerate the perception of delayed development. There was a significant incidence of physical, emotional, and mental disorders, related to the effects of the CKD. An important dilemma is that children who either have had longstanding renal failure, or are inadequately treated from the start, may have a relatively long life expectancy, but are left with significant disability.

MANAGEMENT OF CKD

Following these observations, there has been much emphasis on improving the management of chronic renal failure, in order to minimize the ill effects. Optimal management, which includes careful dietary management, with adequate energy input and appropriate balance of protein, phosphate, salt, water, calcium, bicarbonate, minerals, vitamins, and hormones, can often result in normal growth and development. However, this is difficult to achieve, because it depends on the skill and availability of resources of the treating team, and the compliance of the subject.[6]

Our own experience has been that, with optimal treatment from the first indication of renal disease and with appropriate compliance from the child and family, normal physical development is often

possible.[7] This requires an experienced team, adequate motivation and awareness within the family, and strong extended family and community support. Even when severe renal failure is present from birth, we and others have been able to observe normal brain growth and development, through the sequence of medical management, dialysis and transplantation.[8]

It is particularly important that infants with CKD be managed aggressively from the time that their diagnosis is established. This includes the early incorporation of nasogastric and, ultimately, gastrostomy feeding in infants who do not respond to more conservative measures in order to achieve maximal energy intake and food quality. However, it is also important to encourage the development and maintenance of normal feeding patterns.

This dual approach can be facilitated by establishing the involvement of one or more pediatric nutritionists who have specialized knowledge in the nutritional requirements of children with renal disease. A skilled nutritionist is able to adjust the child's food and drink relevant to the family habits and child's wishes, rather than impose a new diet. It is also important to incorporate professional and other social and psychologic support mechanisms, as described below.

SUPPORT FOR CHILDREN WITH CKD

It has become clear that the ill effects of CKD, coupled with the inherent uncertainties of outcome in patients with this disorder, result in great emotional upheaval to the affected child and her/his family. While accepting that cultural and resource driven issues create individual variations, there are important common principles that are pivotal when addressing the social aspects of kidney disease. The social effects of renal disease can be approached from many viewpoints: the patient, parents, siblings, extended family, staff and community at all levels. Chronic illness has been defined as a disability that restricts a child's ability to perform tasks associated with daily living.[9]

Even if optimal treatment is successful, resulting in acceptable growth and physical and mental development, the rigors of the treatment regime will take their toll. A child with chronic disease has twice the risk of developing a significant psychologic disorder compared with a healthy child and this risk is further increased if there is a recognizable accompanying disability.[10] Studies in children and adolescents with CKD have certainly identified a range of emotional and behavioural problems,[11] even where successful kidney transplantation has been achieved.[12] However, it must also be said that the findings of many studies are inconsistent and may reflect the considerable methodologic challenges that face researchers in this field.[13]

Having a significant illness creates a feeling of 'being different' compared with other children. Children often react adversely to this, with the risk of regressing into isolation or other destructive behavior. Poor growth often has negative consequences for the ego of children with CKD.[14] Being smaller than the peer group and siblings usually exaggerates this feeling of isolation. Since the same factors that reduce growth also affect general fitness and wellbeing, the ill effects are compounded. The treatment to enhance growth and minimize the ill effects of the CKD creates its own problems.

The needs and problems of children with CKD are best examined in three broad age groups. Although there are common features to all of these, some issues are specific to age:

INFANTS AND PRE-SCHOOL CHILDREN

- The management of patients with CKD in this age group is totally dependent on the parents[15]. Providing adequate nutrition is the key to successful treatment. This usually involves feeding a child with a poor appetite, often with consequent stress to the parent, facing frustration and disappointment. The cycle of poor feeding and parental need for a resistant child to eat may create conflict between the child and parent, which may initiate longstanding problems. As stated previously, nasogastric tube feeding is often required, with frequent need for overnight pump feeding. This may create a feeling a failure, which is compounded by the child exhibiting further resistance to normal feeding. When prolonged tube feeding becomes necessary, gastrostomy feeding is recommended. Parents often initially resist this, to avoid the trauma of additional surgery, and because it often exaggerates their feeling of inadequacy as a parent. Once established, however, it is usually clear that, despite the care required for the gastrostomy button, the whole process is simplified. The gastrostomy button is more easily concealed than the nasogastric tube. Another advantage is that it is easier to establish normal feeding patterns from the base of gastrostomy feeds.

- Parents are often required to inflict uncomfortable or even painful procedures on their child. These include bladder catheterization, administering drugs, sometimes by subcutaneous injection and the responsibility, well recognized by the child from an early age, for bringing the child to the hospital/health center for unpleasant procedures inflicted by others.

- Hereditary and congenital conditions are most often recognized during this period and may be associated with guilt feelings in one or both parents. Underlying conflict related to the extended family's disapproval of the matching of the parents may be unmasked and inflict additional stress on the parents.

- The whole process of managing a child with CKD is very time consuming and tiring for the parents and the child. Not only does this add to the potential conflict between parents and child, but also between the parents, sometimes sufficiently severe to be the focal point for failure of their relationship.

- Behavioral disturbances can evolve.

PRIMARY SCHOOL AGE CHILDREN

These patients have reached the age where they are more aware of their differences from other children, are more reactive, and often expected to take more responsibility for their treatment.

- Nutrition remains a key part of the management. The child becomes increasingly aware of the dietary differences between her/his diet and that of peers and siblings. If tube feeding of either type remains necessary, this can be particularly traumatic.
- Issues related to painful and uncomfortable procedures, and resistance to visits to hospitals/ health centers, are likely to be more prevalent than in earlier life.
- The child will often become increasingly aware of differences from the peer group with regards to activity levels and general ability to keep up with the other children.
- The school may not handle the issues related to the child's illness in an appropriate manner.
- Reaction against parents and other authority figures is likely to be compounded and behavioral problems may increase.

ADOLESCENTS

Although there are cultural and individual variations, generally, the adolescent is expected to take increasing responsibility for his/her own illness and its management.

- Schools and even families do not necessarily recognize the adolescent's need for privacy and dignity.
- Adolescents usually become stressed by the amount of time required for their medical needs.
- Nutrition, drugs, and procedures often become more important issues than in childhood.
- Emerging sexuality frequently creates major disturbance.
- Awareness of mortality is important and may result in risk taking behavior.
- Behavior problems may present as antisocial behavior.
- Adolescents with chronic illness have been shown to have twice the incidence of mental disorders compared with their healthy peers.
- Poor compliance is most common in this age group. Tragically, this results in one of the most

common causes of renal transplant graft loss.[16] Our understanding of this issue and our ability to reduce its impact on transplant outcome has been poor. There is a strong argument for a more patient centered approach to research and clinical management in this area for children as well as adolescents.[15,17]

Throughout the full spectrum of these age groups, it is becoming increasingly apparent that there is a major effect on siblings. Recent studies have confirmed important disturbances in a significant number of siblings of subjects with chronic disease, including those with CKD.

It is clear that a long history of CKD in childhood and adolescence is likely to have an adverse impact on an individual's physical and intellectual development. There is ample evidence of disturbed emotional and psychologic wellbeing.[13] All of these factors, even when within the most supportive of social environments, contribute to what appears to be a significant disruption of maturation into adult life. Observations of adult survivors of childhood CKD in several centers in different countries show many positive results, but also highlight failure to achieve educational potential, difficulty in forming lasting intimate relationships, problems in achieving independence and in attaining vocational fulfillment.[18] These maturational problems may be associated with longer periods of CRF and on dialysis. This observation supports the recommendation of the International Pediatric Nephrology Association to offer children priority in cadaveric donor organ allocation systems.

The pediatric nephrologist has a major responsibility in attempting to lessen the psychologic and social burden of renal disease on the child in adolescence, and the family and community. As the medical professional with the ultimate responsibility for the care of the child, the pediatric nephrologist requires skills in communication with the child and family, recognizing the need for a holistic approach to the child's care. In so doing, she/he should work in close association with a number of different professional and other groups:

- Social worker: a competent social worker is a key figure in the team. It is advisable for her/him to be introduced to the family as early as practical. While supporting the family through the disruption to family life, schooling, and commonly, financial affairs, a further role is to provide a mediating role between the family and the medical professionals.
- Psychologist/psychiatrist: requirement is frequently obvious in assessing both mental and emotional development and providing appropriate support and therapy when the patient or family member(s) decompensate. It is desirable for the family, including the patient, to meet with the psychiatrist/psychologist early in the care pathway, so that he/she is able to provide preventive management and to be a familiar figure if intervention is required. As an integral member of the team, her/his expertise can be of great value in advising the other team members on a regular basis. It should be noted that the psyche of the team members needs support, since difficult decisions need to be made on behalf of the child and family.
- Occupational therapists, speech pathologists, physiotherapists.
- Community based: religious organizations, support groups such as service clubs, government agencies.
- Therapeutic camping and peer support group activities.

It is important to stress to the patient, the family, and to the community that the affected child is a normal person with abnormal kidneys. The purpose of the kidneys is to control fluid and electrolytes, maintain normal blood pressure, and excrete toxic substances. The disturbances arising from renal disease can be controlled by judicious use of medical treatment and, when necessary, dialysis and/or transplantation. Meanwhile, such maintenance of renal function allows the whole child to remain effectively normal. Of course, loss of control, or the ill effects of drugs (such as striae and other steroid side-effects, and the disfiguring hirsuitism and gum hypertrophy caused by cyclosporine), polyuria/nocturia and/or bladder disturbances can cause embarrassing urinary incontinence. The plight of children can be improved by increasing public awareness and education of educationalists. Peer pressure is most evident at schools. Other children can reasonably be expected to be ignorant of the needs of affected patients, but it is often surprising and disappointing to observe similar degrees of ignorance shown by teachers. Many of the consequent difficulties at both levels can be diminished by visits to schools, by the 'treating professionals' and appropriate use of the media.

TREATMENT OF CKD

The availability of optimal treatment of CKD varies between different countries and, within each country, between centers. Financial and educational resources are of utmost relevance. Even within specific countries or communities, cultural, racial, and religious differences occur, which determine the attitudes towards treatment of renal disease. In countries with limited resources, facilities, such as dialysis and transplantation, together with the ability to provide optimal medical care of renal failure, can be provided to the wealthy minority, while the majority do not have access to adequate services.

It is too simplistic to view this issue solely in the context of rich and poor countries. Within highly industrialized countries, theoretical access to first-rate medical resources is available to all. Certainly, the majority has access to best possible medical care. However, a recent longitudinal study[19] showed significantly reduced life expectancy in pockets of 'small area deprivation' in New Zealand, a 'first world' country, compared with more highly populated areas. Within these areas of deprivation, there was further reduced life expectancy in the indigenous Maori population and that of the immigrant 'Islanders', compared with the European derived population in the same areas. This inequality translates to healthcare in general, including optimal management of kidney disease.

Conversely a study of Nigerian children with renal failure[20] reviewed the factors that limited their access to dialysis treatment and ways of improvement. Of 81 patients with chronic renal failure, 55 were eligible for dialysis, but only six were dialyzed, thus giving a dialysis access rate of 10.9%. Factors that limited access to dialysis treatment in the patients included financial restrictions of parents (33%) and lack or failure of dialysis equipment (45%). Since most patients could not be dialyzed, preventive nephrology is advocated to reduce the morbidity and mortality from renal failure due to preventable diseases.

The first principle of attaining maximal potential patients with CKD is early recognition and prevention of progression of renal failure. With the increasingly widespread use of intrauterine ultrasound studies, early intervention, may result in improved prognosis for renal development, together with consequent better developmental outcomes. In contrast, this may also result in the survival of a fetus or infant, otherwise non-viable, with the problems of severe renal failure.

Cultural and religious issues create further differences, irrespective of resource availability. Whereas there is general agreement on medical grounds that renal transplantation is the most acceptable treatment for children with end-stage renal failure, the use of cadaver or even live donor kidneys is unacceptable in some communities.

The responsibility of the physician needs to be examined on a wider scale. It is generally found in societies, whatever the availability of resources, that there is continual questioning of priorities of allocation. The management of the individual child with CKD is expensive, particularly if applied at the level required to minimize developmental delay. While valid arguments may suggest that it is of greater general good to divert resources from expensive treatment of small numbers to broader based preventive measures, the physician needs to view the situation from the standpoint of the duty of care to his/her patient, while not abrogating his/her responsibility to the community at large. There are principles of medical ethics, which can be

of assistance. Four such principles are generally accepted by most religious and cultural groups:

- Autonomy (individual freedom to choose).
- Beneficence (being kind).
- Non-maleficence (doing no harm).
- Justice (both to the individual and the wider community).

Beneficence, applied to the individual patient, can be in conflict with non-maleficence and with justice to the community at large. The autonomy of the child is always at risk, particularly at a young age. When all the ethical arguments are applied, the doctor's final decision is usually made simply on the grounds of what is believed at the time, in the circumstances, to be of the greatest benefit to the patient. Whereas the doctor will generally accept responsibility to the community at large in which he/she practices, it is considered by most to be up to that community and those who lead it to make the final decisions about resource allocation, while the doctor considers his/her duty of care to the patient as the most important element. However, the role of the doctor, as a member of the worldwide community is also relevant. It is vital, with increasingly improving worldwide communications, for the world's pediatric nephrologists to recognize their responsibilities to the world's children. The International Association of Pediatric Nephrology addresses this issue as the most important in its charter, with a major focus on education. Doctors from privileged communities should make themselves available to support their colleagues in less resourced societies, while those from these societies should strive to improve the situation from within.

Although legal issues are becoming of increasing universal concern, it appears that if reasonable ethical principles are applied, the doctor is likely to be protected from legal intervention. Although there are vast differences in application and interpretation of the law between different societies, the general principles are remarkably similar. Informed consent is a vital factor in applying the law. An interesting example, which encompasses social factors, ethics, and law, is the approach to a potential live donor. It is critical that the potential donor has a reasonable understanding of the risks, not only of the procedure, but also of the emotional disturbances that may occur if the kidney transplant fails. Although the greatest risk is to the psyche of the donor and recipient, there is a risk of litigation, which might prove that adequately informed consent was not achieved.

Finally, there are positive effects that derive from the difficulties faced by children with renal disease and their families. All the world's great religions teach that great adversity can result in added strength to the individual and to groups. It has been a common observation of our patients that they show marked strength in overcoming their adversities and that they appear to grow into more complete people. We are constantly inspired by the children that we have treated and by their achievements.

SUMMARY

It is hopefully clear to the reader that the social and developmental consequences of CKD in children have now been accepted as very important aspects when children with this disorder are being evaluated and treated. It is no longer appropriate to treat the physical and laboratory disturbances without paying attention to the other concerns that are detailed in this chapter. An optimal approach to this extension of patient management requires a cohesive team attitude and communication between the pediatric nephrologist and primary care physician.

REFERENCES

1. Bernard C. Leçons sur les phénomènes de la vie, communs aux animaux et végétaux. Balleère 1978; 1.
2. Norman LJ, Macdonald IA, Watson AR. Optimising nutrition in chronic renal insufficiency – progression of disease. Pediatr Nephrol 2004; 19(11):1253–1261.
3. McGraw ME, Haka-Ikse K. Neurologic-developmental sequelae of chronic renal failure in infancy. J Pediatr 1985; 106(4):579–583.
4. Crittenden MR, Holliday MA, Piel CF, Potter DE. Intellectual development of children with renal insufficiency and end stage disease. Int J Pediatr Nephrol 1985; 6(4): 275–280.
5. Novello AC, Fine RN. Renal transplantation in children – a review. Int J Pediatr Nephrol 1982; 3(2):87–98.
6. Brouhard BH, Donaldson LA, Lawry KW, McGowan KR, Drotar D, Davis I, Rose S, Cohn RA, Tejani A. Cognitive functioning in children on dialysis and post-transplantation. Pediatric Transplantation 2000; 4(4):261–267.
7. Jureidini KF, Hogg RJ, van Renen MJ, Southwood TR, Henning PH, Cobiac, L, Daniels L, Harris S. Evaluation of long term aggressive dietary management of chronic renal failure in children. Pediatr Nephrol 1990; 4:1–10.
8. Kari JA, Gonzalez C, Ledermann SE, Shaw V, Rees L. Outcome and growth of infants with severe chronic renal failure. Kidney Int 2000; 57:1681–1687
9. Isaacs D, Sewell J. Children with chronic conditions. MJA 2003; 179(5): 235–236.
10. Mrazek A. Psychiatric aspects of somatic disease and disorders. In: Rutter M, Taylor E, (eds.) Child and adolescent psychiatry, 4th edn. Oxford: Blackwell Publishing, 2002; 810–827.
11. Madden SJ, Ledemann SE, Guerrero-Blanco M, Bruce M. Cognitive and psychosocial outcome of infants dialysed in infancy. Child Care Health Dev 2003; 29 (1):55–61.
12. Penkower L, Dew MA, Ellis D, Sereika SM, Kitutu JMM, Shapiro R. Psychological distress and adherence to the medical regimen among adolescent renal transplant recipients. Am J Transplant 2003; 3(11):1418–1425.
13. Feilding D, Brownbridge G. Factors related to psychosocial adjustment in children with end-stage renal failure. Pediatr Nephrol 1999; 13(9):766–770.
14. Reynolds J, Morton M, Garralda M, Postethwaite R, Goh D. Psychosocial adjustment of adult survivors of a paediatric dialysis and transplant programme. Arch Dis Child 1993; 68(1):104–110.
15. Madden S, Hastings R, V'ant Hoff W. Psychological adjustment in children with end stage renal disease: the impact of maternal stress and coping. Child Care Health Dev 2002; 28(4):323–330.
16. Feinstein S, Keich R, Becker-Cohen R, Rinat C et al. Is noncompliance among adolescent renal transplant recipients inevitable? Pediatrics 2005; 115:969–973.
17. Young B, Dixon-Woods M, Windridge K, Heney D. Managing communication with young people who have a potentially life threatening chronic illness: qualitative study of patients and parents. BMJ 2003; 8; 326(7384):305.
18. Henning P, Tomlinson L, Rigden S, Haycock G, Chantler. Long term outcome of treatment of end stage renal failure. Arch Dis Child 1988; 63(1):35–40.
19. Tobias MI, Cheung J. Monitoring health inequalities: life expectancy and small area deprivation in New Zealand. Popul Health Metr 2003(Apr); 1(1):2.
20. Olowu WA. Renal failure in Nigerian children: factors limiting access to dialysis. Pediatr Nephrol 2003(Dec); 18(12):1249–1254.

21. Renal transplantation in childhood

Patrick Niaudet

INTRODUCTION

Dialysis and/or renal transplantation should be considered for children with end-stage renal disease (ESRD) when the glomerular filtration rate falls below 5 ml/minute/1.73 m^2. Although there have been many advances in the conservative treatment of children with ESRD (peritoneal dialysis, hemodialysis, recombinant erythropoietin, and growth hormone), renal transplantation is accepted as the best treatment for children. In recent years, graft and patient survival have increased due to improvements in the care of young patients, and advances in pharmacologic immunosuppression, resulting in a reduction in the frequency and the severity of acute rejection crisis and chronic rejection. This chapter will detail some aspects of renal transplantation in children with ESRD since the primary care physician may encounter such a patient in his/her practice.

In some children with CKD, it is appropriate to plan for renal transplantation before chronic dialysis is needed (pre-emptive transplantation). This is often performed with a living related donor when it is anticipated that dialysis will need to be instituted within the next six months. There are no differences in graft and patient survival, or in the incidence of rejection crisis following pre-emptive transplantation, compared to patients who were treated with dialysis prior to transplant.[1] Therefore, the rate of pre-emptive transplantation has increased during recent years with an improved quality of life for these children.

Renal transplantation is contraindicated in cases of severe brain damage or multi-organ failure. It should be delayed for several months in cases of concomitant infectious disease or if the disease responsible for renal failure is an active disease, which has progressed rapidly, such as hemolytic uremic syndrome or crescentic glomerulonephritis. Pre-existing malignancy is a relative contraindication. Patients with a history of Wilms' tumor may be transplanted if they have been in remission for at least two years. Patients with hepatitis B or C infection should not be excluded unless they have active liver disease.

LIVING RELATED DONOR OR CADAVERIC DONOR?

The results of kidney transplantation with a living related donor (LRD) are better than with a cadaveric donor (CAD). The rate of acute tubular necrosis is lower and the long-term survival is 10% higher with LRD. In addition, the time of transplantation can be decided in advance and the waiting time on dialysis can be shortened, thus limiting the complications observed during this period. Despite the advantages of LRD[2] transplantation, the proportion of them varies greatly from one country to another, from 86% in Scandinavia, to 46% in North America and less than 10% in France. Several factors may explain these differences: the activity of the cadaver transplant program; the criteria for organ allocation to children, which vary among the countries; cultural differences, and the way parents are provided with information about the pros and cons of LRD versus CAD transplantation by doctors.

GRAFT SURVIVAL

As stated previously, the results of renal transplantation have improved during the past 10 years and the results are better with LDR compared to CAD transplants. The current North American data reveal that 1-, 3- and 5-year graft survival are 95, 90, and

83% with living-related donors, respectively, as compared to 91, 82, and 73% with cadaver grafts.[3] However, a cadaver donor may be preferred in settings in which there is a high-risk of recurrent disease leading to loss of the graft, such as focal segmental glomerulosclerosis.

The role of HLA compatibility in cadaveric renal transplantation is controversial, particularly since the introduction of cyclosporine. Most large multicenter studies, however, have found a correlation between the degree of HLA compatibility and graft survival, even among those treated with cyclosporine. The beneficial effect of matching is best observed with respect to long-term outcome. Such results can be estimated using graft half-lives, which is defined as the time needed for half of the grafts functioning at one year to fail. The half-life of HLA identical grafts is 26.9 years, compared to 10.8 years for grafts from a parent matched for one haplotype. Similar results were found for cadaveric-graft recipients in a prospective study: the estimated half-life of HLA-matched grafts was 17.3 years compared to 7.8 years for mismatched grafts.[4]

Optimal HLA matching is therefore preferred, particularly for young recipients, retransplantations, and transplantation in sensitized patients. However, maximization of HLA matching is not entirely beneficial since sharing kidneys based upon such matching increases cold ischemia times and the rate of delayed graft function. This, in turn, may affect long-term graft survival. Lower graft survival is observed in recipients younger than five years of age mainly because of an increased immune reactivity, and an enhanced risk of graft thrombosis.[5] Some investigators have reported a higher incidence of graft failure with kidneys from donors under five years of age and this may be due to a higher incidence of primary non-function and graft thrombosis.

Acute rejection episodes markedly increase the risk of developing chronic rejection, thereby enhancing possible allograft loss over time. In one study of nearly 3,500 children, univariate and multivariate analyses found that the variables most frequently associated with chronic rejection were an acute rejection episode and greater than two such episodes, resulting in relative risks of 3.1 and 4.3, respectively.[6] Given this association, the prevention of acute rejection by providing optimal immunosuppressive therapy is extremely important.

ANTI-REJECTION MEDICATIONS

There are many medications that have been used to prevent or treat rejection episodes in renal transplant units around the world. These will be reviewed briefly here.

CORTICOSTEROIDS

Corticosteroids are used at low doses to prevent acute and chronic rejection and at higher doses to treat acute rejection episodes. The efficacy of corticosteroids is primarily based upon their ability to inhibit the activation and proliferation of T cells. These agents inhibit the transcription of genes that code for several cytokines, such as interleukin-1, interleukin-2, interleukin-6, interferon-gamma, and tumor necrosis factor (TNF)-alpha. Corticosteroids also dampen the activity of monocytes and neutrophils, but have little effect upon the antibody response.

In many transplant centers, corticosteroids are given in association with azathioprine (or mycophenolate mofetil) and cyclosporine (or tacrolimus) (triple therapy) for the prevention of acute rejection. The initial dose is usually given during the transplant procedure as IV methylprednisolone, at doses which vary between 2 to 10 mg/kg BW. The maintenance oral dose varies between 15 to 60 mg/m²/day (0.5 to 2 mg/kg BW/day); this is gradually tapered over time.[7] Some teams stop corticosteroids after 6–12 months. However, withdrawal of steroid therapy has been associated with a high incidence of rejection, which may lead to chronic graft dysfunction and graft loss. Some clinicians prefer alternate day treatment while others administer daily low-dose steroid treatment.

Acute cellular rejection is usually treated with 3–5 intravenous methylprednisolone pulses, at doses of 5–30 mg/kg BW. Following this treatment, the maintenance dose of corticosteroids is often increased, followed by a slow tapering to prerejection doses. Serum creatinine levels may continue to increase for 3–4 days after starting the antirejection therapy, but should decrease after one week and return close to the pretreatment values within one month. Otherwise, the rejection episode is called steroid resistant and other therapies should be entertained.

Corticosteroids have multiple side effects, including growth impairment, susceptibility to infections, cushingoid appearance, acne, hypertension, aseptic bone necrosis, cataracts, hyperglycemia, poor wound healing, and psychologic side effects. One of the most important reasons for stopping corticosteroids, or switching to alternate day treatment, is statural growth impairment, which is frequently observed in patients on daily treatment.

AZATHIOPRINE

Azathioprine is converted in the liver to 6-mercaptopurine, the active metabolite, which is incorporated into DNA. Azathioprine is primarily an antiproliferative agent, which explains why the number of peripheral blood lymphocytes is not affected. Azathioprine is used to prevent rejection but is not effective in the treatment of ongoing rejection.

Azathioprine is given at doses of 2–3 mg/kg BW when used in conjunction with only corticosteroids. In the triple therapy regimen, the azathioprine dose is lower, ranging from 1–2 mg/kg BW. Azathioprine is usually well tolerated. The main side effect is myelotoxicity, with leukopenia, and less frequently thrombocytopenia, or megaloblastic anemia. Other side effects include hepatotoxicity, pancreatitis, interstitial pneumonitis, increased risk of viral infections, alopecia and neoplasia.

Azathioprine and 6-mercaptopurine are both metabolized in the liver. Allopurinol interferes with the metabolism of 6-mercaptopurine, which in part involves xanthine oxidase. Thus, 6-mercaptopurine accumulation and possibly severe bone marrow toxicity may ensue with concurrent use of these agents. Allopurinol should therefore generally be avoided in patients treated with azathioprine.

MYCOPHENOLATE MOFETIL (MMF)

MMF, the prodrug of the active immunosuppressant mycophenolic acid, is an inhibitor of inosine 5-phosphate dehydrogenase and guanosine monophosphate synthetase, which reduces de novo purine synthesis in T and B lymphocytes. The use of MMF appears to be safe and beneficial among children. Eighty-six patients receiving MMF in combination with cyclosporine and prednisone without induction were compared with a historic control group of 54 children receiving azathioprine instead of MMF. Patient survival after three years was 98.8% in the MMF group and 94.4% in the azathioprine group (NS). Cumulative acute rejection episodes occurred in 47% of patients in the MMF group versus 61% in the azathioprine group ($P<0.05$).[8]

The recommended dose of MMF is 1200 mg/m^2 per day divided in two oral doses. Adverse effects include diarrhea, vomiting, leukopenia, anemia, and infectious complications.

CYCLOSPORINE

Cyclosporine is a metabolite of the fungus, *Tolypocadium inflatum*. It acts at an early stage of T lymphocyte activation, mainly the T helper cells. It inhibits the transcription of interleukin-2, other cytokines, proto-oncogenes, and receptors for cytokines. The new oral preparation of cyclosporine A, cyclosporine microemulsion (Neoral) has an improved pharmacokinetic and pharmacodynamic profile when compared to the standard oral preparation.

The metabolism of cyclosporine occurs in the liver where it is transformed by the enzyme, cytochrome P-450. Cyclosporine and its metabolites are mainly excreted through the biliary tract while urinary excretion concerns only 6% of the drug. Several factors may alter cyclosporine metabolism. Of interest are the drugs which interfere with cytochrome P-450. Phenobarbital, phenytoin, rifampin induce enzyme activity and decrease cyclosporine blood levels, thereby increasing the risks of rejection. Ketoconazole, erythromycin and IV methylprednisolone inhibit cytochrome P-450 activity and therefore increase cyclosporine blood levels. This may result in toxic side effects. Measurements of blood cyclosporine levels are therefore useful when giving a drug that may interfere with cyclosporine metabolism.

The use of cyclosporine has resulted in enhanced allograft survival. The European Dialysis and Transplant Association (EDTA) registry reported overall renal graft survivals of 75 and 57% at one and five years, respectively, for children less than 15 years old who were transplanted since 1985. By comparison, if only those who received cyclosporine in this registry are assessed, graft survival was 82 and 73% at two and three years, respectively.

Unfortunately, cyclosporine has several side effects. The most worrying is acute and/or chronic nephrotoxicity. Acute nephrotoxicity is related to the vasoconstrictive effect of cyclosporine on the afferent arteriole resulting in a decreased renal blood flow. As a result, cyclosporine may increase ischemic graft damage and affect the graft outcome in patients with delayed graft function. Chronic nephrotoxicity results in a permanent impairment of renal function with histologic alterations of the renal parenchyma consisting of tubular atrophy and interstitial fibrosis. The other side effects include hypertension, hyperkalemia, hypomagnesemia, neurotoxicity, hepatotoxicity, hirsutism, and gum hypertrophy.

TACROLIMUS (FK506)

Tacrolimus is a cyclic peptide which acts in a similar way to cyclosporine. The in vitro immunosuppressive effect of tacrolimus on lymphocyte activation is 50- to 100-times higher than cyclosporine.

Recent trials in adults have shown similar graft survival outcomes with tacrolimus when compared to cyclosporine-based regimens; however, the incidence of acute rejection and requirement for intensive immunosuppression may be less with tacrolimus. In children, some evidence suggests that similar graft survival rates are observed with tacrolimus- and cyclosporine-based regimens.

The side effects of tacrolimus on the kidney are similar to those of cyclosporine. Neurotoxicity appears to be more common with tacrolimus than with cyclosporine. Diabetes mellitus may develop. In children, special attention should be given to patients who develop primary Epstein–Barr Virus (EBV) infection, as there is an increased risk of lymphoproliferative syndrome, which is reversible after discontinuation of tacrolimus.

RAPAMYCIN

Rapamycin, the product of a fungus, has immunosuppressive properties through the inhibition of the cytosolic enzyme TOR, which regulates the differentiation and proliferation of lymphocytes. Rapamycin, as well as a similar compound RAD, may be used in combination with other immunosuppressants.[10] The main side effects include hyperlipemia, thrombocytopenia, leucopenia, and delayed wound healing.

ANTILYMPHOCYTE ANTIBODIES

Antilymphocyte antibodies recognize T cell surface receptors. They block lymphocyte functions by binding to cell surface receptors or kill lymphocytes. They are used to reverse acute rejection episodes, also during the early post-operative period to prevent rejection.

Polyclonal antilymphocyte preparations consist of antisera raised in animals (horse, rabbit) immunized with human lymphocytes, thymocytes, or lymphoblasts. They contain a wide variety of antibodies directed against many hematopoietic antigens. Unwanted antibodies can be responsible for neutropenia, thrombopenia, or serum sickness. One such commonly utilized antibody is antithymocyte globulin or ATG. The prophylactic use of polyclonal antilymphocyte preparations has been shown to improve graft survival by 10–15% compared to conventional treatment. Polyclonal antilymphocyte preparations are also used in the treatment of acute rejection episodes.

Monoclonal antibodies have been produced to inhibit a number of different T-cell surface receptors. The first used in clinical transplantation was OKT3, which is an anti-CD3 antibody that binds to the δ chain of the T-cell receptor and is a potent inhibitor of almost all T-cell functions. OKT3 is very effective in the treatment of acute rejection, of steroid resistant rejection, and also in the prophylaxis of rejection. However, its use is limited by the formation of anti-OKT3 antibodies.[11] The most serious side effect is the so-called 'first-dose reaction' which occurs in more than two-thirds of the patients after their first dose of OKT3, and consists of fever, chills, headache, vomiting, diarrhea, hypotension, and sometimes pulmonary edema, particularly if the patient is overloaded with fluids. These symptoms are related to the activation of T-cells and the release of several cytokines. They are partially controlled by corticosteroids, pentoxifyllin, or anti-TNF monoclonal antibodies. Other side effects include anaphylaxis, aseptic meningitis, seizures, thrombosis, and acute graft dysfunction.

Monoclonal antibodies against the interleukin-2 receptor have been shown to reduce the incidence of early acute rejection. There are two chimeric or humanized antibodies (basiliximab and daclizumab) which are both safe and effective. There is no comparative study between these two antibodies. Nowadays, more than half of the children who are undergoing renal transplantation receive an IL-2 receptor antibody as induction therapy.

COMPLICATIONS OF RENAL TRANSPLANTATION

DELAYED GRAFT FUNCTION

Patients who do not require dialysis during the first week after kidney transplantation have better graft survival rates than those with delayed graft function due to acute tubular necrosis. The long-term graft survival rate is 15–25% lower in recipients with delayed graft function.

VASCULAR THROMBOSIS

Vascular thrombosis (renal artery or renal vein) is the second cause of early graft failure. The main risk factor for the development of thrombosis is the combination of young age in both donor and recipient. Other risk factors include multiple arteries, bench surgery of graft vessels, venous malformation in the recipient, hypercoagulability status of the recipient, and a hypotension episode during or after surgery. In order to prevent graft thrombosis, careful hemodynamic monitoring is most important. Furthermore, preventive treatment with low molecular weight heparin has been shown to be very effective.[12]

REJECTION

Hyperacute rejection occurring within the first minutes following transplantation is due to preformed anti-HLA antibodies that bind to vascular endothelial cells and activate the complement cascade. The aggregation of platelets on the damaged endothelium leads to fibrin deposition and vascular thrombosis.

Acute rejection is the most frequent complication. It may occur several days or weeks after transplantation and is characterized by cellular infiltration of the graft. The classical clinical signs of acute rejection are fever and graft tenderness. However, these signs are less commonly observed with current immunosuppressive regimens that include cyclosporine. With these new regimens, acute rejection episodes are often only manifested by a rise of plasma creatinine and occur several weeks after transplantation.

Chronic rejection is the most common cause of graft loss. Acute rejection and low cyclosporine doses are two major risk factors for chronic rejection and subsequent graft loss.[13] The role of cyclosporine and FK 506 in the histologic changes observed in patients with chronic graft dysfunction is still a matter of discussion.

HYPERTENSION

Hypertension is frequent after renal transplantation and represents a significant cause of morbidity.[14] Moreover, it has a detrimental effect on allograft survival. The incidence of hypertension decreases with time. ACE inhibitors should be used with caution, especially if a renal artery stenosis is suspected, following Doppler examination. In such cases, angiography is performed and angioplasty may be needed to overcome renal artery stenosis in selected cases. During the early postoperative period, hypertension may be due to fluid overload, to acute rejection, to hypercalcemia, or to the use of corticosteroids and/or cyclosporine or tacrolimus. Later, the main causes of hypertension are chronic rejection, renal artery stenosis, recurrence of primary disease, urinary tract obstruction and high renin production by native kidneys if pretransplant nephrectomy has not been performed.

INFECTIONS

Infections are a permanent risk in patients receiving immunosuppressive drugs.[15] Urinary tract infections with *Staphylococcus aureus* or *Escherichia coli* and pulmonary infections are frequent during the early post-operative period. Prophylactic treatment with trimethoprim-sulfamethoxazole may prevent urinary tract infection and also reduce the incidence of *Pneumocystis carinii* infections.

Viral infections, particularly with viruses from the herpes virus group, are frequent and may be life-threatening. Cytomegalovirus (CMV) infection may occur in a seronegative patient receiving a graft from a CMV-positive donor or in seropositive recipients either as a result of reactivation or reinfection with the donor's strain. CMV infection may present with clinical symptoms including fever, leucopenia, thrombopenia, pneumonitis, hepatitis and allograft dysfunction. The incidence of clinical disease is higher in seronegative recipients with primary CMV infection. Prophylactic treatment with acy-

clovir may reduce the severity of the disease. The treatment of CMV disease includes gancyclovir and decrease of immunosuppressive treatment.[16]

Varicella infection may be responsible for severe disease with encephalitis, pneumonitis, hepatic dysfunction, and death. A transplanted child exposed to varicella should receive varicella-zoster immune globulin within 72 hours of exposure. If clinical symptoms of the disease develop, intravenous acyclovir should be administered and immuno-suppressive drugs should be withdrawn. Immunization with the live varicella vaccine is recommended prior to transplantation for all children without varicella antibodies.[24] This procedure prevents severe varicella.

Epstein-Barr virus (EBV) infection is frequent but usually asymptomatic. However, in patients receiving strong immunosuppression, including antilymphocyte antibodies, there is a risk of lymphoproliferative syndrome. Discontinuation of immunosuppression and anti-B lymphocyte antibodies are recommended in this setting.

Herpes simplex virus often causes labial ulcerations and oral acyclovir is effective. Warts due to papilloma viruses are common in patient transplant. BK virus infection may cause renal allograft dysfunction.[19,20]

RECURRENCE OF PRIMARY DISEASE

Recurrence of primary disease is responsible for graft failure in 5–15% of cases in pediatric series.

Among the glomerular diseases which may recur in the graft, the most frequent is focal segmental glomerular sclerosis (FSGS). The overall risk of recurrence of nephrotic syndrome after transplantation is estimated to be around 25%.[21,22] Graft failure occurs in about 60% of patients with recurrence, versus 23% of those without recurrence.[23] Some patients may show good renal function for several years despite persistent nephrotic syndrome. The treatment remains controversial: plasma exchanges and cyclosporine are the most often advocated. We recently reported that iv cyclosporine at doses that maintain blood levels higher than 200 ng/ml may be effective.[24]

Apart from FSGS, membranoproliferative glomerulonephritis often recurs in the graft and approximately 20% of grafts are lost from recurrence. In IgA nephropathy and Henoch-Schönlein purpura nephritis, the recurrence of IgA deposits in the graft is very common, but clinical recurrence and histologic glomerular involvement are quite uncommon. The same is true for lupus nephritis which rarely recurs in the allograft.

In patients with hemolytic uremic syndrome, there is no risk of recurrence when the disease has occurred after a prodromic diarrhea (typical HUS). By contrast, recurrence can occur in atypical forms of HUS with a high incidence of graft failure.[25]

In patients with Wilm's tumor, the risk of recurrence or metastasis is negligible after two years of complete remission. Renal transplantation can be performed safely after this delay.

In patients with primary hyperoxaluria, recurrence of oxalate deposits in the graft is constant, leading in most cases to graft failure. Therefore, the best approach, at least in children, seems to be a combined liver and kidney transplant performed as soon as the patient reaches end-stage renal disease, in order to prevent systemic oxalosis.[26] Care should be taken to prevent oxalate deposition in the graft as long as hyperoxaluria is present.

MALIGNANCY

Immunosuppressive therapy in renal transplant recipients is associated with an increased risk of malignancies. Lymphoma is the most common form of malignancy observed in children with renal allografts. Penn reported 208 malignancies in children, 31% of which were lymphomas, 29% skin cancers, 6% carcinomas of the vulva or perineum, 5% primary liver tumors, 5% sarcomas, 3% thyroid cancer, 3% Kaposi's sarcoma, 3% carcinomas of uterine cervix, and 15% other tumors.[27] In the NAPRTCS report, cancer developed in 12 out of 1,550 children who received 1667 kidney grafts. Six had lymphoproliferative disorders, five had sarcomas, and one had a thyroid cancer.

NON-COMPLIANCE

Several reports have emphasized the high incidence of non-compliance with treatment, especially in adolescents and young adults.[28] Some authors found a rate as high as 50%. Non-compliance is a major cause of late graft loss or permanent graft dysfunction. Graft failure due to non-compliance is estimated to range between 5–10%. This can be partially prevented with educational programs.

GROWTH AFTER RENAL TRANSPLANTATION

Although most children have improvement in statural growth after successful renal transplantation, catch-up growth is not often observed. The most important factors that may interfere with statural growth after renal transplantation are renal graft function and the dose/duration of corticosteroid therapy.[29] Catch-up growth is only observed when the renal function is normal or nearly normal. Growth is impaired when the dose of corticosteroids is above 5 mg/m^2/day. Alternate day steroid therapy has been shown to improve growth velocity. The best results are observed when corticosteroids are withdrawn. However, this is not possible in all cases and acute rejection episodes or progressive chronic rejection has been observed in some patients following cessation of corticosteroids. Growth after transplantation is better in young children.

Recombinant GH has been given to children with growth failure after renal transplantation with subsequent improvement in growth velocity. Growth velocity was significantly higher with GH than with placebo in a controlled, double-blind trial.[30] However, several studies have shown significant alteration in renal function following GH therapy, due to acute rejection episodes or a worsening of chronic rejection. This may be secondary to the effects of GH on the immune system. In our experience, the risk of acute rejection is significantly increased with GH therapy if the patient has experienced more than one acute rejection episode after transplantation.[31]

PREPARATION FOR RENAL TRANSPLANTATION

Since recombinant erythropoietin is available, blood transfusions are rarely needed for patients on dialysis. In the pre-cyclosporine era, it was clear that pretransplant blood transfusions improved allograft survival, although the mechanisms are still poorly understood. Most transplantation teams do not perform systematic pretransplant blood transfusions as these can induce the development of cytotoxic anti-HLA antibodies, and because of the potential hazards of blood transfusions.

Anti-HLA antibodies may result not only from previous blood transfusions but also from pregnancies or previous renal transplants that have failed. They are detected by a cytotoxic assay on a panel of lymphocytes from different donors. Before considering transplantation with a given donor, the recipient's serum is incubated with the donor's lymphocytes in the presence of complement. A positive reaction with donor T lymphocytes, due to the presence of anti-class I HLA antibodies, is an absolute contraindication to transplantation with that donor (positive cross match). The significance of a positive B lymphocyte cross match when the T lymphocyte cross match is negative is controversial. It is probably harmful in patients who are candidates for retransplantation. Some patients develop IgM anti-HLA antibodies, which are not deleterious for the graft.

An evaluation of the lower urinary tract with voiding cystography is important and correction of urinary tract abnormalities should be performed before transplantation, as these abnormalities may be responsible for a ureterohydronephrosis in the graft, increasing the risk of graft loss. Patients with massive vesicoureteric reflux or permanent urinary infection should undergo nephroureterectomy, in order to avoid sepsis in the recipient receiving immunosuppressive drugs. Patients with lower tract uropathies e.g. (posterior urethral valves, prune-belly syndrome, neurogenic bladder) and abnormalities of bladder function should be assessed with urodynamic studies.[32,33]

Immunizations should be updated as described in detail in chapter 19. Live vaccines, such as varicella or measles, should be given at least two months before transplantation. In patients with severe renin-dependent hypertension, a left nephrectomy should be performed before transplantation and the right kidney may be removed at time of transplantation. Investigations should be performed to exclude thrombophilia, which may increase the risk of early graft thrombosis.

SUMMARY

The ultimate outcome for children with ESRD depends on the successful donation of a CAD or LRD renal transplant. In this chapter, many aspects of the care of transplant patients have been discussed. It is also important to stress that there are many patients, both children and adults, who wait for considerable periods after being cleared to be an allograft recipient. It is vital that primary care physicians and pediatric nephrologists work closely together to maintain the patients' health until transplantation is achieved. It is also important that increased effort toward the goal of providing more cadaveric allografts be made by physicians and other interested parties, so that more children can be transplanted within weeks or months of reaching ESRD.

REFERENCES

1. Flom, LS, Reisman, EM, Donovan, JM et al. Favorable experience with preemptive renal transplantation. Pediatr Nephrol 1992; 6: 258–261.
2. McEnery, PT, Stablein, DM, Arbus, GS, Tejani, A. A report of the North American Pediatric Renal Transplant Cooperative Study. N Engl J Med 1992; 326:1727–1732.
3. Seikaly M, Ho PL, Emmet L et al. The 12th annual report of the North American Pediatric Renal Transplant Cooperative Study : renal transplantation from 1987 through 1998. Pediatr Transplant 2001; 5:215–231.
4. Cecka, JM, Terasaki, PI. The UNOS Scientific Renal Transplant Registry – 1991. In: Terasaki PI, editor. Clinical transplants 1991. Los Angeles: UCLA Tissue Typing Laboratory, 1991: 1–11.
5. Hwang AH, Cicciarelli J, Mentser M et al. Risk factors for short- and long-term survival of primary cadaveric renal allografts in pediatric recipients: a UNOS analysis. Transplantation 2005; 80:466–470.

6. Tejani A, Cortes L, Stablein D. Clinical correlates of chronic rejection in pediatric renal transplantation. A report of the North American Pediatric Renal Transplant Cooperative Study. Transplantation 1996; 61:1054–1058.

7. Hricik DE, Almawi WY, Strom TB. Trends in the use of glucocorticoids in renal transplantation. Transplantation 1994; 57:979–989.

8. Jungraithmayr T, Staskewitz A, Kirste G et al. Pediatric renal transplantation with mycophenolate mofetil-based immunosuppression without induction: results after three years. Transplantation 2003; 75:454–461.

9. Kahan, BD. Drug therapy: Cyclosporine. N Engl J Med 1989; 321:1725–1738.

10. Hoyer PF, Ettenger R, Kovarik JM, Webb NJ, Lemire J, Mentser M, Mahan J, Loirat C, Niaudet P, VanDamme-Lombaerts R, Offner G, Wehr S, Moeller V, Mayer H. Everolimus in pediatric de nova renal transplant patients. Transplantation 2003; 75:2082–2085.

11. Niaudet, P, Jean, G, Broyer, M, Chatenoud, L. Anti-OKT3 response following prophylactic treatment in paediatric kidney transplant recipients. Pediatr Nephrol 1993; 7:263–277.

12. Broyer, M, Mitsioni, A, Gagnadoux, MF et al. Early failures of kidney transplantation: a study of 70 cases from 801 consecutive grafts performed in children and adolescents. In Grünfeld JP, Bach JF, editors. Advances in Nephrology. St Louis: Mosby Year Book, 1993: 169–189.

13. Guyot, C, Nguyen, JM, Cochat et al. Risk factors for chronic rejection in pediatric renal allograft recipients. Pediatr Nephrol 1996; 10:723–727.

14. Broyer, M, Guest, G, Gagnadoux, M-F, Beurton, D. Hypertension following renal transplantation in children. Pediatr Nephrol 1987; 1:16–21.

15. Rubin, RH. Infectious disease complications of renal transplantation. Kidney Int 1993; 44: 221–236.

16. Harbison, MA, De Girolami, PC, Jenkins, RL, Hammer, SM. Ganciclovir therapy of severe cytomegalovirus infections in solid-organ transplant recipients. Transplantation 1988; 46:82–88.

17. Zamora, I, Simon, JM, Da Silva, ME, Piqueras, AI. Attenuated varicella virus vaccine in children with renal transplants. Pediatr Nephrol 1994; 8:190–192.

18. Shroff R, Trompeter R, Cubitt D, Thaker U, Rees L. Epstein-Barr virus monitoring in paediatric renal transplant recipients. Pediatr Nephrol 2002; 17:770–775.

19. Ginevri F, De Santis R, Comoli P et al. Polyomavirus BK infection in pediatric kidney-allograft recipients: a single-center analysis of inci-

dence, risk factors, and novel therapeutic approaches. Transplantation 2003; 75:1266–1270.

20. Haysom L, Rosenberg AR, Kainer G et al. BK viral infection in an Australian pediatric renal transplant population. Pediatr Transplant 2004; 8:480–484.

21. Tejani, A, Stablein, DH. Recurrence of focal segmental glomerulosclerosis posttransplantation: a special report of the North American Pediatric Renal Transplant Cooperative Study. J Am Soc Nephrol 1992; 2:S258–263.

22. Gagnadoux, MF, Niaudet, P, Broyer, M. Nonimmunological risk factors in pediatric renal transplantation in children. Pediatr Nephrol 1993; 7:89–95.

23. Baum MA. Outcomes after renal transplantation for FSGS in children. Pediatr Transplant 2004; 8:329–333.

24. Salomon R, Gagnadoux MF, Niaudet P. Intravenous cyclosporine therapy in recurrent nephrotic syndrome after renal transplantation in children. Transplantation 2003; 75:810–814.

25. Loirat C, Niaudet P. The risk of recurrence of hemolytic uremic syndrome after renal transplantation in children. Pediatr Nephrol 2003; 18:1095–1101.

26. Broyer, M, Jouvet, P, Niaudet, P, Daudon M, Révillon Y. Management of oxalosis. Kidney Int 1996; 49: S93–98.

27. Penn, I. Malignancies in children. In Tejani A, Fine RN, (eds). Pediatric Renal Transplantation. New York: Wiley-Liss, 1994: 462–467.

28. Shaw RJ, Palmer L, Blasey C, Sarwal M. A typology of non-adherence in pediatric renal transplant recipients. Pediatr Transplant 2003; 7:489–493.

29. Bereket, G, Fine, R. Pediatric renal transplantation. Pediatric Clinics of North America 1995; 42: 1603–1628.

30. Fine RN, Stablein D, Cohen AH, Tejani A, Kohaut E. Recombinant human growth hormone post-renal transplantation in children: a randomized controlled study of the NAPRTCS. Kidney Int 2002; 62:688–696.

31. Guest G, Berard E, Crosnier H, Chevallier T, Rappaport R, Broyer M. Effects of growth hormone in short children after renal transplantation. French Society of Pediatric Nephrology. Pediatr Nephrol. 1998;12:437–446.

32. Theodorou C, Katsifotis C, Bocos J, Moutzouris G, Stournaras P, Kostakis A. Urodynamics prior to renal transplantation—its impact on treatment decision and final results. Scand J Urol Nephrol 2003; 37:335–338.

33. Franc-Guimond J, Gonzalez R. Renal transplantation in children with reconstructed bladders. Transplantation 2004; 77:1116–1120.

22. Transition of children with renal diseases into adulthood

J Stewart Cameron

INTRODUCTION

McDonagh[1] and others have emphasized that the formal transfer of the care of an adolescent patient from a pediatric clinic to one based in internal medicine is but a single step in the gradual progress of transition from childhood to adulthood within a setting of ongoing management, sometimes accompanied by evident disabilities and stresses, always by medical supervision and intervention. Despite the obvious and recognized importance of the topic of transition, until recently it has received remarkably little attention in writing either from pediatricians, or especially internists and surgeons. Some general articles have appeared,[1–8] and in the United Kingdom some general clinical guidelines for the process have been discussed and drafted.[9] However, as I noted in a review in *Pediatric Nephrology* in 2001,[10] it is disappointing to find that many of the points made about this process as it takes place within nephrology when I first wrote about the topic 20 years ago,[11] remain apposite today,[8] although awareness of the problem has apparently increased and a number of articles have appeared on the subject as it applies to nephrology, here in the United Kingdom principally from Alan Watson.[5,6,13]

Little written material is available for those undergoing transition,[1,14,15] which perhaps reflects the relative neglect of adolescent medicine in general,[1,18] but the topic of continuing effective and humane care of children as they become adults is a much broader one than the care of adolescents alone. All of us may aim at care of the whole patient, but in practice patients are divided into groups, not by their individual needs but by those of service organization.[19]

First, individuals in need of chronic medical care ('patients') are divided according to their main complaint or disease into various specialities, even though they may have many problems outside their 'main' complaint, a problem outside the scope of this chapter. Then they are cross-cut again by age-defined services, from neonatology through pediatrics, to internal medicine, and finally to geriatrics. The adolescent patient meets the difficulties of transfer of care just when he or she is already struggling with the usual problems of identity, independence, self-image, burgeoning sexuality, and the need to define his or her goals in life, against a background of the additional burdens of his or her chronic illness and its multifarious treatments and restrictions.

The importance of children growing up with chronic complaints requiring continued management is part of the change of emphasis in pediatrics during the past 50 years in developed countries, as other chapters of this book testify. While in the still-developing world acute infections, electrolyte problems, diarrheas and similar 'classical' pediatric problems dominate the clinical scene, in developed countries more and more time is taken up in dealing with children who have continuing problems. This is especially true of the pediatric specialities, for example, pediatric oncology, cardiology,[20] endocrinology, including the care of juvenile-onset diabetics,[21] cystic fibrosis,[22,23] and the care of patients with mental or physical handicaps such as Down syndrome. In all of these groups, survival of patients into their 40s and 50s or even beyond is becoming common; pediatric nephrology is no exception. There is much to be learned from the experience of caregivers in these areas, and exchange of information needs to be increased.

Thus today the work of pediatricians is largely concerned not only with initiating management decisions, but also preparing children and adolescents for a journey through life encumbered by the effect of their malady, together with all the apparatus of management by medicines, surgical operations, physical treatments, and restrictions in diet and lifestyle; but above all the continuing need for attendance at hospital clinics and interaction with medical personnel of all types.

If we take a recent edition of a standard text of pediatric nephrology,[24] 35 of forty chapters, deal with chronic conditions requiring continuing management into adult life, and only five with what could by any stretch of the imagination be called self-limiting diseases: acute glomerulonephritis, the nephritis of Henoch-Schönlein purpura, uncomplicated urinary tract infections, acute renal failure, and renal trauma – and even these conditions may have some long-term consequences, e.g. children with acute glomerulonephritis[25] or acute renal failure.[26] Of course some conditions such as isolated uncomplicated proteinuria and hematuria are common in schoolchildren, but even this list will encompass a proportion of children with ongoing problems, as any nephrologist knows. These conclusions are borne out by the long-term data reviewed in other chapters of this book. Thus today, the pediatric nephrologist in the developed world overwhelmingly sees children who will require care for many years, usually through adolescence and beyond.

The result is that the responsibility of a pediatric nephrologist today for the majority of his or her patients is to initiate, for each infant or child, a plan of treatment for decades and not for years, which may well last a lifetime and include in its targets independence, employment, sexual and social maturity, and possibly pregnancy. Already there are patients under the care of adult units for renal diseases whose management began in childhood more than 40 years ago and some themselves now have families. This perspective may not be easy to bear in mind when faced with a sick infant or child for the first time! Nevertheless, as McDonagh writes 'transition is a process which ideally should begin on the day of diagnosis'.[1] Management decisions with long-term consequences, especially if irreversible, must be taken with extreme care and with an eye on

the future; for example, the use of drugs capable of inducing sterilization, the removal of precious remnant renal tissue, the care of vascular access in those in end-stage renal failure, and any procedure (including transplantation itself) likely to lead to allo-immunization.

SOME SPECIFIC CLINICAL PROBLEMS IN RENAL MEDICINE

These are variously reviewed in other chapters of this book, but will be summarized here. Obviously children undergoing treatment for end-stage renal failure come first to mind. Their contract with their medical attendants is truly one for life, with only the death of one or the other (or retirement in the case of the physician) capable of terminating it. Sadly, despite the very encouraging results of dialysis and especially living-related donor transplantation in children in recent years, kidneys placed into pediatric recipients are subject to the same slow attrition as those in adults following the first year.[27] The half-life of the average cadaver donor kidney remains obstinately around 7.5 years, and a moment's calculation shows that of 100 kidneys, after 25 years – when the former child will still be no more than a young adult – only some 10–15% of grafts will still be functioning. Thus planning for transplantation in children needs to take account of the near necessity for further transplantation in future, perhaps with a period of intercalated dialysis. Clearly this has implications as to which HL-A mismatches or other allo-sensitizing procedures may or may not be acceptable. For the unfortunate minority in whom transplantation is or has become impossible, perhaps because of disease recurrence, but more often allo-sensitization, the future is even more complicated. At least today through recombinant growth hormone we can offer statural growth to those trapped on dialysis or still growth-retarded following transplantation,[28] but this is only one aspect of all-round physical, social, and psychologic development.

Sadly also, we do not achieve nearly as much as we would like to believe we do for our children in long-term renal failure with regard to either psychologic adjustment, educational attainment, or the establishment of an individual identity as judged by employment or independent living away from home, or the development of interpersonal relationship as judged by marriage.[29–31] That this is strongly determined by local cultural patterns is emphasized by the geographical variation in the data of Ehrich et al.[29] between various countries. In general, children with renal failure who are now adults in Northern Europe showed a higher level of social rehabilitation as judged by these criteria. A recent analysis from the Netherlands of Groothoff and colleagues[32] found 20 years later a near-normal quality of life in surviving patients with end-stage renal disease treated by transplantation, although like those treated first while already adult, these pediatric survivors showed poorer quality of life if still remaining on dialysis. Of interest was that the mental components of the instrument used (Rand SF 36) were normal whichever treatment was in use in the childhood survivors, in contrast to those treated during adulthood in which it was poor in those on dialysis.

Although some truly can be said to heal, many children with glomerulopathies require very long-term follow-up.[33] Few children with mesangiocapillary glomerulonephritis can be expected to go into complete remission, although the opposite is true for those with membranous nephropathy. Although the majority of children with steroid-sensitive relapsing nephrotic syndrome (see Chapter 7) go into remission within 5–10 years, a substantial minority may continue relapsing and not establish persisting stable proteinuria or complete remission even after 30 years' disease. These unfortunates share with their transplanted brothers and sisters all the problems of long-term treatment with corticosteroids, with the additional risk of subfertility or even sterility with the use of mustard-like drugs, especially the boys. Great care needs to be exercised in the use of drugs which can impair or eliminate fertility in children with renal disease. Growth retardation from the corticosteroid treatment, although often present, was rarely severe even in those treated for prolonged periods in several, now

historical series,[34] and today recombinant growth hormone treatment is available if needed.

Children with lupus nephritis now usually survive, but almost always have a prolonged course; in our own series, only about 10% of childhood-onset lupus patients achieved complete and stable remission off all treatment, even after three decades or more of follow-up.[35] Again this group of children is exposed to all the problems of long-term corticotherapy including growth retardation, as well as the renal and systemic effects of the disease, to create an especially difficult mix of problems. Most of these patients are girls, and problems of the effect of the disease, its complications and the drugs used to treat it on fertility, contraception, and pregnancy are especially large. Compliance with treatment is commonly – and understandably – a major problem.

THE DILEMMA OF DISEASE APPARENTLY 'IN REMISSION'

It is even more difficult to know what to do about children whose renal disease has apparently healed. Long-term follow-up of a number of groups shows that later some of these apparently 'healed' patients may suffer from late secondary manifestations, particularly hypertension. This may occur following hemolytic–uremic syndrome[36,37] or acute glomerulonephritis,[38] and less commonly in the nephritis of Henoch-Schönlein purpura.[39,40] It is difficult to justify follow-up attendances at clinic or hospital first to the parents, and later to the adolescents themselves, when nothing is apparently amiss and nothing active is being done.[39,40] There is no consensus either in pediatric or adult medicine as to what is best for such patients

The largest group of children in end-stage renal failure have reflux nephropathy,[18] but in those with reflux only and good renal function, clear markers of likely chronicity and/or progression have been identified: hypertension and proteinuria. Such children will need indefinite follow-up, and many will have had or will require surgical intervention. Combined adult-pediatric clinics have been established to cope best with these young patients[41] as has been done in some countries for example for patients with cystinosis.

Children with hypertension not arising from a specific treatable cause clearly will require lifelong management (see Chapter 10), and the necessity of preventing the many consequences of high blood pressure by adequate hypotensive management from the beginning scarcely needs emphasis. The internists who inherit these children from pediatric clinics are often unaware even today, however, of the lower target pressures which adolescents require since the majority of their hypertensive patients are middle-aged or elderly.

Special problems arise with diseases which have systemic manifestations outside the kidney as well as causing renal damage. Cystinosis[42] and oxalosis[43] immediately come to mind. Although both are rare inherited disorders, both have a prominent place in most pediatric nephrology services and extra-renal problems come to dominate the picture as time goes by. Although it looks now as though very early treatment of cystinosis by oral phospho-cysteamine may be preventive, a number of children remain whose disease runs its course into renal failure from infancy to early adult life. These children often receive successful transplants, with 'recurrence' of disease in the grafted organ limited to harmless microchimerism of vascular cells and infiltrating monocytes. However, the ability of phospho-cysteamine to arrest deteriorations in pancreatic endocrine, thyroid, and above all cerebral function remains uncertain. Growth in these patients is also poor in the majority of cases.

Oxalosis[43] also presents its problems. In the United States, treatment has overwhelmingly been by kidney transplantation in isolation, but one advantage of combined hepatic and renal transplantation as in Europe is the cure of the disease in the whole body. Otherwise, deterioration in vascular structures through oxalate infiltration takes place. Isolated renal transplantation in oxalosis could be regarded as a short-term solution only.

The management of all inherited conditions affecting the kidney is, of course, lifelong,[44] from inherited stone disease to the variety of cystic diseases of the kidney, tubulopathies[45] together

with other systemic diseases affecting the kidney amongst many organs – such as Fabry's disease.

THE MANAGEMENT OF THE TRANSITION FROM THE PEDIATRIC CLINIC IN PRACTICE

The biggest danger of transition is the avoidable loss to follow-up and care of a young patient who has potentially containable or reversible disease,[46,47] and the biggest problem is the gap which exists in many parts of the world between pediatric and adult services. Even if there is no gap and no problem, we have to ask how we can minimize the disturbance of a change in caregivers and their attitude to the adolescent and his or her family when the change does take place.

How the problem is to be handled in detail will depend very much upon the local units' history, geography, and the personalities and personal relationships – and it must be said prejudices – of staff working within both units. The first step is to perceive that a problem may be present. Sadly, in many places, communications between the various arms of the pediatric and adult nephrologic services are less than ideal. As pediatrics evolved during the nineteenth century, the special needs of children were recognized in the creation of many hospitals distinct from the general run of fever, maternity, and general adult hospitals. This arrangement, which had advantages in the days when most pediatrics involved acute care, now has grave disadvantages when the majority of pediatric hospital patients have life-long problems. The difficulties are particularly great when the children's renal unit is sited within a special children's hospital, which is geographically separated from, or even remote from, the adult renal unit in a community district or university hospital. In this case, there will be a transfer of place as well as of nursing and medical staff, which is bound to have profound effects on the adolescent and his or her family. Treatments regarded as standard in the pediatric unit, such as automated peritoneal dialysis and growth hormone, or some dietary supplements, may not readily be available in the adult unit for financial or administrative reasons. The adolescent and the parents will quickly sense the rapport – or lack of it – between the two units.

In many cases, whatever the site involved, there will be profound differences in policies with regard to (say) living donor transplantation, dietary advice, drug preferences or physical activity, and a new set of instructions and new advice are given, which may conflict with that given hitherto. The adult unit will, in general, tend to treat the patient as an autonomous adult, whose preferences are paramount, and relegate the parental presence (if any) to a supportive role only. They may minimize disability and emphasize independence. Many parents find this very difficult to accept, especially when issues of confidentiality arise in someone – aged 16 or over in the United Kingdom, 18 or over in the USA – when permission of the young patient must be sought before any information can be transmitted to parents.

What can be done to minimize this disruption of care ? (Table 22.1). Most of the answers to this question are simple common sense,[1–14] but it is surprising how often they are ignored in day-to-day practice in many parts of the world.

First, the transfer must be foreseen and planned well in advance, and held up and discussed as a positive goal with the young patient, rather than suddenly sprung on patients as a new event. Obviously care is best if the pediatric and adult teams work together with agreed treatment protocols, get on well together, and work under the same roof. However, whatever the geographical and administrative relationship between the pediatric and adult unit, the opportunity must be given for the patient to meet medical, nursing, dietetic, and other staff from the adult unit, and to visit and become familiar with the physical unit itself, especially important for patients on chronic dialysis. Second, the transfer should not be a sudden, once-and-for-all-time, immediate affair; there is good reason for some continued visits to the children's unit which are gradually phased out. Depending upon the degree of his or her previous involvement, the family physician can provide a nucleus for continued care as well. A corollary here is that it carries obvious advantages if pediatricians spend some time training in adult units, concentrating on the youngest patients, and studying their entry into the new environment. Equally, adult nephrologists must spend some time in pediatric nephrology units, and it is good to see that this is included in recognized training programs in a number of countries. All of this remains true for nursing and other staff caring for young patients.

The timing of such a transfer has been – and remains – the subject of continuing debate.[1–14] The only firm conclusion which can be drawn is that the decision has to made with each individual young patient, based less upon their chronologic age than upon their degree and rate of development in terms of psychosocial functioning, independence, and general maturity. If the timing is right, the

---

Table 22.1 Facilitating the transfer: action points

- Pediatric unit should foster independence.
- Care should be taken to inform and involve the young patients as well as parents in all discussions and transfers of fact.
- Written information on the disease and its consequences, immediate and remote, should be available and discussed with both child and parents.
- Transfer to the adult unit should be a positive part of a long-term plan discussed and agreed with the patient.
- Early personal contact with members of staff from the adult unit while still under pediatric care should be routine.
- Site/clinic visits with information well in advance should be routine.
- Joint adult-pediatric clinics and joint adolescent in-patient facilities should be available.
- Policies on management should be agreed in advance.
- Extra initial support in the adult clinic and unit should be provided.
- Feedback from young patients who have undergone the transition to both pediatric and adult units should be sought, with appropriate action.
- As part of routine training pediatric nephrologists should spend some time in adult renal units and vice versa.

parents will rapidly cease to attend the adult clinic visits, communication can be directly with the young patient, their visits are often soon replaced by a boy- or girl-friend. It is often forgotten that, unlike other patients in the adult unit, because previous communication has been almost exclusively with the parents, the background and details of their condition may be unknown to the young patient him- or herself, and this gap in knowledge needs to be assessed and addressed.

There are of course dangers in getting the timing of transfer wrong. Too long a stay in the pediatric unit leads to a resentful non-compliant adolescent who complains that no-one ever talks to *him* rather than to his parents, and who feels increasingly out of place in an environment often visibly directed at the needs of smaller children, with fluffy or plastic toys, and other reminders of infancy prominent. There may be an unmet need to discuss matters relating to developing sexuality, including contraceptive advice, which are next to impossible to deal with in the context of interviews including the parents, and a need to plan continued education and/or employment. Problems are faced by parents as well, in helping their child to gain independence after a decade or more of chronic illness, medical intervention, and understandable anxiety on their part, which may require great tact from the internist to unravel.

Equally it may be dangerous and frightening to launch an immature child – even one over the age of 15 chronologic years – into a new, frightening, and apparently uncaring environment where he or she is expected to assume responsibilities with which they cannot yet cope. It must not be forgotten that almost all adult renal units are much bigger than the average children's unit, and there may be a strong feeling that what has been intensive, personal, and highly supportive care has been withdrawn at transfer, especially if self-reliance and independence are being emphasized at the same time. One pediatric unit is likely to serve many adult units, so on transfer, contact with other young patients with whom bonds have been developed may be lost. In adult chronic renal failure units, the median age of patients is likely to be over 60, and

young patients a minority: in a recent European study of 15,000 patients on dialysis,[48] the 20–30 year old prevalent cohort was smaller than the 80–90 year old cohort! In contrast to dialysis units, in adult transplant units the age of recipients will be lower, but the adult unit even though further away than the dialysis unit, may well be nearer home than the specialist pediatric nephrology unit. Transfer needs to be considered from the age of about 14 years onwards; but how and when, and over what period, must be individualized.

The previous paragraphs are, of course, a strong argument for a jointly staffed unit of adolescent renal medicine, especially for in-patient care, with jointly run transitional clinics for patients approaching transfer. However, the blunt fact is that only a minority of renal centers have such a unit at the present time.[49]

A sentence above includes the words '*with* each individual patient' rather than '*for* each individual patient'. The two teams need to discuss the timing of transfer with the young patients, and let them have a major voice as to when: sometimes the response will surprise the team members.

CONCLUSION

When, after discussion and cooperation, the young patient finally reaches the point of transfer, at whatever age between about 14 and 20 years that seems best for him or her, then the pediatrician should be able to heave a sigh of relief that another individual has been launched successfully into adult life with a life-plan in place, not too much damaged or limited by actions that may have been temporarily necessary during childhood. Despite the many special problems encountered by children with their chronic renal diseases, their treatments, and their caregivers, almost all make the transition to adult life successfully, although the indicators of independence leave much to be desired. They are a resolute and toughened group, in a word survivors; a group of young people who should command our respect as well as our care. For their caregivers, there is much to research in this area since opinion is rife and data few.

ACKNOWLEDGMENT

I would like to thank Dr Alan Watson for helpful discussion during the preparation of this paper.

REFERENCES

1. McDonagh. The adolescent challenge. Nephrol Dial Transplant 2000; 15:1761–1765.
2. Schidlow DV, Friel SB. Life beyond pediatrics: transition of chronically ill adolescents from pediatric to adult health care. Med Clin N Amer 1990; 74:1113–1120.
3. Court JM. Outpatient-based transition services for youth. Paediatrician 2000; 18:150–156.
4. Bowes G, Sinnema G, Suris J-C, Buhlmann U. Transition health services for youth with disabilities: a global perspective. J Adolesc Health 1995; 17:23–31.
5. Watson AR (rapporteur). Adolescents and chronic illness: crossing the paediatric/adult divide. Report of a conference held in Nottingham, October 1996. Paediatrics Today 1997; 5:18–19.
6. Viner R. Transition from paediatric to adult care. Bridging the gap or passing the buck ? Arch Dis Child 1999; 81:271–275
7. White PH. Success on the road to adulthood. Issues and hurdles for adolescents with disabilities. Rheum Dis Clin N Amer 1997; 23:697–707.
8. David TJ. Transition from the pediatric clinic to the adult services. J Roy Soc Med 2001; 94:373–374.
9. Kurtz Z, Hopkins A, editors. Services for young people with chronic disorders in their transition from childhood to adult life. Royal College of Physicians; London. 1996.
10. Cameron JS. The continued care of children with renal disease into adult life. Pediatr Nephrol 2001; 16:680–685.
11. Cameron JS. The continued care of pediatric patients with renal disease into adult life. Am J Kidney Dis 1985; 2:91–95 .
12. Watson AR, Phillips D, Argles J. Transferring adolescents from paediatric to adult renal units. Br J Renal Med 1996; 1:24–26.
13. Watson AR, Shooter M. Transitioning adolescents from pediatric to adult dialysis units. Adv Perit Dial 1996; 12:176–178.
14. Tips to ease the transfer to adult care: Movin'on. Pediatric renal group, Tri-state renal network, Indianapolis. No date given.
15. Collier J, Pattison H, Watson A, Sheard C. Parental information needs in chronic renal failure and diabetes mellitus. Europ J Pediatr 2001; 160:31–36.
16. Moore EA, Collier J, Evans JHC, Watson AR. The need to know: information needs of parents of children with the nephrotic syndrome. Child Health 1994; 2:147–149.
17. Watson A. Meeting the information needs of children and their families. In Clinical Paediatric Nephrology. 3rd edn. eds. Webb NJA, Postlethwaite R. Oxford, Oxford University Press, chp 25, 2003.
18. Bennett-Richards K, Neild GH. Adolescent nephro-urology. J Roy Coll Physcns Lond 2000; 34:153–158.
19. Chambers J. Some hazards of growing up. J Roy Soc Med 1997; 90:121.
20. Somerville J. Near misses and disasters in the treatment of grown-up congenital heart patients. J Roy Soc Med 1997; 90:124–127
21. Savage MO, Besser GM. When and how to transfer patients from pae-

diatric to adult endocrinologists: experience from St Bartholomew's hospital. Acta Pediatr Scand Suppl 1997; 423:117–126.
22. Walshaw MJ. The transfer of adolescents with cystic fibrosis to an adult clinic. Paediatr Resp Med 1996; 4:16–18.
23. Webb AK, Jones AW, Dodd ME. Transition from paediatric to adult care: problems that arise in the adult cystic fibrosis clinic. J Roy Soc Med 2001; 94[suppl 40]:5–7.
24. Holliday MA, Barratt TM, Avner ED, editors. Pediatric Nephrology. 3rd edn. *Passim* Williams and Wilkins, Baltimore, 1994.
25. Hertelius M, Berg U. Renal function during and after childhood acute poststreptococcal glomerulonephritis. Pediatr Nephrol 1999; 13:907–911.
26. Georgaki-Angelaki HN, Steed DB, Chantler C, Haycock GB. Renal function following acute renal failure in childhood; a long term follow up study. Kidney Int 1989; 35:84–89.
27. Broyer M, Chantler C, Donckerwolke R, Ehrich JHH, Rizzoni G, Schärer K. The paediatric registry of the European Dialysis and Transplant Association: 20 years' experience. Nephrol Dial Transplant 1993; 7:758–768.
28. Hokken-Koelega ACS, Stijnen MAJ de R, de Muink Keizer Schrama SMPF, Wolff ED, De Jong MCJW, Donckerwolcke RA, Groothoff JW, Blum WF, Drop SLS. Growth hormone treatment in growth-retarded adolescents after renal transplant. Lancet 1994; 343;1313–1317.
29. Ehrich JHH, Fassbinder W, Rizzoni G, Geerlings W, Selwood N, Broyer M, Tufveson G, Brunner FP, Wing AJ, Brynger H. Rehabilitation of young adults during renal replacement therapy in Europe. 2. Schooling, employment and social situation. Nephrol Dial Transplant 1992; 7:579– 586.
30. Henning P, Tomlinson L, Rigden SPA, Haycock GB, Chantler C. Long term outcome of treatment of end stage renal failure. Arch Dis Child 1988; 63:35–40.
31. Reynolds JM, Morton MJS, Garralda ME, Postlethwaite RJ, Goh D. Psychosocial adjustment of adult survivors of a paediatric dialysis and transplant programme. Arch Dis Child 1993; 68:104–110.
32. Groothoff JW, Grootenhius MA, Offringa M, Gruppen MP, Korevaar JC, Heymans HAS. Quality of life in adults with end-stage renal disease since childhood is only partially impaired. Nephrol Dial Transplant 2003; 18:310–317.
33. Cameron JS. The long-term outcome of glomerular diseases. In Strauss and Welt's Diseases of the Kidney, 6th edn. editors: Schrier RW, Gottschalk CW. Boston: Little Brown: 1996; 1919–1981.
34. Trompeter RS, Lloyd BW, Hicks J, White RHR, Cameron JS. Long term outcome for children with minimal change nephrotic syndrome. Lancet 1985; i:365–370.
35. Cameron JS. Lupus nephritis in childhood and adolescence. Pediatr Nephrol 1994; 8:230–249.
36. Fitzpatrick MM, Shah V, Trompeter RS, Dillon MJ, Barratt TM. Long term renal outcome of haemolytic uraemic syndrome. Br Med J 1991; 303:489–492.
37. Small G, Watson AR, Evans JHC, Gallagher J. Hemolytic-uremic syndrome: defining the need for long term follow-up. Clin Nephrol 1999; 52:352–356.
38. Schacht RG, Gluck MC, Gallo GR, Baldwin DS. Progression to uremia after remission of acute post-streptococcal glomerulonephritis. N Engl J Med 1976; 295;977–981.
39. Goldstein AR, White RHR, Akuse R, Chantler C. Long term prognosis of Henoch-Schönlein purpura. Lancet 1992; 339:280–282.
40. Koskimies O, Mir S, Rapola J, Vilska J. Henoch-Schönlein nephritis:

Long-term prognosis of unselected patients. Arch Dis Child 1981; 56:482–484.

41. Woodhouse CRJ. Hazards of growing up. J Roy Soc Med 1997; 90:356.

42. Ehrich JHH, Brodehl J, Byrd DI, Hossfeld S, Hoyer PF, Leipert K-P, Offner G, Wolff G. Renal transplantation in 22 children with nephropathic cystinosis. Pediatr Nephrol 1991; 5:708–714.

43. Marangella M, Ramello A. (eds). Fourth workshop on primary hyperoxaluria. J Nephrol 1998; 11 [Suppl 1]: 3–74.

44. Morgan SH, Grünfeld J-P. (eds) Inherited Disorders of the Kidney. Oxford, Oxford University Press: 1998.

45. Watson AR. Non-compliance and transfer from pediatric to adult transplant unit. Pediatr Nephrol 2000; 14:469–472.

46. Cochat P, de Geest S, Ritz E. Drug holiday: a challenging child–adult interface in kidney transplantation. Nephrol Dial Transplant 2000; 15:1924–1927.

47. Haffner D, Weinfurth A, Manz F, Schmidt H, Bremer HJ, Mehls O, Schärer K. Long-term outcome of pediatric patients with hereditary tubular disorders. Nephron 1999; 83:250–260.

48. Valderrábano F, Hörl WH, Jacobs C, et al. Patients and methods. In: European Study of Anaemia Management (ESAM). Nephrol Dialysis Transplant, 2000, 15 [supplement 4]: 7

49. A show of hands from the plenary audience of the IPNA meeting in London in 1998 suggested that at the most, only 40% of pediatric nephrology units represented at that meeting had contact with such a unit.

Since this manuscript was prepared, a paper has appeared which covers a lot of the same ground:

Watson A. Problems and pitfalls of transition from paediatric to adult renal care. Pediatr Nephrol 2005; 20:113–117.

Index

Note – Page numbers in *italic* refer to tables; page numbers in **bold** indicate figures.

abdominal masses *55*
abdominal palpation 55
ACE inhibitors *see* angiotensin converting
    enzyme (ACE) inhibitors
acid-base handling in proximal tubular cell
    171
acquired diseases 62–5
acute glomerulonephritis (AGN) 95, 25–45
    common types/causes *95*
    impaired renal function 100
    natural history 98–9
    pathology and pathophysiology 95–6
acute nephritis 95–102, 187
    definition 95
    renal biopsy *99*
acute post-infectious glomerulonephritis
    (APIGN) 95
    ß-hemolytic streptococcal strain 98
    clinical features 97–8
    differential diagnosis 97–8
    epidemiology 96–7
    expected rate of normalization of
        laboratory and clinical features *98*
    infections precipitating *97*
    laboratory abnormalities *98*
    long-term course and outcome 100–1
    management options 99–100
    renal function 100
    triggering factors 96–7
acute renal failure (ARF) 30, 47, 60–2, 93,
    181–7, 254
    causes 61, *181–2*
    classification 181–3
    diagnosis 61, 181, *183*, 184
    dialysis 191
    etiology 60–1, 181–3
    hemolysis-associated 186
    history 182–3
    intrinsic *182*
    management **62**, 190
    nutritional support 190–1
    pathogenesis 185
    pharmacological treatment 190
    physical examination 182–3
    pigment-induced 186
    postoperative 186
    post-renal *182*, 189–90
    pre-renal *181*
    prevention 190
    prognosis 62, 191–2
    recovery phase 191
    specific disorders associated with
        intra-renal 185–7
    stages 182, *183*
    treatment 61
    urine studies 183–5

acute renal replacement therapy 62
acute tubular necrosis (ATN) 185
acute tubulo-interstitial nephritis (ATIN) 95
adrenal androgens 211
adrenal hormone axis 211–12
    clinical findings 211–12
adrenal insufficiency 212
adrenocorticotropic hormone (ACTH)
    211–12
albumin and protein to creatinine
    concentration ratio *57*, 81, 85
ambulatory blood pressure monitoring
    (ABPM) 119–23, 199
    oscillometric mean *123*
amiloride 127, 172–3, *177*
aminoglycoside nephrotoxicity 185–6
amlodipine 99
amphotericin B nephrotoxicity 186
amplitude coded CDS (aCDS) 16
androstendione 211–12
anemia in chronic renal failure (CRF)
    198–9, 220
angiography 22
angiotensin converting enzyme (ACE)
    inhibitors 66, 92, 99, 112, 126–7, 135,
    199, 248
angiotensin II (AT2) 135, 194
antegrade pyelography 184
antenatally detected urinary tract
    abnormalities (AUTAs) 35–9
    antenatal intervention 36–7
    counseling 37
    investigations 37
    management points 37
    scheme for postnatal investigations **38**
antibiotics 65, 227–9
    appropriate dosing **230**
    for abnormal kidney function 229–31
    optimal use 227
    pharmacokinetic considerations *229*
    prophylactic *232*
    urinary tract infection (UTI) 231–2
    use with dialysis 231
    with active metabolites normally
        excreted by kidney *230*
antidiuretic hormone (ADH) 85
anti-HLA antibodies 250
antihypertensive drugs *60*
antilymphocyte antibodies 246–7
anti-microbial therapy 225
anti-muscarinic therapy 157
antistreptolysin O (ASO) 98
aquaporin (AQP) 177
aquaporin-2 (AQP2) **178**
arteriography 184

ascites 55
asymptomatic bacteriuria (ABU) 142
atherosclerosis 131
atrial natriuretic peptide (ANP) 86
autonomy 240
autosomal dominant medullary cystic
    kidney disease 51
autosomal dominant polycystic kidney
    disease (ADPKD) 50
autosomal recessive polycystic kidney
    disease (ARPKD) 48–50
    clinical features 49
    diagnosis 49–50
    outcome 50
azathioprine 112, 245

bacterial infections 92–3
bacteriology 63
bacteriuria 57
Bartter's syndrome 54, 64, 171–2
behavioural problems 237
beneficence 240
ß-blockers 127
bicarbonate 58
bioelectrical impedance (BIA) 217
bladder
    dysfunction 139, 148
    dyssynergia 4
    neurogenic 4
    neuropathic 47–8
    percutaneous puncture 143
bladder function, *see also* nocturnal enuresis
    (NE)
bladder instability 28
bladder puncture, ultrasonography **143**
bladder-sphincter dysfunction 28, **158**,
    160–3
blood pressure 58, *58*, 118, 127
    birth until 1 year of age
        for boys **121**
        for girls **122**
    by percentiles of height
        for boys **119**
        for girls **120**
    casual 117
    evaluation 117–25
    methodological issues 117–23
    normative data 117–18
    see also hypertension
blood tests 57, 144–5
blood urea nitrogen (BUN) 182
blood urea nitrogen (BUN):serum
    creatinine ratio 184, *184*

CAKUT problems 35
calcitriol in chronic renal failure (CRF) 196

calcium
  in chronic renal failure (CRF) 195
  in renal osteodystrophy 197
calcium channel blockers 126, 199
cardiac arrest 131
cardiac arrhythmia 131
cardiovascular disease (CVD)
  epidemiology 131–3
  hypertension 117
  kidney disorders 131–7
  modification 135
  natural history 135
  non-traditional risk factors 135
  preventive therapy 135–6
  risk factors 133–6, **134**
  schematic of **133**
cardiovascular mortality in ESRD **132**
cellular casts 97
cephalosporins 65
chlorambucil 90
chronic glomerulonephritis (CGN) 95, 193
chronic kidney disease (CKD) 131
  adolescents 238–9
  adult survivors 238
  attaining maximal potential 240
  classification system 6–8
  clinical picture in children 235
  immunization 225
  infants and pre-school children 237
  management 236
  primary school age children 237–8
  responsibility of physician 240
  social and developmental consequences
    235–41
  stages defined by ranges of GFR 7
  staging 6–7
  support 236–9
  treatment 239–41
  urine abnormalities 7
chronic nephritis 103–15
  common histopathologic patterns *103*
  definition 103
chronic progressive renal disease 71
chronic renal failure (CRF) 30, 35, 193–201
  anemia 198–9, 220
  calcitriol in 196
  calcium in 195
  dialysis in 200–1
  endocrine abnormalities 221
  etiology 193
  GH-IGF-1 homeostasis 207–8
  growth in 199–200, 217–18, 221
  height curve 218
  hypertension 199
  incidence 71, 193
  malnutrition 194, 219–20
  management 221, 236
  nutrition 194, 219–20
  pathophysiology 193–6
  phosphate in 195–6
  pre-endstage **208**
  prognosis 200
  renal anemia 198–9

thyroid disorders 210–11
  thyroid hormone action 209–10
  treatment *194*
chronic renal insufficiency 71
circumcision 149
collecting duct
  aldosterone action **174**
  disorders 173–7
  hereditary tubulopathies *174*
  transport pathways **174**
color Duplex sonography 16
complement factor measurement 98
complement fractions *96*
computed tomography (CT) 19–20, 184
  angiography 20
  nephro-urologic applications 20
congenital abnormalities
  kidney 35–52
  urinary tract 35–52
congenital conditions 237
congenital hydronephrosis 22–6
congenital nephrotic syndrome 64
congenital urinary tract malformations 26
congenital uropathy 22–6
congenital VUR or PUV, suspected **24**
continuous ambulatory peritoneal dialysis
    (CAPD) 201
continuous renal replacement therapies
    (CRRT) 191
contrast agents 66
convulsions 61–2
cortical necrosis 64
corticosteroids 89, 244–5
cortisol 211
creatinine 57
  changes in *57*
  clearance 4
  concentrations *58*
C-reactive protein 144
Cushing's syndrome 212
cyclophosphamide 90, 100
cyclosporine 245–8
cyclosporine A 91
cystic disease of the kidney 56
cystinosis 256
cystitis, definition 142
cytinuria 166–8
  clinical manifestations 166
  diagnostic approach 167
  general characteristics 166–7
  phenotypes I, II and III 167
  presentation 166
  transport pathways **167**
  treatment 167–8
cytomegalovirus (CMV) infection 248

dehydroepiandrosterone (DHEA) 211
dehydroepiandrosterone (DHEA)-sulfate
    211
Dent's disease *see* X-linked hypercalciuric
    nephrolithiasis (XLHN)
Denys-Drash syndrome 89
desmopressin (DDAVP) 156–7

dialysis 131, 134
  access to treatment 240
  acute renal failure (ARF) 191
  antibiotics use with 231
  chronic renal failure (CRF) 200–1
diastolic blood pressure 118, 127
dietary assessment 216
diffuse mesangial IgA deposits, diseases
    associated with *110*
diffuse mesangial proliferation (DMP) 87,
    106
dilated vesicoureteral reflux 148
dimercaptosuccinic acid (DMSA) 18, **40**, **46**,
    125, 146, 149–50
dipyridamole 100, 112
distal convoluted tubule, transport
    mechanisms **173**
distal renal tubular acidosis (dRTA) 175–7
  clinical features 176
  general characteristics 175–6
  treatment 176
dethylene-triamine pentaacetic acid (DTPA)
    19
diuretics 127, 190
dopamine 65, 190
Doppler sonography **16**
drug dose
  adjustment *231*
  calculations 230–1
  interval prolongation regimen 231
  modified reduction regimen 231
  reduction regimen 230
drug loading dose 230
drug maintenance 230
drugs
  and neonatal kidney 65–6
  elimination by kidneys 228
DTP vaccine 226–7
Duplex Doppler sonography (DDS) 16
duplex kidneys
  clinical features 40
  management 40–1
duplex systems 40–1
dysfunctional voiding 28, 158, 161–2
dyslipidemia 133–5

echogenic kidney **49**
ectopic kidney 39–40
edema 55
  causes *56*
  pathogenesis 85–6
educational resources 239
electrolyte metabolism 220
emotional problems 237
enalapril 127, 199
end stage renal disease (ESRD) 87–9,
    99–100, 103, 131, 196, 204, 235, 243
  cardiovascular mortality in **132**
endocrine abnormalities
  chronic renal failure (CRF) 221
  mechanisms 203–4
endocrine system, effects of kidney
    disorders 203–13

eosinophilic nodular 'fibrinoid' mesangial deposits **111**
epithelial Na⁺ channel (ENaC) 173
eplerenone 127
Epstein–Barr virus (EBV) infection 246, 248
equinovarus deformity **39**
erythrocyte sedimentation rate (ESR) 145, 201
erythropoietin (EPO) 198–9
Escherichia coli 140, 144, 187, 248
ethylene-diamine tetraacetic acid (EDTA) 19
European Dialysis and Transplant Association (EDTA) 246

Fabry's disease 256
familial nephronophthisis (NPH) 50–1
fat-free mass (FFM) 217
fibrocellular crescent (PAS) **107**
fibromuscular dysplasia 125
financial resources 239
FK 506 247–8
fluoroscopy 22
focal mesangial proliferation 106
focal segmental glomerulosclerosis (FSGS) 87–9, 248
follicle-stimulating hormone (FSH) 205
fractional protein binding 228
frequent relapses 86, 90
functional bladder capacity (FBC) 154, 156
furosemide 65

gentamicin 65
GH-IGF-1 homeostasis in chronic renal failure (CRF) 207–8
giggle incontinence 163
Gitelman's syndrome 171–2
  treatment 172
glomerular filtration rate (GFR) 3, 53, 95, 181, 185, 203, 215, 228
  adults 5
  children and adolescents 5
  compromised *65*
  infant and child *3*
  limitations of serum creatinine to estimate 4–5
  maturation **53–4**
  measurement 3–4
  stages of CKD defined by *6, 7*
glomerular function 53–4
glomerular lesion 106
glomerulonephritis (GN)
  natural history 99
  primary *95*
  secondary *95*
glucocorticoids 212
glucosuria 57
gonadal hormones 204
gonadotrophin releasing hormone (GnRH) 205
gonadotropic hormone axis 204–6
gonadotropins 205–6
gross hematuria, evaluation **11**
growth aspects 215–23, 237

after renal transplantation 249
chronic renal failure (CRF) 199–200, 217–18, 221
failure etiology **219**
percentage of children with height < 3rd percentile 215
growth assessment 216
growth hormone (GH) 206–8
  neuroendocrine control of release 206
  serum concentrations and kinetics 206
growth hormone (GH) receptor signaling and tissue action 206–7
growth hormone-releasing hormone (GHRH) 206
growth retardation 217
  etiology 218–21
  in chronic renal failure (CRF) 199–200

H. influenza type b vaccine (Hib) 226
heart rate 127
height curve in chronic renal failure (CRF) 218
hematuria 9–11, 71
  causes *56*
  colorants in urine 75–6
  definition 75–80
  diagnostic workup **79**
  differential diagnosis 77–8, *78*
  glomerular origin 77
  gross 11–12, 56
  imaging protocol 28–9
  microscopic 9–11, 57
  non-glomerular origin 77–8
  painful 12
  undetermined origin 78
  workup 78–80
hemoglobinuria 75, 186
hemolysis 186
hemolytic uremic syndrome (HUS) 187–8, 249, 255
  anticipation of Stx *187*
  cardiopulmonary features 189
  clinical findings 188–9
  epidemiology 187
  etiology 187
  gastro-intestinal features 188
  hematologic features 188
  neurologic features 189
  non-diarrhea-associated 189
  outcome 189
  pathogenesis 187
  renal features 188
  treatment 189
Henoch-Schönlein purpura (HSP) 97, 100, 110, 249, 254–5
heparin 210–11
heparin-warfarin 112
hepatitis B vaccine 226
hepatorenal syndrome 187
hereditary conditions 237
hereditary isolated glycosuria 168–9
  general characteristics 168–9
  molecular pathophysiology 169

transport pathways for glucose at luminal and basolateral membranes of proximal convoluted tubular cell **168**
herpes simplex virus 248
hormone action disorders 203–4
hormone-binding plasma proteins 204
hormones, loss in urine 93
horseshoe kidney **40**
human chorionic gonadotropin (HCG) 204
hydronephrosis, prenatally recognized **23**
hydrops fetalis 55
hyperkalemia 61
hyperparathyroidism 196–8
hypertension 30, 58, 117–29, 135, 255–6
  cardiovascular disease 117
  causes *59, 124*
  chronic renal failure (CRF) 199
  clinical diagnosis 123
  clinical manifestation 59
  common oral drugs and dosage regimens *126*
  monitoring 123
  patient history *123*
  pharmacologic treatment 126–7
  physical abnormalities and specific disorders leading to *124*
  prevalence of 134
  renal transplantation 248
  therapy 125–7
  treatment 59
hypervolemia, control of 199
hyponatremia 58, 61

idiopathic nephrotic syndrome (INS)
  alternative forms of therapy 90
  classification 87–9
  disease associated with *88*
  initial treatment 89–93
  symptomatic treatment 92
IgA nephropathy 103–15, 249
  clinical features 107–9
  differential diagnosis 110
  electron microscopy 107, **108**
  epidemiology 103–4
  etiology 104
  findings at presentation 107–9
  immunofluorescence **104**
  laboratory investigation 109
  light microscopy findings 105–7
  mechanism of progression 105
  mesangial proliferation **107**
  natural history 110
  pathogenesis 104, **106**
  pathology 104, 111
  predisposing genetic factors 104–5
  primary 100
  prognosis 103, **109**, 110–11
  progression 106–7, 112
  sequential renal biopsies **113**
  treatment 111–13
IgA1 molecule with hinge region O-glycosylation sites **105**

IgG 98
IgM 98
imipramine 157
immunization
    chronic kidney disease (CKD) 225
    current recommendations 225–7
    post-transplant patients 227
    pre-transplant patients 225–6
    renal transplantation 250
immunofluorescence 96
    IgA nephropathy **104**
immunoglobulins *96*, 98
inactivated poliovirus vaccine (IPV) 226
incomplete responder 87
indomethacin 66, 177
inherited conditions, management of 256
insulin-like growth factors (IGF) 200, 204,
    207
    binding protein concentrations **208**
    molar concentrations **208**
    plasma binding and tissue action 207
    serum concentrations 207
insulin-mediated glucose metabolism **204**
interventional procedures 22
intravenous urography (IVU) 17, **17**, **41**
inulin clearance 3
iron supplementation 198
isohormone spectrum shifts 203–4
isotope studies of urinary tract 18–19

kidney
    congenital abnormalities 35–52
    echogenic 42, **42**
    maldevelopment 41–2
    normal development and function 1–5
kidney damage/dysfunction, evidence of
    7–8
kidney disorders, cardiovascular disease in
    patients with 131–7
kidney function
    estimation 6
    prevalence of abnormalities at each level **8**
kidney malformation syndromes 56
kidney transplantation *see* renal
    transplantation
Korotkoff sounds 118
Kunin method 231

late responder 87
lazy bladder syndrome 162
left ventricular hypertrophy (LVH) 131, 134
left ventricular mass index (LVMI) **132**
legal issues 240
Leydig cell 204–5
Liddle syndrome 173–5
lipid metabolism, abnormalities 92
lisinopril 127
loop of Henle, transport pathways in thick
    ascending limb **172**
loop of Henle/distal tubule *166*, 171–2
lower urinary tract, functional disorders 28
luteinizing hormone (LH) 205
lymphoproliferative syndrome 248

MAG 3 renogram 19, **45**
magnetic resonance angiography (MRA),
    urinary tract 20–1
magnetic resonance imaging (MRI) 29
magnetic resonance-urography (MRU) 15,
    21
malnutrition **216**, 219–20
    see also nutrition
mass screening 67–73
    abnormal findings 69
    arguments in favour 72
    clinical picture 69–72
    final pathologic diagnosis 69
    international attitudes 67–9
    theoretical merits 72
maturation 53–4
    during fetal life 53
    glomerular filtration rate (GFR) **53–4**
    postnatal 53
maximal urine concentrating ability 144
MDRD (Modified Diet in Renal Disease) 5
medical ethics, principles of 240–1
medullary cystic disease 50–1
medullary necrosis 64
medullary sponge kidney 51
membranoproliferative glomerulonephritis
    71, 249
mental development 235
mercapto-acetyl-triglycine (MAG3) 19, **45**
6-mercaptopurine 245
mesangial cell proliferation 87, 106
metabolic abnormalities 215
metabolic acidosis 221
metabolic clearance rate (MCR) **206**
metabolic disorders 235
methyl prednisolone 91, 112
metoprolol 127
microscopic hematuria *10*, 69, *70*, 80
mictiograms, patterns of **161**
micturition 54
minimal change disease (MCD) 87–9
MMR vaccine 226–7
monoclonal antibodies 247
monosymptomatic nocturnal enuresis
    (MNE) 153
multicystic dysplastic kidney (MCDK) 42,
    43, 51–2
mycophenolate mofetil (MMF) 91, 245
myelomeningocele 47, **48**
myoglobinuria 75, 186

National Kidney Foundation's Chronic
    Kidney Disease Outcomes Quality
    Initiative (NKF K/DOQI) guidelines 5
neonate
    imaging 31
    kidney problems 53–66
    renal disease in 54–6
    urinary tract infection (UTI) 231–2
nephritic syndrome 29
nephrogenesis, schematic representation **2**
nephrogenic diabetes insipidus (NDI) 65
    clinical diagnosis 177

general characteristics 177
molecular pathophysiology 177
therapy 177
nephron formation 35
nephron number 65
nephrotic syndrome (NS) 29, 85–94
    clinical features 85
    complications 92
    definitions 86–7
    diseases associated with *89*
    etiology *64*
    idiopathic form (INS) 85
    laboratory findings 85
    steroid dependent (SDNS) 86
    steroid resistant (SRNS) 86–7, 91–2
    thromboembolic complications 93
nephro-urological imaging, diagnostic
    algorithms 22–31
neurofibromatosis 125
neurogenic bladder 4
neuropathic bladder 47–8
neuropathic incontinence 162–3
newborn and young infant 3
nifedipine 99
nitrofurantoin 147
nocturnal enuresis (NE)
    bladder function 154–5
    conditioning alarms 157
    definition 153
    desmopressin (DDAVP) 157
    diversity of population **153**
    epidemiology 153
    evaluation 155, **156**
    genetics 155
    hereditary component 155
    pathophysiology **154**
    sleep/psychology 155
    treatment **156**, 157
    urine production 154
NPH *see* familial nephronophthisis (NPH)
nutritional aspects 215–23, 236–8
    see also malnutrition
nutritional score 217
nutritional status 216

obstructive uropathy, imaging algorithm **25**
OKT3 247
oligoanuria 188
oligohydramnios *39*, 54
oligonephropathy 65
oliguria 181
oliguric renal insufficiency **60**
oxalosis 256
oxybutinin 157

papillary necrosis 64
parathyroid gland hyperplasia 196
parathyroid hormone (PTH) 195, 197–8
pediatrics, common kidney problems in,
    and choice of laboratory studies 8–13
pelviureteric junction (PUJ) obstruction
    43–4, **44–5**
percutaneous bladder puncture 143

percutaneous nephrostomy 184
perinatal problems 54
peritoneal dialysis 62, 201
pharmacokinetics, basic concepts 227–8
pheochromocytoma 125
phosphate
    in chronic renal failure (CRF) 195–6
    in renal osteodystrophy 196
physical development 235
physical examination 55
pituitary-adrenal disorders, diagnosis and
    management 212
placenta 54
plain film of kidney, ureters, and bladder
    (KUB) 16–17
plasma hormone concentrations
    decreased 203
    increased 203
plasma insulin concentration **204**
plasmapheresis 91–2
platelet-derived growth factor (PDGF) 105
pneumococcal infections 93
pneumococcal vaccine 226
Pneumocystis carinii 248
polyhydramnios 54
post-streptococcal glomerulonephritis
    (PSGN) 12
posterior urethral valves (PUV) 47
    congenital **24**
Potter facies 55, **55**
prednisone 89, 93, 100, 112
primary hyperoxaluria 249
primary IgA nephropathy 100
primary systemic vasculitis 97
prohormones, conversion to hormones 203
proteinuria 29, 57, 71, 80–3
    asymptomatic 8–9
    benign persistent 82
    causes *57*
    children/adolescents *8*, **9**
    definition 80–1
    diagnostic workup *83*
    differential diagnosis 81–2, *82*
    intermittent 81
    orthostatic (postural) 81
    persistent or fixed 82
    workup 82–3
proximal renal tubular acidosis (pRTA)
    clinical features 170–1
    general characteristics 170
proximal tubule *166*
proximal tubule disorders 166–71
pseudohypoaldosteronism type I (PHAI)
    175
psychological problems 236
psychologist/psychiatrist involvement 239
puberty 205
pulse responder 87
pyelonephritis 140–2
    acute changes visualized by different
        techniques **146**
    definition 142
    follow-up investigation *147*

symptoms *142*
    ultrasonography 145–6

radiocontrast nephropathy 186–7
radiographic studies 15–33
radionucleotide scans 184
rapamycin 246
recombinant erythropoietin (EPO) 220, 250
recombinant human growth hormone
    (rhGH) 200, 216, 220, 249
recommended daily allowance (RDA) 219
red blood cells 75, 97
    morphology 76, **76–7**
reflux nephropathy 255
renin dependent hypertension 250
relapse 86, 90
renal agenesis 39
renal biopsy *99*, 185
renal catabolism 203
renal cystic disease 48
renal cystic disorders 30–1, *48*
renal dysplasia 41–2, **46**
renal failure (RF) 30
renal fusion 39–40
renal hypoplasia 41–2
renal osteodystrophy 195, 220
    calcium in 197
    phosphate in 196
    PTH in 197–8
    skeletal lesions 196
    treatment 196–8
renal parenchymal disease 29
renal plasma flow (RPF) 228
renal replacement therapy (RRT) 193
renal stone disease 20
renal tract development 35
renal transplantation 31, 201, 212, 236, 241,
    243–51
    anti-rejection medications 244–7
    complications 247–9
    contraindicated 243
    delayed graft function 247
    graft survival 243–4
    growth after 249
    HLA compatibility 244
    hypertension 248
    immunization 250
    infections 248
    living related donor vs. cadaveric donor
        243
    malignancy 249
    non-compliance with treatment 249
    preparation 250
    recurrence of primary disease 248–9
    rejection 247–8
    vascular thrombosis 247
renal trauma 254
renal tubular cell injury 185
renal tubular disorders 165–80
    clinical manifestations 165
    presentation 165
    subdivisions 165
renal vascular disease 20, 30, 125

renal venous thrombosis (RVT) 63
resources, availability of 240
respiratory disorders 59
rhabdomyolysis 186
rocker bottom feet **39**

screening 26
serum albumin concentration 217
siblings, major effect on 238
social development 235
social problems 236
social worker involvement 239
sodium concentration 184
sodium restriction 126
sodium wasting 58
somatotropic hormone axis 206–8
sphincter bypass 163
spironolactone 127
staccato voiding 161–2
Staphylococcus aureus 248
static renal scintigraphy 19
steroid resistant nephrotic syndrome
    (SRNS) 86, 91–2
    primary 87
    secondary 87
structural incontinence 163
support staff involvement 239
suprapubic aspiration *145*
systemic lupus erythematosus (SLE) 97
systolic blood pressure 118, 127

tacrolimus (FK506) 246
target tissue sensitivity 204
thiazide 177
thromboembolic complications in
    nephrotic syndrome (NS) 93
thyroid disorders in chronic renal failure
    (CRF) 210–11
thyroid hormone action in chronic renal
    failure (CRF) 209–10
thyroid hormone axis 208–11
    clinical findings 208–11
thyroid hormones 208–9
    binding proteins 209
thyroid-stimulating hormone (TSH)
    209–10
thyroid suppression, failure of **210**
thyrotrophin-releasing hormone (TRH) 206
thyroxin administration, failure **210**
Tolypocadium inflatum 245
total body water (TBW) 217
transforming growth factor ß (TGFß) 105
transition of children into adulthood
    253–60
    action points *257*
    dilemma of disease apparently in
        remission 255–6
    management of 256–8
    specific clinical problems in renal
        medicine 254–6
transplantation *see* renal transplantation
transtubular reabsorption and secretion
    228–9

tricyclic antidepressants 157
trimethoprim 147
trisomy syndromes 56
tuberculosis 20
tuberous sclerosis complex (TSC) **49**, 51
tubular basement membrane (TBM) 50
tubular function 53
tumors, role of imaging 30–1

ultrasonography 184
    bladder puncture **143**
    pyelonephritis 145–6
    vesico-ureteral reflux (VUR) 151
ultrasound studies, urinary tract 15–16
ureterohydronephrosis 250
urge incontinence 160–1
urinalysis 57, 183
urinary incontinence 157–63, 239
    classification 158
    definition 157–8
    epidemiology 157–8
    evaluation and treatment strategy
        158–60, **159**
urinary protein/creatinine ratio 57, 81, 85
urinary remission 86
urinary sediment 76–7, 97
urinary tract
    antenatally detected abnormalities *36*, **36**
    congenital abnormalities 35–52
    isotope studies 18–19
    magnetic resonance angiography (MRA)
        20–1
    obstruction 163
    trauma 20
    ultrasound (US) studies 15–16
urinary tract colic, imaging protocol 28–9
urinary tract infection (UTI) 12–13, 62,
    139–52, 158, 254
    antibacterial treatment 146–7
    antibiotics 231–2
    antimicrobial agents *64*
    bacterial virulence factors 140
    clinical features 141–2
    definitions 139

diagnosis 62
etiology *144*
febrile infants and young children **12**
future directions 150–1
global scope of problem 140–1
imaging algorithm 27, **27**
imaging protocols 26–7
investigation and follow-up 146
IVU 41
laboratory investigations 142–5, *143*
level of infection – lower or upper 142
long-term course and outcome 149–50
malformations 140
management options 146–8
morphologic evaluation *145*
natural history 141–2
neonates 231–2
pathophysiology 139
predisposing factors 139–40
prophylaxis 63, 147
radiological investigation 145–6
risk factors for renal scarring 140
signs and symptoms *63*, 141–2
treatment according to location, severity
    and age *147*
treatment of acute infections 63
types *139*
urine cultures 147
urine culture 143
    storage influence on outcome **144**
    urinary tract infection (UTI) 147
urine diagnostic indices 183–4
urine formation 53
urine investigation 142–4
urine storage and transport 144
urine volumes 55
uroflowmetry **162**
urosepsis 47, **47**

vaginal voiding 163
varicella
    infection 93, 248
    vaccination 226–7
vascular thrombosis 247

venography 184
vesico-amniotic shunt 37
vesico-ureteral reflux (VUR) 4, 16, 19, 22,
    28, 45–6, **46**, 140, 158
    congenital **24**
    conservative treatment *149*
    course after diagnosis **148**
    grading **140–1**
    malformations 140
    neoimplantation of ureter *150*
    reimplantation of ureter using Cohen's
        method **149**
    risk factors for renal scarring 140
    surgical treatment 148
    transurethral injection treatment *150*
    treatment and follow-up 151
    ultrasonography 151
vesico-ureteric junction (VUJ) obstruction
    45
viral infections 93
vitamin D metabolism 220
vitamins, loss in urine 93
voiding, vaginal 163
voiding cystography 250
voiding cystourethrogram (VCUG) 13, 16,
    18–19, 23, 125
voiding dysfunction 28, 158, 161–2

water disturbances 220
white blood cells 97
Wilms' tumor 243, 249

xanthine oxidase 245
xanthogranulomatous pyelonephritis
    (XPN) 20
X-linked hypercalciuric nephrolithiasis
    (XLHN)
    general characteristics 169
    interplay between H^+-ATPase and CIC5
        channel in the process of acidification
        170
    molecular pathophysiology 169
    treatment 169

T - #0503 - 071024 - C8 - 246/189/14 - PB - 9780367391294 - Gloss Lamination